Marine Pharmacognosy

ACTION OF MARINE BIOTOXINS AT THE CELLULAR LEVEL

CELL BIOLOGY: A Series of Monographs

EDITORS

D. E. BUETOW

Department of Physiology
and Biophysics
University of Illinois
Urbana, Illinois

I. L. CAMERON

Department of Anatomy
University of Texas
Medical School at San Antonio
San Antonio, Texas

G. M. PADILLA

Department of Physiology and Pharmacology
Duke University Medical Center
Durham, North Carolina

G. M. Padilla, G. L. Whitson, and I. L. Cameron (editors). THE CELL CYCLE: *Gene–Enzyme Interactions,* 1969

A. M. Zimmerman (editor). HIGH PRESSURE EFFECTS ON CELLULAR PROCESSES, 1970

I. L. Cameron and J. D. Thrasher (editors). CELLULAR AND MOLECULAR RENEWAL IN THE MAMMALIAN BODY, 1971

I. L. Cameron, G. M. Padilla, and A. M. Zimmerman (editors). DEVELOPMENTAL ASPECTS OF THE CELL CYCLE, 1971

P. F. Smith. THE BIOLOGY OF MYCOPLASMAS, 1971

Gary L. Whitson (editor). CONCEPTS IN RADIATION CELL BIOLOGY, 1972

Donald L. Hill. THE BIOCHEMISTRY AND PHYSIOLOGY OF *TETRA-HYMENA,* 1972

Kwang, W. Jeon (editor). THE BIOLOGY OF AMOEBA, 1973

Dean F. Martin and George M. Padilla (editors). MARINE PHARMACOGNOSY: Action of Marine Biotoxins at the Cellular Level, 1973

In preparation

Joseph A. Erwin (editor). LIPIDS AND BIOMEMBRANES OF EUKARYOTIC MICROORGANISMS

A. M. Zimmerman, G. M. Padilla, and I. L. Cameron (editors). DRUGS AND THE CELL CYCLE

MARINE PHARMACOGNOSY

ACTION OF MARINE BIOTOXINS AT THE CELLULAR LEVEL

EDITED BY

DEAN F. MARTIN

Department of Chemistry
University of South Florida
Tampa, Florida

GEORGE M. PADILLA

Department of Physiology and Pharmacology
Duke University Medical Center
Durham, North Carolina

ACADEMIC PRESS   New York and London   1973

QP
631
M37

ACADEMIC PRESS, INC.
111 Fifth Avenue, New York, New York 10003

United Kingdom Edition published by
ACADEMIC PRESS, INC. (LONDON) LTD.
24/28 Oval Road, London NW1

LIBRARY OF CONGRESS CATALOG CARD NUMBER: 72-84374

PRINTED IN THE UNITED STATES OF AMERICA

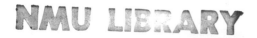

Contents

Chapter I   **Marine Bioactive Agents: Chemical and Cellular.Correlates**

Marion T. Doig, III, Dean F. Martin, and George M. Padilla

Chapter II   **Biochemistry of Nemertine Toxins**

William R. Kem

List of Contributors

Numbers in parentheses indicate the pages on which the authors' contributions begin.

M. A. BURKLEW, Florida Department of Natural Resources, Marine Research Laboratory, St. Petersburg, Florida (179)

MARTIN T. DOIG, III, Department of Chemistry, University of South Florida, Tampa, Florida (1)

ANGELA F. DULHUNTY, School of Physiology and Pharmacology, University of New South Wales, Kensington, Australia (85)

PETER W. GAGE, School of Physiology and Pharmacology, University of New South Wales, Kensington, Australia (85)

MIYOSHI IKAWA, Department of Biochemistry, University of New Hampshire, Durham, New Hampshire (203)

R. M. INGLE,* Florida Department of Natural Resources, Marine Research Laboratory, St. Petersburg, Florida (179)

WILLIAM R. KEM, Department of Pharmacology and Therapeutics, The J. Hillis Miller Health Center, University of Florida College of Medicine, Gainesville, Florida (37)

DEAN F. MARTIN, Department of Chemistry, University of South Florida, Tampa, Florida (1, 265)

TOSHIO NARAHASHI, Department of Physiology and Pharmacology, Duke University Medical Center, Durham, North Carolina (107)

* Present address: Conservation Consultants, Inc., Tallahassee, Florida.

ix

GEORGE M. PADILLA, Department of Physiology, and Pharmacology, Duke University Medical Center, Durham, North Carolina (1, 265)

ZVI PASTER, Department of Zoology, Tel-Aviv University, Tel-Aviv, Israel (241)

JOHN J. SASNER, JR., Zoology Department and Jackson Estuarine Laboratory, University of New Hampshire, Durham, New Hampshire (127)

K. A. STEIDINGER, Florida Department of Natural Resources, Marine Research Laboratory, St. Petersburg, Florida (179)

RICHARD F. TAYLOR, Department of Biochemistry, University of New Hampshire, Durham, New Hampshire (203)

Preface

The science of marine pharmacognosy—the study and utilization of marine drugs—is in many respects in a state of infancy. This statement must be tempered, however, with the acknowledgment that marine organisms and materials have been used from ancient times to cure or relieve various illnesses, ranging from stomachache to more exotic diseases. We also recognize that research in the field of marine pharmacognosy is accelerating and has attracted scientists trained in a range of disciplines, including agriculture, bacteriology, botany, chemistry, oceanography, pharmacology, physiology, and zoology. The marine bioactive substances being studied include a group that is among the most ubiquitious, the most potent, and the most diverse in its range of activity known to man. And yet its activity is, in many instances, poorly understood.

It appears timely, therefore, to bring together the present state of knowledge concerning the activity of selected marine drugs. The unifying theme of this volume—the use of marine biotoxins as probes of cellular functions—constitutes a useful means of understanding the information that has been obtained as well as the techniques and methods being used.

The contributions to this volume have three features. First, the contributors have presented details of procedures they have found useful. These include methods of isolation and characterization of bioactive agents, voltage-clamp techniques, kinetics of toxin-induced hemolysis, measurement of muscle contraction, toxin-induced alterations, bioassays, and microcalorimetry. Second, the contributions, individually and collectively, demonstrate the use and usefulness of marine bioactive agents as research tools. The uses may be one or more applications from a diverse range including removal of or binding to specific components of membranes, agents that block specific physiological processes (cholinesterase inhibitors, general depolarizing agents, sodium pump blockers, etc.), antibiotics, and pesticides. Finally, the contributions help extend application of the techniques, procedures, and results to other relevant problems in physiology, pharmacology, and other fields. In a more general sense, this information will prove to be invaluable to scientists engaged in biological oceanography and comparative physiology.

We are grateful to Mrs. Susan Padilla for technical assistance.

Dean F. Martin
George M. Padilla

CHAPTER I

Marine Bioactive Agents: Chemical and Cellular Correlates

MARION T. DOIG, III, DEAN F. MARTIN,
and GEORGE M. PADILLA

I. Introduction

A. Concept of Biodynamic Compounds

A natural compound from the sea usually comes to the attention of biologists because it exerts a striking (and most often toxic) effect on other organisms in the marine community. Greater emphasis has thus been

1

TABLE I

REPRESENTATIVE BIOACTIVE SUBSTANCES ISOLATED FROM MARINE ANIMALS

Taxonomic group	Genus and species	Compound(s)	Activity[a]	Reference
Porifera				
Sponges	*Microciona prolifera*	Ectyonin	Antibiotic	Nigrelli *et al.* (1959)
Coelenterata				
Hydroids	*Physalia physalis*	5-HT, low MW protein, and polypeptides	CNS, RS, NMS, ANS, CVS, GI	Lane *et al.* (1961)
Jellyfish	*Aurelia aurita*	—	CNS	Barnes and Horridge (1965)
Sea anemones	*Rhodactis howesii*	—	CNS, anticoagulant	E. J. Martin (1966)
Annelida				
Segmented worms	*Lumbriconereis heteropoda*	Nereistoxin	NMS, ANS, CVS, GI, anesthetic	Okaichi and Hashimoto (1962)
Mollusca				
Gastropods	*Haliotis* spp.	Paolin I Paolin II	Antibiotic Antiviral	C. P. Li *et al.* (1962, 1965)
Bivalves	*Mercenaria mercenaria*	Mercene	Antitumor	Schmeer (1966)
Octopus	*Octopus* spp.	Cephalotoxin, 5-HT, tyramine, octopamine	CNS, RS, NMS, ANS, CVS, GI, hemolytic	Hartman *et al.* (1960)
Arthropoda				
Lobsters	*Homarus americanus*	Homarine	CNS	Gasteiger *et al.* (1960)

Echinodermata				
Starfish	*Asterias* spp.	Saponins	CVS, hemolytic, sperm immobilization	Yasumoto et al. (1964)
Sea urchins	*Tripneustes gratilla*	Protein	CNS, RS, NMS, ANS, CVS	Alender et al. (1965)
Sea cucumbers	*Actinopyga agassizae*	Holothurin A	NMS, hemolytic, antitumor	Nigrelli and Jakowska (1960)
Chordata				
Hagfish	*Eptatretus stoutii*	Eptatretin	CVS	Jensen (1963)
Sharks	*Hexanchus grisseus*	Ciguatera toxin	CNS, NMS, GI	der Marderosian (1968)
Stingrays	*Urobatis halleri*	Protein	CNS, RS, ANS, CVS, GI	Russell (1965)
Puffers	*Tetraodontidae*	Tetrodotoxin	CNS, RS, NMS, ANS, CVS, GI	Murtha (1960)
Mullet	*Mugil cephalus*	—	CNS, NMS, GI	der Marderosian (1968)
Weeverfish	*Trachinus vipera*	Protein venom, 5-HT	CNS, ANS, CVS	Russell and Emery (1960)
Scorpion fish	*Dendrochirus* spp.	Protein venom	CNS, RS, NMS, CVS	Russell (1965)
Newts	*Taricha torosa*	Tetrodotoxin	CNS, RS, NMS, ANS, CVS, GI	Mosher et al. (1964)
Turtles	*Chelonia mydas*	—	CNS, GI	der Marderosian (1968)
Snakes	*Pelamis platuras*	Protein	CNS, RS, NMS, ANS	der Marderosian (1968)

[a] Abbreviations: CNS, central nervous system; CVS, cardiovascular system; NMS, neuromuscular system; ANS, autonomic nervous system; RS, respiratory system; GI, gastrointestinal tract; 5-HT, 5-hydroxytryptamine.

placed on biotoxins or venoms than on any other class of compounds derived from the sea. This treatise is an attempt to compile studies on biotoxins. Yet the definition of compounds of interest to the scientific community must be widened beyond the area of toxicology to include whatever "bioactive compounds" may occur within natural products. This follows the suggestion of E.P. Chain (as cited by Halstead, 1968b) who used the similarly general term "biodynamic substance" to prompt the discovery of new drugs and toxins in what may be termed systematic toxinology. A bioactive substance is, therefore, any substance other than food that affects the structure and function of another organism in the marine environment. Biotoxins represent a somewhat more restrictive category, partly obscuring the fact that many "toxins" ultimately lead to the production of useful drugs, particularly after careful isolation, characterization, and alteration by synthetic means (Baslow, 1969, 1971). The term "drug" need not be limited to its strictly medical usage, but should be synonymous with the term "bioactive compound," as it also denotes any chemical substance that affects a specific physiological function (Fingl and Woodbury, 1965).

The main purpose of this chapter is to focus attention upon specific cellular effects of representative bioactive compounds and to correlate such pharmacological activities with the chemical uniqueness they possess. We have also sought to include other bioactive compounds not fully described in this volume in an attempt to acquaint the reader with new and, as yet, not fully investigated sources of pharmacological materials.

B. Pharmacology of Natural Products

A wide range of useful drugs has been isolated from plants (and animals). Although it is impossible to compile a full inventory, these drugs include analgesics, antibiotics, anticoagulants, antileukemic agents, cardioactive agents, enzymes, hormones, narcotics, and vitamins. The utility of these drugs was documented by a recent survey; more than 47% of new prescriptions contained drugs of natural origin as either the sole ingredient or as a component (der Marderosian, 1968).

The record of success in isolating new drugs from terrestrial plants is moderately impressive. At least 10,000 of the more than 400,000 species of plants have been screened chemically and/or pharmacologically to some degree. The successes are even more significant when we consider how many plant substances may have been less than thoroughly screened and prematurely rejected.

By comparison, the potential array of marine bioactive agents should be even more impressive. For example, approximately 80% of the earth's

TABLE II

REPRESENTATIVE BIOACTIVE SUBSTANCES ISOLATED FROM MARINE PLANTS

Taxonomic group	Genus and species	Compound	Activity[a]	Reference
Schizophyta (Bacteria)	*Flavobacterium piscicida*	—	CNS, antifugal, antiyeast	Halstead (1965)
Eumycophyta (Fungi)	*Cephalosporium acremonium*	Cephalothin	Antibiotic	Abraham (1962)
Cyanophyta (Blue-green algae)	*Nostoc rivulare*	—	Carcinogenic	Schwimmer and Schwimmer (1964)
Chlorophyta (Green algae)	*Chlamydomonas reinhardtii*	Fatty acids	Antibiotic	Starr (1962)
Chrysophyta (Golden algae)	*Prymnesium parvum*	Prymnesin	CNS, NMS, hemolytic, cytolytic, antispasmodic	Parnas (1963)
Pyrrophyta (Dinoflagellates)	*Gonyaulax catenella*	Saxitoxin	CNS, RS, NMS, ANS, CVS, GI	Bull and Pringle (1968)
Phaeophyta (Brown algae)	*Laminaria* spp.	Laminarin	Anticoagulant	Dewar (1956)
Rhodophyta (Red algae)	*Digenea simplex*	Kainic acid	Anthelmintic	Murakami *et al.* (1955)

[a] Abbreviations: CNS, central nervous system; CVS, cardiovascular system; NMS, neuromuscular system; ANS, autonomic nervous system; RS, respiratory system; GI, gastrointestinal tract.

PRELIMINARY ISOLATION
Drug suggested by analogy or
general screening program

SCREENING AND DISCOVERIES
Unique or potentially useful
biological activity is found

SOURCE MATERIALS
Obtain enough material for
isolating and characterizing
the active compound(s)

EFFECTIVE CHEMOTHERAPY
Test for efficiency in treatment of animals

CHARACTERIZATION AND SYNTHESIS

MASS SCALE SYNTHESIS

PHARMACOLOGICAL STUDIES
Testing for drug activity and safety

GOVERNMENTAL APPROVAL

1. Disclosure of complete drug source,
   manufacturing information
2. Preclinical results disclosed
3. Future research plans and other
   supporting data

CLINICAL EVALUATION

1. Testing with human volunteers to determine
   metabolism, absorptions and elimination,
   side effects, safe dose range, preferred
   method of administration. Obtain therapeutic index (value versus hazards).
2. Initial diagnosis test
3. Outside controlled tests

MASS PRODUCTION
Economic, governmental, technical limitations apply

MARKETING PROCEDURES
Economic, governmental limitations also apply

FIG. 1. Flow diagram for the isolation and production of drugs from marine sources.

animal life lives in the ocean and comprises 500,000 species in 30 phyla. And, according to Halstead (1965, 1967, 1968a), biotoxins are found throughout the entire phylogenetic series of marine animals (Table I). Of all these biotoxins, perhaps less than 1% have been examined for pharmacological activity. Probably, fewer than two dozen have been fully evaluated as to their chemical and pharmacological properties.

This paucity of known drugs from marine sources is surprising considering the potential value of plant sources alone (Table II). There are some explanations for this lack of substances. One problem is economic; it costs, on the average, about $40,000 to isolate an active agent and about $7,000,000 to develop and market from it a useful drug (D. F. Martin, 1970). A second problem is the lack of an interdisciplinary team (except in a few isolated situations) for isolating, screening, and developing the product. Other obstacles include those common to isolating drugs from terrestrial sources: harvesting and patent problems (Fig. 1).

Harvesting may be a formidable obstacle if an analogy to terrestrial organisms is valid. The useful drugs in these organisms (alkaloids, enzymes,

TABLE III

Useful Bioactive Compounds Isolated from Benthic Algae

Compound	Source	Uses
Kainic acid (Fig. 4)	*Digenia simplex*	Anthelmintic against parasitic round worm (*Ascaris lumbricodes*), whip worm (*Trichuris trichura*), tapeworm (*Taenia* spp.)
Domoic acid (Fig. 6)	*Chondria armata*	Exterminates *Oxyics* and *Ascaris* worms
Laminine (Fig. 9)	*Laminaria augustata* (and about 20 species of Laminariaceae)	Hypotensive agent
Laminarin sulfate (Fig. 10)	*Laminaria caloustonii* and other spp.	Anticoagulant, heparinlike activity, antilipemic properties
Alginic acid (Fig. 11)	Kelp, brown seaweeds, *Fucus* spp., *Macrocystis* spp.	Tablet-disintegrating agents, derivative, blood anticoagulant sodium salt, inhibits strontium uptake from gastrointestinal tract
Carrageenan (Fig. 2)	*Chondrus crispus*	Antiviral activities, antiulcer properties, anticoagulant, antithrombic activity

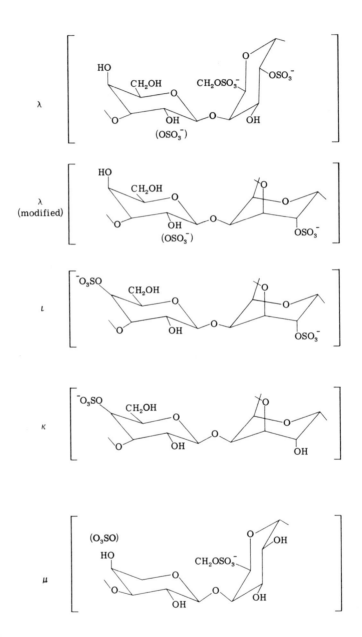

Fɪɢ. 2. Idealized structures of carrageenans. (After Mueller and Rees, 1968.)

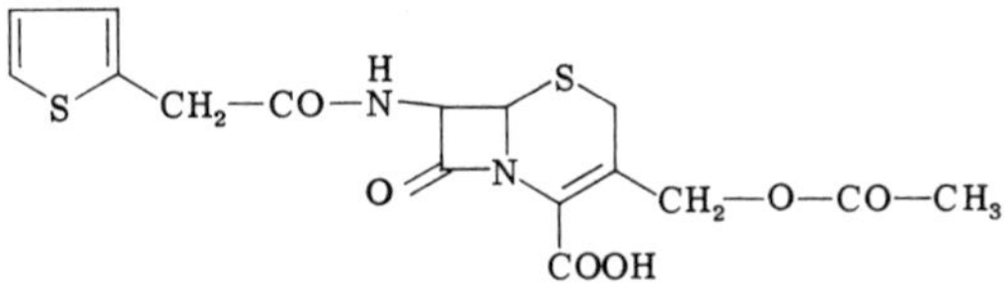

Fig. 3. Structure of cephalothin.

glycosides, steroids, terpenoids, etc.) rarely constitute more than a fraction of 1% by weight (Youngken, 1968), and, typically, several kilograms of dried material are required for the initial extraction. Obviously, there are exceptions; with dinoflagellates, investigators have isolated interesting bioactive substances with much less material (cf. Schantz et al., 1966).

Classic drugs, however, have been obtained from marine sources, chiefly, but not exclusively, from benthic algae (Table III). For example, red seaweed polysaccharides (carrageenan, Fig. 2) have been used as laxatives since Roman times. Cod-liver oil from the codfish *Gadus morrhua* is another notable product. Other examples include spermaceti from the head of the sperm whale and protamine sulfate from the sperm of salmon.

Numerous pharmacological agents of marine origin have been developed in recent years. Cephalothin (Fig. 3) (marketed as Keflin by Lilly Pharmaceutical Co.; Osol et al., 1967) is an antibiotic that is active against a number of penicillin-resistant staphylococci and some gram-negative species of bacteria. Kainic acid (Fig. 4) in combination with santonin is marketed as Digesan (Takeda Pharmaceutical Industries, Ltd., Osaka), and is a useful anthelmintic or vermifuge against tapeworm *Taenia* spp., the parasitic roundworm *Ascaris lumbricoides*, and the whipworm *Trichuris trichura* (Tanaka et al., 1957). Carrageenan (see Fig. 2), as isolated from *Chondrus crispus* and various species of *Gigartina*, causes growth of connective tissues (Robertson and Schwartz, 1953; McCandless, 1965, 1967). Sodium alginate from brown seaweeds is able to remove radiostrontium (^{90}Sr) from the body without affecting calcium metabolism (Waldron-Edward, 1968). Tetrodotoxin (see Fig. 11) (from for example, the porcupine fish *Diodontidae* and the puffer fish *Tetraodontidae*) is a neurotoxin that causes respira-

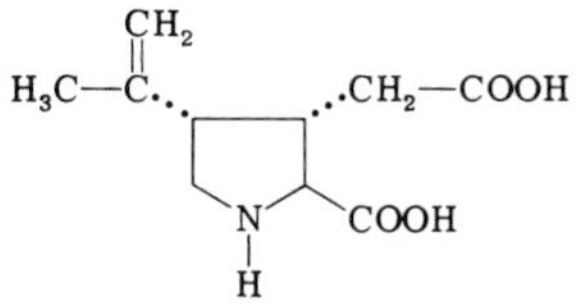

Fig. 4. Structure of α-kainic acid.

TABLE IV

RELATIVE TOXICITIES OF SELECTED MARINE AND NONMARINE BIOTOXINS

Toxin	Source	Toxic dose in mice[a] ($\mu g/kg$)	Reference
Botulinus toxin A	Bacterium, *Clostridium botulinum*	0.00003 (MLD, IP)	Mosher *et al.* (1964)
Tetanus toxin	Bacterium, *Clostridium tetani*	0.0001 (MLD, IP)	Mosher *et al.* (1964)
Palytoxin	Zoanthid, *Palythoa*	0.15 (LD_{50}, IV)	Moore and Sheuer (1971)
Cobra neurotoxin	Snake, *Naja naja*	0.3 (MLD, IP)	Mosher *et al.* (1964)
Batrachotoxin	Frog, *Phyllobates aurotaenia*	2 (LD_{50}, IV)	Albuquerque (1972)
Saxitoxin	Dinoflagellate, *Gonyaulax catenella*	3.4 (LD_{50}, IV)	Wiberg and Stephenson (1960)
Tetrodotoxin	Puffer fish, *Sphoeroides rubripes*	8 (MLD, IV)	Russell (1965)
Sea snake venom	Sea snake, *Laticauda semifasciata*	130 (LD_{50}, IV)	Tu (1971)
Ciguatoxin	Moray eel, *Gymnothorax javanicus*	500 (MLD, IP)	Scheuer *et al.* (1967)
Curare	Plant, *Chondodendron tomentosum*	500 (MLD, IP)	Mosher *et al.* (1964)
Strychnine	Plant, *Strychnos nux-vomica*	500 (MLD, IP)	Mosher *et al.* (1964)
Prymnesin	Golden algae, *Prymnesium parvum*	1,400 (LD_{50}, IP)	Paster (1968)
Holothurin A	Sea cucumber, *Actinopyga agassizi*	10,000 (MLD, IP)	Nigrelli and Jakowska (1960)
Ostracitoxin	Boxfish, *Ostracion lentiginosus*	200,000 (MLD, IP)	Thomson (1964)

[a] Abbreviations: MLD, minimum lethal dose; IV, intravenous; IP, intraperitoneal; LD_{50}, 50% mortality.

tory failure and neuromuscular blocking (Kao, 1966, 1967; Russell, 1967); in smaller doses, it has been used clinically as a palliative drug in terminal cancer (Burkholder, 1963).

Utilization of other marine biotoxins may require smaller doses because, typically, marine biotoxins appear to be more powerful than their pharmacologically comparable terrestrial counterparts. Perhaps they have a repellent or defensive function in many instances that would offer an evolutionary advantage. As an example of potency, saxitoxin has about 10^6 times the potency of cocaine in blocking action potentials (Shanes *et al.*, 1959). The lethal dosage for man, based on studies of accidental death, may be as low as 0.54 mg (Schantz, 1970). The toxic doses of some representative marine biotoxins are listed in Table IV together with those for terrestrial poisons for comparison.

Comparisons of LD_{50} for mice are valid, but these may not be revealing. For example, ostracitoxin (pahutoxin, see Fig. 12) from the Hawaiian boxfish is not impressively potent because it is only weakly toxic to mammals, but it is impressively ichthyocidal (Thomson, 1964, 1968). The toxin is assumed to serve a repellent function since other fish could not survive in aquaria that contained freshly captured boxfish (Brock, 1955).

The potential for utilization of bioactive agents of marine origin is great, and a thorough understanding of the structure–activity relationships of these agents will certainly lead to the synthesis of new drugs with highly selective actions. It is not within the scope or purpose of this chapter to review the properties of all marine bioactive agents. This has been done by others (Halstead, 1965, 1967, 1968a; Russell, 1965, 1967; der Marderosian, 1968; Baslow, 1969, 1971). It is our hope, however, that by reviewing the chemical and cellular correlates of representative biotoxins we can suggest useful approaches to a better understanding of the action of marine biotoxins at the cellular level and thus enhance their utilization by researchers in the fields of pharmacology.

C. Factors Affecting Distribution and Occurrence of Bioactive Agents

1. SEASONAL FACTORS

Seasonal dependence of bioactivity has been noted in several instances. Some available examples should indicate the pattern involved and may suggest some basis for the fluctuations.

A tentative correlation between toxicity and reproductive cycle was established for some puffer fish (Yudkin, 1944). Studies of males and females at different stages of maturation would prove interesting, although

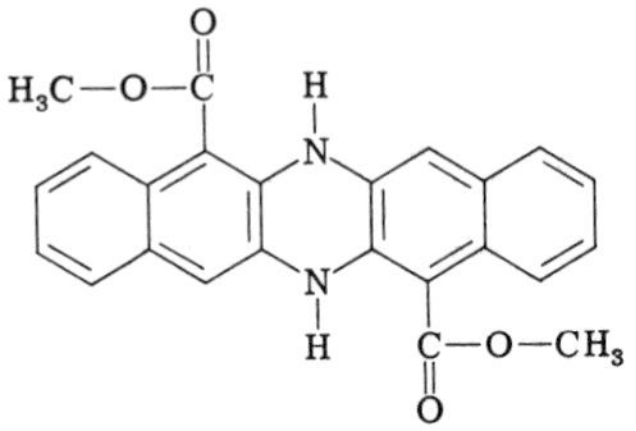

Fig. 5. Structure of caulerpin.

the seasonal fluctuation of toxicity of the fish may have an origin other than in the reproductive cycle.

A second example of seasonality of bioactivity is seen in the benthic algae *Caulerpa*, which is perhaps the most popular edible alga in the Phillipines. It becomes poisonous during rainy months probably because of agitation: an injury to the plant thallus causes extrusion of caulerpin (Fig. 5) (Doty and Aguilar-Santos, 1966, 1970). Also, Pratt and co-workers (1951) reported that the greatest antibacterial activities were found in California seaweed during fall and spring; others (e.g., Roos, 1957) have observed winter or summer maxima depending upon the periods of active growth.

A type of seasonal pattern is also observed with the sand crab, *Emerita analoga*, which is toxic because of a type of paralytic shellfish poisoning, and with the king crab, *Tachypleus tridentatus*, which is toxic during reproductive seasons (Halstead, 1965).

2. VARIATIONS IN SOURCE MATERIAL

Some marine bioactive agents show a constancy of properties despite the fact that they have been isolated from different sources. With other agents, the source material, as well as the locale, season, and the species, may be critical. Some examples may indicate both patterns.

Ostracitoxin (pahutoxin) was originally isolated from dermal mucous secretions of Hawaiian boxfish *Ostraction lentiginosus*, and ostracitoxin-like substances are evidently widely distributed throughout the trunkfish (Thomson, 1964). The specific toxin, however, has not been identified in all species. Skin mucous secretions from three Hawaiian fish (two species of cowfish, *Lactona fornasini* and *L. diaphanus*, and *Rhynocostracion sp.*) were much less toxic than was *O. lentiginosus*. The toxic secretions from *L. fornasini* were much less stable, though the secretory cells seemed to be similar to those of *O. lentiginosus* (Thomson, 1964, 1968). Finally, the Atlantic boxfish, *Lactophrys triqueter*, may have the same toxin, but the fish appears to be much more toxic (Thomson, 1968). Whether these differences in toxicity are due to differences in concentration of ostracitoxin or to more fundamental differences remains to be demonstrated.

Tetrodotoxin is a common term designating several toxins from various sources. Over 50 of some 100 species of puffers or pufferlike fish are responsible for tetrodon poisoning through tropical and some temperate waters (Russell, 1965). Generally, the toxin has been isolated from puffer fish of Japan ("fugu" fish) and other countries around the South China Sea (Kao, 1966). An identical toxin was isolated from the skin of the newt, *Taricha torosa* (Buchwald *et al.*, 1964). A toxin (called spheroidin) from eggs of *Spheroides rubripes* was found to be identical to tetrodotoxin (Kao, 1966).

No adequate explanation is presently available for the appearance of tetrodotoxin in some but not all species of one suborder of fish (cf. Halstead, 1965). The toxin is also found in one family of amphibians in different species of newts and salamanders. To further complicate the problem, a given species may be toxic in the same season in one area, but not in another. Also, the infestation appears to pass from one fish to another in the same location. Obviously, further studies of the biogenesis of tetrodotoxin are needed.

In contrast, E. A. Rees "experienced extreme variations in carrageenan extractives with changing species, season, and locale," despite great care to standardize methods of extraction of these bioactive materials from red algae (cf. Mueller and Rees, 1968). Different (idealized) carrageenans are

TABLE V

Variation of Kappa Carrageenan with Source[a]

Kappa carrageenan source	Sulfation ratio[b]
Chondrus crispus standards	
REX 5103	7
REX 5104	20
REX 5105	4
Gigartina stellata	4
G. acicularis	4
G. pistillata	25
G. radula	2
Eucheuma cottonii	20
E. spinosum	0.05

[a] Mueller and Rees (1968).
[b] Ratio of 3,6-anhydrogalactose units to 3,6-anhydrogalactose 2-sulfate units.

shown in Fig. 2. The simplest form was thought to be kappa, and devia-
tions from the idealized structure, are indicated by the progressive sulfation of 4,6-anhydrogalactose moieties (Table V). The technique consists
of methylation followed, successively, by oxidation hydrolysis of the
glycoside linkage, then complete acid hydrolysis accompanied by disulfa-
tion; appropriate galactonic acids in esters are isolated by means of chromatography. The effect of sulfation relative to ideal kappa carrageenan is
indicated by the *Chondrus crispus* standards (Table V). REX 5103 contained an excess of sulfate over "ideal" kappa, but further fractionation
yielded material that had higher gelling forms (higher sulfate, REX 5104)
and lower gelling forms (lower sulfate, REX 5105) than the parent. The
data in Table V indicate the three different carrageenan types: ideal kappa
(from *Eucheuma cottonii*), forms with intermediate metabolism (*Chondrus*
and *Gigartina* spp.), and iota (fully sulfated 3,6-anhydrogalactose units,
Eucheuma spinosum).

3. EFFECT OF DEPTH

Few have studied the effect of depth on the toxicity of marine organisms.
Presumably, the effects would be due to changes in bathymetry (changes
in temperature, salinity, pH, and nutrient composition). Changes in depth
should also be paralleled by changes in species dominance, e.g., three species
of Gulf puffer, encountered in Florida west coast waters, have different
toxicities and can be separated bathymetrically: *Spheroides nephelus* (completely nontoxic), 10 fathoms or less; *S. spengleri* (extremely toxic in all
parts), 10–30 fathoms; and *S. dorsalis* (variably toxic), 30–50 fathoms
(Burklew and Morton, 1971). Though bathymetry is a useful correlation
parameter, it must be recognized that it is only a gross one. Factors such
as food source, seasonality of food supply, and feeding habitat may be
significant in the production of biotoxins. Nevertheless, bathymetry can
be a good starting point to attempt to survey variations in toxicity for
various species. It is likely that this gross correlation parameter will help
account for variations in the toxicities of other fish as well as coelenterates.
[See also Chapter 6 (Steidinger *et al.*) for examples in estuarine species.]

II. Major Characteristics

A. Physical and Chemical Properties

1. SOLUBILITY

The solubility characteristics of a bioactive substance may be an asset
and/or a limitation in its utilization as a drug, a drug model, or any related

TABLE VI

CHEMICAL PROPERTIES OF SELECTED MARINE BIOTOXINS

Toxin	Source	Empirical formula	Molecular weight	Chemical classification	Reference
Saxitoxin	Dinoflagellate, *Gonyaulax catenella*	$C_{10}H_{17}N_7O_4 \cdot 2$ HCl	372	Purine base with 3-carbon bridge linking positions 3 and 9 and a methyl carbamate at position 6	Schantz (1963)
Prymnesin	Chrysomonad, *Prymnesium parvum*	$C_{15}H_{15}N_7O_3$ —	281 23,000	Fatty acids, protein, sugars, and phosphate	Wong *et al.* (1971) Paster (1968)
Palytoxin	Zoanthid, *Palythoa* sp.	$C_{145}H_{264}N_4O_{78}$	3,300	Steroidal, saponinlike	Moore and Scheuer (1971)
Anabaseine	Hoplonemertine, *Paranemertes peregrina* Coe	$C_{10}H_{12}N_2$	160	Alkaloid	Kem *et al.* (1971)
Holothurin A	Sea cucumber, *Actinopyga agassizi*	$C_{50-52}H_{81-85}O_{5-6}SNa$	—	Steroidal saponin	Nigrelli (1955)
Ciguatoxin	Moray eel, *Gymnothorax javanicus*	$C_{35}H_{65}NO_8$	627	Lipid containing quaternary nitrogen and carbonyl moieties	Scheuer *et al.* (1967)
Tetrodotoxin (Tarichatoxin)	Puffer, *Spheroides rubripes*	$C_{11}H_{17}N_3O_8$	239	Amino perhydroquinazoline	Kao (1966)
Ostracitoxin	Boxfish, *Ostracion lentiginosus*	$C_{23}H_{46}NO_4Cl$	435	Choline chloride ester of a fatty acid	Thomson (1964)

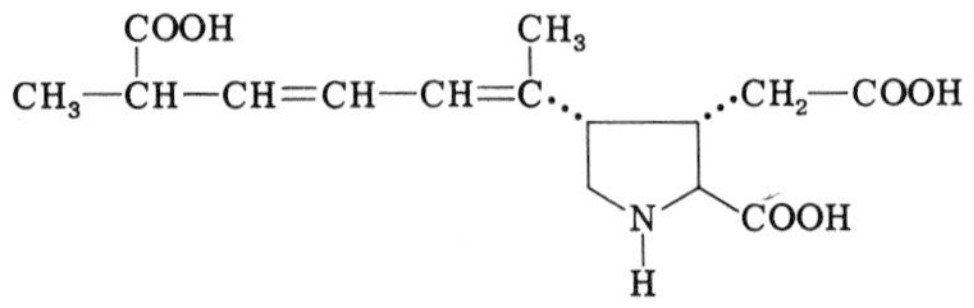

COOH   CH₃
CH₃—CH—CH=CH—CH=C...   ...CH₂—COOH

                              N   COOH
                              |
                              H

FIG. 6. Structure of domoic acid.

application. Saxitoxin (see Fig. 8), which is very soluble in water (Section III,A,4), if eliminated rapidly via the kidney would have a short duration of action (Bull and Pringle, 1968). Should excretion of the material be too rapid, however, vasoconstrictors could be used in conjunction with saxitoxin to extend the duration of action and to localize the action (Bull and Pringle, 1968).

2. MOLECULAR WEIGHTS

Potent marine biotoxins that have been characterized to date fall into two molecular weight categories: the majority have molecular weights of less than 700, and a minority have molecular weights far in excess of this value (Table VI). The toxins in the first category were isolated from a range of phyla. Not enough purified toxins are available to suggest a correlation between molecular weight and phyletic level. In fact, there is an overlap of the two categories within the phylum. For example, *Gonyaulax catenella* and *Gymnodinium breve* have toxins in the first category, while the reported molecular weight for the toxin from *Prymnesium parvum* places it in the second category. It is possible that with additional purification toxic components with lower molecular weights may be derived.

There appears to be no correlation between molecular weight and potency. For example, saxitoxin and palytoxin are among the most potent marine biotoxins, yet the molecular weights differ by a factor of five, and they fall into two different categories.

Finally, no comparison between terrestrial and marine counterparts can be made in terms of molecular weight. Sea snake venoms may be a possible exception. Venoms from sea snakes are complex mixtures of polypeptides that are highly active. In this respect, they show strong similarities to land

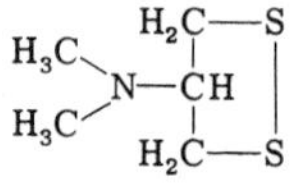

        H₂C—S
H₃C |
    N—CH
H₃C |
        H₂C—S

FIG. 7. Structure of nereistoxin.

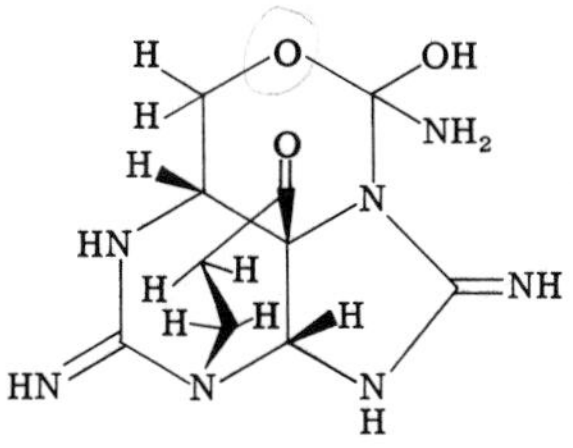

FIG. 8. Structure of saxitoxin. (As reported by Wong *et al.*, 1971.)

snake venoms. The lethal toxin of *Laticauda semifasciata* has a molecular weight of about 6800.

3. FUNCTIONAL GROUPS

Analysis of functional groups and classification as to compound type are significant steps in the characterization of marine bioactive agents. Arranging these substances by compound types is useful, if only to demonstrate the diversity of molecular species represented. Some examples of the types of compound presently recognized are listed in Table I. Compounds isolated from marine sources include acids (Fig. 6) (fatty and acrylic acid), amines (primary and polyamines), amino acids, disulfides (nereistoxin, see Fig. 7 and Chapter IV), enzymes (including amine oxidases, thiaminases, phospholipases), guanidine derivatives [saxitoxin (Fig. 8), tetrodotoxin], nucleic acid derivatives (spongouridine and spongothymidine), polysaccharides [carrageenan and laminarin (Figs. 9 and 10)], saponins, sterols (cholesterol, fucosterol), steroidal glycosides (holothurin A), terpenoids (crassin), and vitamins (thiamine, cyanocobalamine).

However, more specific applications of functional group analysis await further investigation, and tetrodotoxin is a particularly useful example. Tsuda and co-workers (1964) who attempted to correlate structure and toxicity of this compound noted that the hemilactal link (oxygen bridge between C-5 and C-10, Fig. 11) is essential for biological activity; the derivative in which the link is missing (tetrodonic acid) is completely inactive. In addition, Kao and Nishiyama (1965) suggested the guanidinium moiety may also be responsible for biological activity for reasons that are summarized elsewhere (Section III,A).

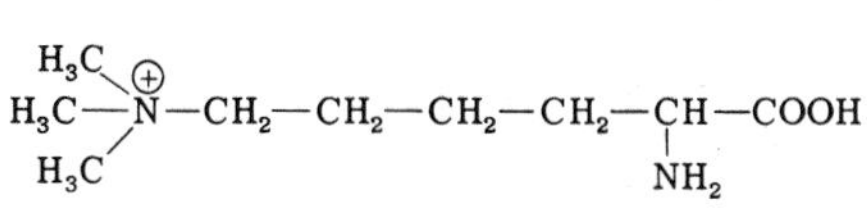

FIG. 9. Structure of laminine.

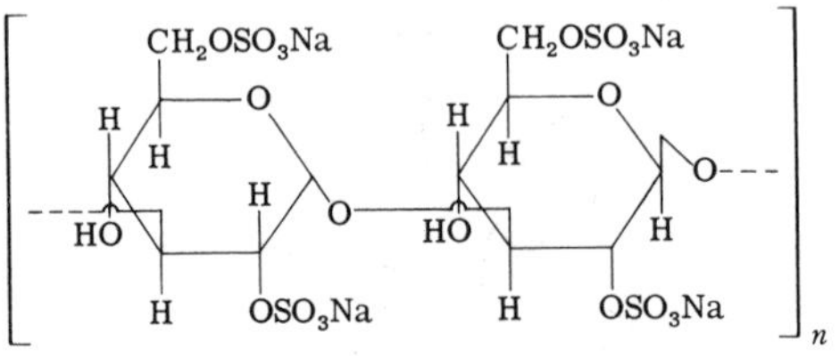

Fig. 10. Structure of sodium laminarin sulfate.

A tryptophan residue is responsible for the toxicity of sea snake venom (*Erabu unagi* and *Laticauda semifasciata*), though it may not be necessary for the antigenicity of purified venom (Tu, 1971). Detoxification occurs when the venom is treated with reagents that attack the indole group of tryptophan (2-nitrophenylsulfenyl chloride, *N*-bromosuccinamides, and 2-hydroxy-5-nitrobenzyl bromide). The toxins from *L. semifasciata* have arginine as the N-terminal amino acid. Modification of the arginine (with 1,2-cyclohexanedione) has no effect on the toxicity. The toxins have four identical disulfide bridges that evidently contribute to stability of the molecular configuration and, thus, to the physical stability. For example, no loss of toxicity occurs when the toxin solution is heated to 100°C for 30 minutes or when the pH is changed from 1 to 11.

B. *Physiological Properties*

1. Membrane-Modifying Agents

A. Specific Ion Transport. Several biotoxins evidently affect transport of ions across a membrane, but a systematic study of this problem has not been made. Some standard systems used include transport across the squid giant axon membrane by measuring conductances (Narahashi *et al.*, 1966) with the voltage clamp technique (see Chapter IV), by studying transport

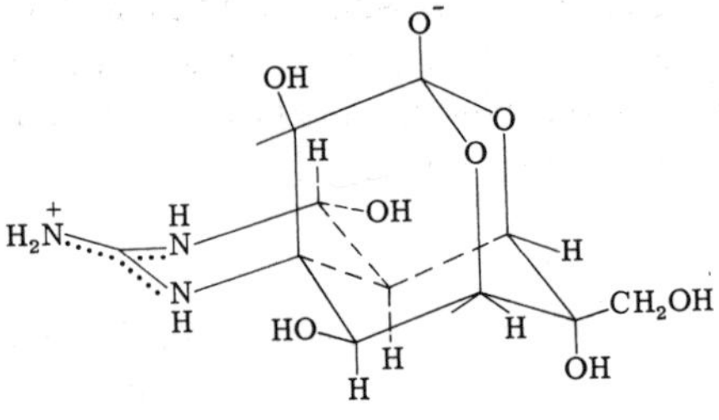

Fig. 11. Structure of tetrodotoxin.

across frog skin (see Chapter V), or by investigating transport in red blood cells (D. F. Martin *et al.*, 1971). Evidently, the more recent model lipid bilayer system has not been used (cf. Gutknecht and Tosteson, 1970). The artificial membrane system and the frog skin apparatus have much to recommend them for screening tests. The use of the turtle bladder has been suggested also (Gennaro and Meszler, 1968) because it does transport sodium ions, although it is not an excitable tissue.

Tetrodotoxin reduces membrane permeability to sodium (see Section III,A). Isolated nerve preparations have been used with great success to elucidate the mechanisms of tetrodotoxin action. The toxin inhibits nerve conduction, but does not depolarize the membrane (Kao and Nishiiyama, 1965), and, more specifically, it eliminates or blocks inward movement of sodium, although the movement of potassium is unaffected (Narahashi *et al.*, 1966). The blocking action is highly specific: sodium movement is blocked only when the toxin is placed on the outer membrane surface; no significant effect was noted when tetrodotoxin was placed inside the squid axon (Narahashi *et al.*, 1966). Saxitoxin has a similar blocking effect on sodium transport, and does not affect the potassium or chloride transport (cf. Dettbarn *et al.*, 1965; see also Chapter III).

Tetrodon and taricha nerves are highly resistant to tetrodotoxin, but saxitoxin is just as potent to these nerves as it is to frog nerve (cf. Kao, 1967). The specific resistance to tetrodotoxin may be related to the known inability of tetrodotoxin to block the calcium spike in certain tissues, or it may be related to a sparse distribution of sodium channels in these nerves (Narahashi *et al.*, 1966).

Larsen and Lane (1966) suggested that the cardiovascular effect of toxin from nematocysts of *Physalia* is due to interference with the sodium and potassium pump. The suggestion that the true toxin alters permeability of capillary walls has been made (cf. Larsen and Lane, 1966), but alterations of fine structures in cell or capillary walls have not yet been observed. The toxin is not a hemolysin.

The venoms of some vermivorous species of mollusks produce hemorrhage in mammals, presumably indicating gross membrane disruption (Russell, 1965).

2. Hemolytically Active Biotoxins

Several marine biotoxins are both ichthyocidal and hemolytically active, though there is no compelling evidence to suggest that the two activities are directly linked *in vitro*. Ostracitoxin (pahutoxin, see Fig. 12), holothurin A, prymnesin (see Table IV), asterotoxin (a starfish toxin; Hashimoto and Yasumoto, 1960), and one component of *Gymnodinium breve*

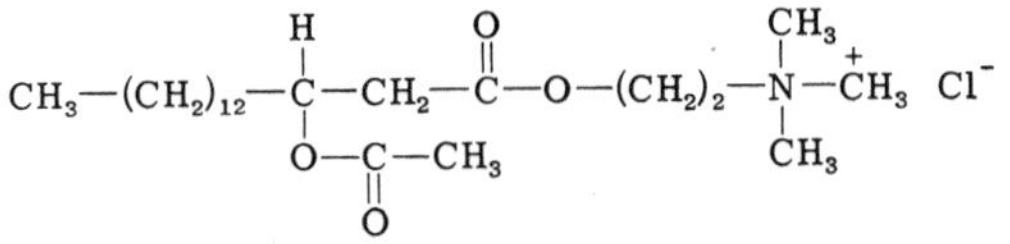

$$CH_3-(CH_2)_{12}-\overset{\overset{\displaystyle H}{|}}{\underset{\underset{\displaystyle O}{\overset{|}{O-C-CH_3}}}{C}}-CH_2-\overset{\overset{\displaystyle O}{\|}}{C}-O-(CH_2)_2-\overset{\overset{\displaystyle CH_3}{|}}{\underset{\underset{\displaystyle CH_3}{|}}{\overset{+}{N}}}-CH_3 \quad Cl^-$$

Fig. 12. Structure of ostracitoxin (pahutoxin).

toxin (Paster and Abbott, 1969) are hemolytically active, though they differ greatly in specific hemolytic activity.

In a few instances, some of the hemolytic properties have been quantified, as the following examples indicate. Ostracitoxin, either natural or synthetic, was found to be a strong hemolysin (Thomson, 1968; Boylan, 1966) even at 0.1 ppm (citrate buffer) and when tested against amphibian, fish, and mammalian erythrocytes. Ostracitoxin also caused strong agglutination reactions at a concentration greater than 50 ppm in fish (eleven species) or with rabbit erythrocytes, though not with mouse or human erythrocytes. In contrast, saponin (Merk) or crude holothurin, though hemolytically active, did not produce agglutination in the erythrocytes tested (Thomson, 1968). Boylan (1966) found that a decrease in chain length by four carbons of the synthetic toxin, choline 3-acetoxyhexadecanoate, produced a marked decrease in hemolytic activity.

The hemolytic activity of prymnesin has also been studied in some detail, as discussed in Chapters VIII and IX. It may be noted that the hemolytic activity is maximum at a pH of about 5.5 (Padilla, 1970), that the kinetics of hemolysis of rabbit erythrocyte suspension have been measured, and that the variation of hemolytic rate with concentration follows a Michaelis-Menten pattern (D. F. Martin and Padilla, 1971). Hemolytic and ichthyocidal activity of prymnesin is lost rapidly when the toxin is maintained at alkaline pH or when heated above 35°C (cf. Shilo, 1967). Saxitoxin, though not a strong lysin, causes passive hemagglutination. This latter property is a more sensitive assay than a mouse bioassay if fresh antigen is prepared each day (Johnson and Mulberry, 1966; see also Chapter VI).

It may be reasonably assumed that strong lysins attach to the membrane, remove a specific component, and produce a destructive effect. The action of other substances has a more subtle effect, but, possibly, it is as deleterious in impairing other membrane functions (e.g., antigen–antibody interactions).

3. METABOLIC INHIBITORS

A. CHOLINESTERASE ACTIVITY. The inhibition of cholinesterase activity by a marine biotoxin should be a useful diagnostic tool, particularly since the methodology by potentiometry is described in useful detail (Jensen-Holm *et al.*, 1959). Impurities can produce an inhibiting effect not found in the purified toxin, or the effect may not be sufficient to account for the toxic activity. Few if any purified marine biotoxins have demonstrated toxicity due to cholinesterase inhibition. Some examples can illustrate the problem (see Chapter VII).

The respiratory depressive action of saxitoxin was ascribed to a demonstrated inhibition (with impure toxin) of cholinesterase in the caudate nucleus (Pepler and Loubser, 1960). More recent research with purified toxin suggests that the affinity of saxitoxin for cholinesterase is too slight for this to be a viable mechanism (Dettbarn *et al.*, 1965).

Acetylcholinesterase was inhibited by saxitoxin (1.3×10^{-5} M), and choline acetylase was also inhibited (4.4×10^{-7} M), but, again, the affinities do not account for the toxicity (Kuriaki and Nagano, 1957).

Dettbarn and co-workers (1965) also found that holothurin A does not compete for the acetylcholine receptor.

"Ciguatoxin" (see Tables IV and VI) was reported to inhibit cholinesterase activity in animals (K. M. Li, 1965). Scheuer and co-workers (1967) were unable to crystallize ciguatoxin isolated from the Moray eel. They concluded that this toxin is a "lipid containing a quaternary nitrogen atom, one or more hydroxyl groups, and a cyclopentanone moiety." The observed anticholinesterase activity still needs explanation.

A purified ichthyocidal toxin islated from *Gymnodinium breve* did not inhibit cholinesterase activity (D. F. Martin and Chatterjee, 1970), and this was confirmed by others (Trieff and co-workers, 1970).

B. PROSTAGLANDINS. *i. Structure.* Prostaglandins are a family of C_{20} carboxylic acids with a wide range of biological activities. These fatty acids are among the most potent of all known biological substances, and slight changes in structure are responsible for distinct changes in biological activity. All prostaglandins have a prostanoic acid skeleton (Fig. 13), and there are four basic ring structures (Fig. 14). The structures of some of the more interesting prostaglandins (i.e., those with potential pharmacological uses) are shown in Fig. 15. The subscripts 1, 2, or 3 refer to the number of double bonds in each molecule.

ii. Marine source. A pharmacologically inactive prostaglandin deriva-

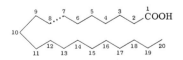

FIG. 13. Prostanoic acid structure.

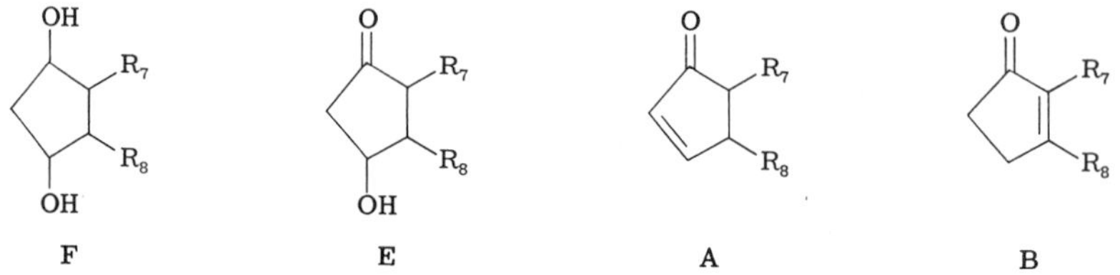

FIG. 14. The basic ring structure of prostaglandins. (After Andersen, 1971.)

TABLE VII

POTENTIAL USES OF SELECTED PROSTAGLANDINS[a]

Potential use	Isomer	Specific effects
Birth control	PGF$_2$-alpha	Reduces secretion of progesterone which is necessary to insure implantation of a fertilized ovum in the wall of the uterus; may induce regression of the corpus luteum
Induced childbirth	PGE$_2$ and PGF$_2$-alpha	Uterine contractions are stimulated at very low doses; have been used to induce childbearing labor in several thousand women
Abortion and induction of menstruation	PGE$_2$ and PGF$_2$-alpha	Mechanism unknown, but process is probably more complex than stimulation of uterine contraction
Prevention of peptic ulcers	PGE$_1$ and PGE$_2$	Inhibit gastric secretions of acid and pepsin in dogs; prevent gastric and duodenal ulcers in rats
Treatment of asthmatics	PGE$_1$	Breathing an aerosol preparation can improve airflow; relaxes smooth muscle of bronchial tubes
Nasal decongestant	PGE$_1$	Clears nasal passages by constricting the blood vessels
Regulate blood pressure	PGA$_1$ and PGE$_2$	Lower blood pressure
	PGF$_2$-alpha	Raises blood pressure
Metabolic regulation	PGE$_1$	Counteracts effects of many hormones which stimulate metabolic processes
	PGE$_2$	Inhibits releases of norepinephrine in response to nerve stimulation in isolated cat spleen and rat heart

[a] Pike (1971).

tive, 15-*epi*-PGA$_2$ (Fig. 16), has been isolated from the gorgonian *Plexaura homomalla*, which is found in coral reefs off the coast of Florida (Weinheimer and Spraggins, 1969). This inactive isomer has been converted to more useful compounds (PGE$_2$ and PGF$_2$-alpha) by inversion of the carbon atom at position 15 and by alteration of the ring substituents. The very high concentration of the inactive isomer in the cortex of gorgonian soft corals (up to 1.3% on a dry weight basis) enhances the possibility of commercial production of active prostaglandins from this source (until synthetic methods become competitive). The biological significance of prostaglandins in marine sources is speculative at this time.

iii. Pharmacological activities. The pharmacological potential of the prostaglandins is interesting because of their ubiquity, potency, and pharmacological diversity. Ramwell and Shaw (1971) have suggested that

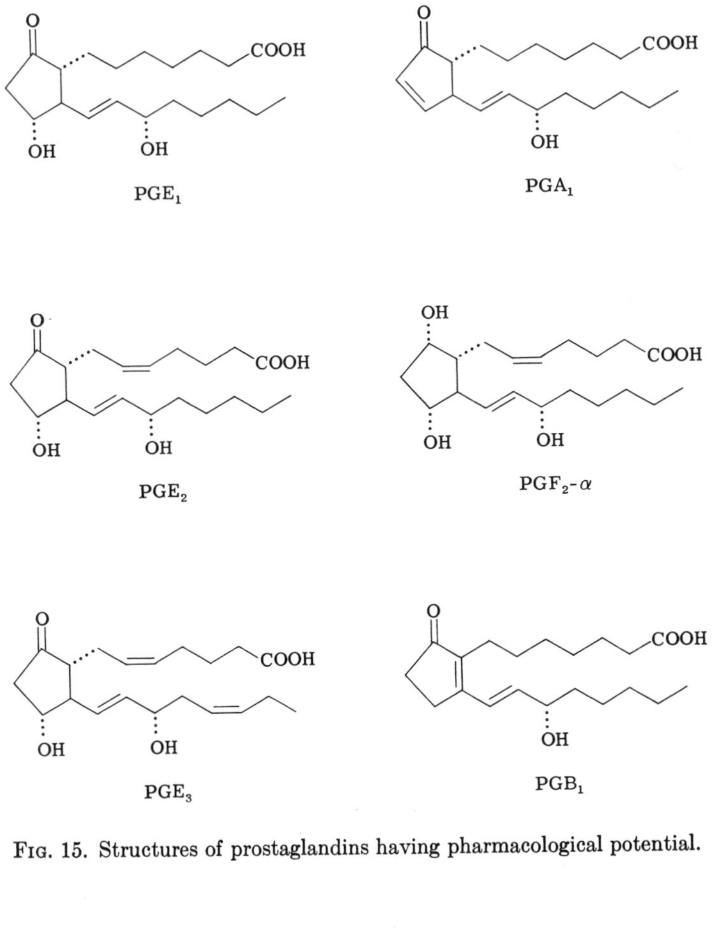

FIG. 15. Structures of prostaglandins having pharmacological potential.

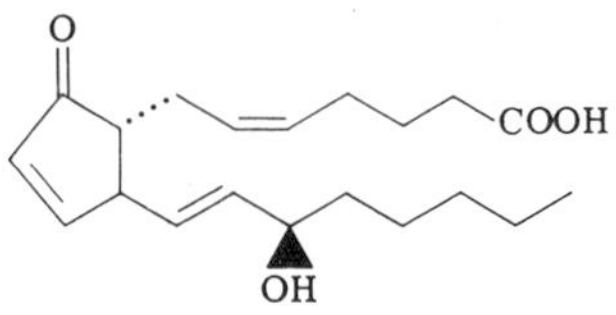

FIG 16. Structure of the prostaglandin isolated from the gorgonian *Plexaura homomalla* (15 - *epi*-PGA₂).

the diversity of action of prostaglandins is due to effects on a regulatory system such as the adenyl- or guanylcyclases. The effects of selected prostaglandins are summarized in Table VII along with their potential therapeutic uses. The most promising areas for prostaglandin applications in physiology and medicine include abortion, birth control, asthma, hypertension, decongestion, stomach ulcers, and study of cyclic AMP formation. In addition, the anti-inflammatory action of aspirin may be due to blockage of prostaglandin synthesis, and prostaglandin antagonists could be useful in the treatment of inflammation. Structural analogs of the known prostaglandins may have new activities, and will certainly be important in the study of structure–activity relationships.

III. Chemical and Cellular Correlates

A. Saxitoxin–Tetrodotoxin

The value of any discussion on the action of saxitoxin is improved by concomitant discussion of tetrodotoxin. The similarity in chemical and pharmacological perperties and in systemic effects has long been noted. Both toxins block excitation of nerve and skeletal muscle, without depolarization (cf. Kao, 1966, 1967; Narahashi *et al.*, 1967, and references cited therein). Both toxins are more selective in their activity on conduction than common local anesthetics. Both are specific inhibitors of sodium currents (Dettbarn, 1971).

1. DIFFERENCES

Despite these similarities, some differences deserve review.

A. PHYSICAL PROPERTIES. First, the solubilities are different. Both are highly polar and hydroscopic, but tetrodotoxin is only sparingly soluble in acidified water. Saxitoxin is very soluble in water, insoluble in nonpolar solvents, and sparingly soluble in methanol and ethanol. Both compounds have basic functions. Saxitoxin has two, with pK's of 8.3 and 11.5. Tetrodotoxin exhibits only a pK of 8.5; the hydroxyl group on C-4 masks the pK of the guanidinium group.

These differences in physical properties may account for longer recovery times noted for tetrodotoxin in isolated nerves and intact animals (Kao and Fuhrman, 1963; Kao and Nishiyama, 1965). Physical properties may also account for differences in actions on isolated nerves, particularly the concentration dependence and reversibility. The conductance block in isolated nerves is reversible up to 300 μM with saxitoxin, but with tetrodotoxin it is often irreversible at 0.3 μM (Dettbarn *et al.*, 1960).

A second difference in physical property may be significant in understanding the palliative action of tetrodotoxin. The masking of one pK by the hydroxyl group in tetrodotoxin could have a significant cellular effect. Tetrodotoxin should be able to penetrate the lipid sheath in the nonionic form, and yet, because of the masking effect, a sufficient concentration of the active cationic form would be available for effecting action (mimicking) as a local anesthetic.

B. SYSTEMIC ACTIONS. The two toxins are similar in systemic actions, and characteristically produce a rapid and progressive muscular weakness. They differ in a significant respect—the effect on blood pressure (Kao and Nishiyama, 1965). With tetrodotoxin, hypotension and action on the central nervous system (CNS) always accompanies paralysis; with saxitoxin, no hypotension accompanies paralysis (at low doses). Bull and Pringle (1968) attributed this significant difference to "differences in physical properties and the non-myelinated postganglionic fibers of the sympathetic nervous system." Kao (1966) notes that if the mechanism of hypotension involves a block of vasomotor nerves, at least to some extent, the hypotension difference described may indicate saxitoxin's greater selectivity of action on somatic motor nerves.

Two differences in CNS activity have appeared in animal testing and clinical reports. Tetrodotoxin, but evidently not saxitoxin, is a unique hypothermic agent as well as a potent emitic agent. The former action is thought to be exerted on the hypothalamus; the latter is believed to be exerted on the medullary chemoreceptor trigger zone (cf. Kao, 1966).

C. NEURORESPONSE OF DIFFERENT SPECIES. Differences in the actions of the two toxins on nerves from taricha newts (*Taricha torosa*) and tetrodon fish (*Spheroides madulaties*) has already been mentioned (Section II,B). Replacement of external sodium by choline, an inert ion, reduced action potential amplitude, which indicates the dependence on external sodium for activity. This observation, coupled with the known resistance of this preparation to tetrodotoxin poisoning, suggests that the action of this toxin is membrane specific, not ion specific. The doses of saxitoxin needed

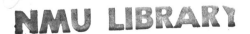

to block desheathed taricha and tetrodon nerves are only slightly higher than for desheathed frog nerve, a more common excitable membrane. This response would suggest that there are gross similarities between the three membranes; some peculiar features must be present in the taricha and tetrodon nerves that preclude effective association with tetrodotoxin, as evidenced by the resistances of the two nerves (1000 and 30,000 times, respectively, relative to frog nerve).

D. DIFFERENCES IN LOSS OF POTENCY. Loss of potency of the two toxins can be achieved by molecular changes, though not of the same type. As noted earlier, loss of a hemilactal link destroys the potency of tetrodotoxin; such a link is absent in saxitoxin. This latter toxin exists in two tautomeric forms that have slightly different toxicities. Reduction (using 1 mole of hydrogen) destroys the toxicity of saxitoxin. The optical activity is not destroyed, however, indicating the center of optical activity is not involved in the toxicity (cf. Schantz, 1970).

2. SIMILARITIES DUE TO EFFECTS OF GUANIDINIUM MOIETIES

The cellular effects of tetrodotoxin and saxitoxin may be understood better in terms of known properties of guanidinium compounds (Kao and Nishiyama, 1965). Guanidinium ion, $(H_2N)_2C=NH^+$, in isotonic concentration can restore the ability of sodium-deficient cells to conduct impulses (cf. Tasaki *et al.*, 1966). Guanidinium ion, because of its size, may act as a current carrier and substitute for sodium. In contrast, N-substituted guanidines have three different effects: (1) the ability to restore excitability may be reduced; (2) they may inhibit the ability of guanidinium ion or sodium ion to restore excitability; (3) the antagonistic effects develop without depolarization (Larramendi *et al.*, 1956).

The general similarities of the two toxins thus seem to be due to the presence of N-alkyl-substituted guanidinium ions on both molecules. Such ions typically would be able to substitute for sodium, and could pass through the sodium channels in the membrane, although, obviously, their movement would be slower because of steric and other interactions. This has been demonstrated by slow rising phases on their action potential spikes (Kao, 1967). In the instances of the two toxins, however, the nitrogen substituents that constitute the rest of the molecules are bulky, and not only limit passage of the guanidinium ion, but inhibit the movement of sodium as well.

3. MECHANISM OF TETRODOTOXIN ACTION

Four modifications of the above scheme were postulated with particular reference to tetrodotoxin. First, some type of complementary structural feature of the membrane around the sodium channels was assumed to account for the potency and specificity of either tetrodotoxin or saxitoxin (Kao and Nishiyama, 1965).

Second, with tetrodotoxin, it was postulated that membrane components are bound by the molecule in such a way that membrane calcium cannot be displaced by depolarization (Narahashi *et al.*, 1964). This would account for the strong and selective action of tetrodotoxin, and may be consistent with observations that the toxin does not block the calcium spike observed for certain excitable tissues (cf. Hagiwara and Nakajima, 1966).

Third, the potency of the toxin was ascribed to a relatively sparse distribution of sodium channels on the membrane surface (Narahashi *et al.*, 1966). In contrast, the lower potential of a more common local anesthetic such as procaine, which is a lipid-soluble blocking agent, is ascribed to this agent's diffusion into the phospholipid layer of the nerve membrane, thus reducing its effective concentration.

Finally, it would seem that the site of action of tetrodotoxin–membrane association must be a "gate" of the sodium channel on the outer membrane surface, in view of the nonblocking action of the toxin when internally perfused in the squid giant axon.

B. Alginic Acid

Alginic acid is a polyuronide (Fig. 17) found in brown seaweeds (see Table III). The alginates find a wide range of uses resulting in production of over 10,000 tons annually in the United States, Britian, Japan, France, and Norway. The uses depend upon a combination of unique properties including (1) polyelectrolytic behavior in solutions, (2) viscosity enhancement for dilute solutions, (3) gell formation by chemical reaction, and (4) base-exchange properties. For example, alginic acid and the alginates are used in foods as stabilizers, probably a successful combination of properties (1) and (2), and in dentistry, because of property (3). The last property is exploited in prevention and treatment of radiostrontium toxicity.

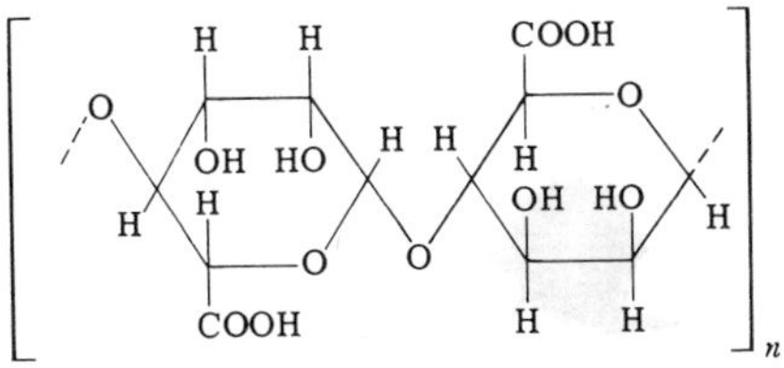

FIG. 17. Structure of alginic acid.

1. PROPERTIES OF ALGINIC ACID

A. DISSOCIATION CONSTANT. The dissociation constant of alginic acid
varies with the source because of different proportions of mannuronic and
guluronic acid. In 0.1 M NaCl solution, the pK value for alginic acid from
Laminaria hyperborea is 3.74; the acid from *L. digitata* has a pK of 3.12.

B. SOLUBILITY. Alginic acid is insoluble in water, and can be precipitated
from a solution of alginates by addition of mineral acids. Alginates of alkali
metals and magnesium are water soluble; those of most divalent and
polyvalent metals are insoluble in water and in organic solvents.

The structure of the alkaline earth alginates is uncertain. Suggestions
that calcium (and presumably strontium or barium) may form cross-links
between chains through adjacent carboxyl groups (Schweiger, 1962) have
been made, though they may not be very satisfying structurally. Molecular
models indicate the links would be possible, though the chains would be
distorted, and the degree of crystallinity indicates the proportion of these
links must be small (Percival and McDowell, 1967).

The equilibrium [Eq. (1)] can be defined in terms of a selectivity coefficient K [Eq. (2)]. Here, the concentrations in the gel phase are expressed
as equivalent fractions, while those in the liquid are expressed as normali-
ties (Haug, 1961).

$$
\begin{array}{cccc}
\text{M(Alg)}_2 + & 2\,\text{Na}^+ \rightleftharpoons & 2\,\text{NaAlg} + & \text{M}^{2+} \\
\text{(gel)} & \text{(liquid)} & \text{(gel)} & \text{(liquid)}
\end{array}
\tag{1}
$$

$$
K = \frac{[\text{M}_{gel}]\ [\text{Na}^+\ aq]^2}{[\text{Na}_{gel}]^2[\text{M}^{2+}\ aq]}
\tag{2}
$$

The selectivity constants depend upon the divalent metal ion and upon
the general observed coordinating tendency of the divalent metal ions,
with some exceptions. First, the selectivity coefficients for a given metal
pair do vary with source, which is a reflection of the mannuronic/guluronic
ratios. The values for the calcium–sodium selectivity coefficient are 7.5
for *Laminaria digitata* and 20 for *L. hyperborea* stipe. A second exception
is that strontium has a high affinity for alginates, particularly those with
a major proportion of guluronic acid (Haug, 1961).

2. APPLICATION TO TREATMENT AND PREVENTION OF RADIOSTRONTIUM
   TOXICITY

The known preference of alginates for calcium has stimulated research
in the use of alginates to control or prevent radiostrontium activity,

specifically to inhibit absorption of ^{90}Sr into the bloodstream. A review of ^{90}Sr properties may be useful before considering the application of alginic acid.

A. PROPERTIES OF RADIOSTRONTIUM. Currently radiostrontium is present at low levels in the atmosphere, and the trend is a downward one, though, prior to the test ban treaty, contamination levels were increasing. Atmospheric ^{90}Sr is deposited in crops, passes through the food chain, and appears in cereals and meats, (although it appears mainly in dairy products). Like its congener, calcium, strontium is absorbed into the blood stream from the gastrointestinal tract, and is deposited in skeletal tissue. The half-life is about 30 years, and the long-term danger from bone tumors or from leukemia is ever present. Removal of ^{90}Sr from bone without extensive bone demineralization is impossible, and methods of treatment have been tried to prevent absorption from the bloodstream.

B. USE OF ALGINATES. Alginates offer several advantages in the treatment and prevention of radiostrontium poisoning. First, they have the characteristics of satisfactory binding agents; they are effective, palatable, nontoxic, and available; they do not interfere with normal growth of rats (up to 24% of diet; Waldron-Edward, 1968). Second, the overall calcium metabolism in animals is barely altered, according to studies of growth curves and chemical balance (Waldron-Edward, 1968), even though sodium freely exchanges with calcium ion. Finally, sodium alginate has a differential effect in binding strontium *in vivo*.

The discrimination effect has a chemical and a physiological basis. The former is simple: strontium ion is able to replace sodium in alginates, and this can be enhanced by using calcium alginate instead of the sodium form. The preference for strontium enhances a natural physiological discrimination of the mammalian body in favor of strontium and against calcium.

This discrimination can be described in radiological assays for *in vivo* experiments using equal specific activities of radiostrontium and radiocalcium in ligated duodenal loops, both without and with alginates. After a defined time, about 30 minutes, the femurs were removed and assayed (Waldron-Edward, 1968).

The discrimination ratio (DR, the ratio of radio strontium to radio calcium) gives the discrimination against strontium. Obviously, a DR value of 1 would represent no discrimination. In early experiments, the DR value for controls was 0.72, and there was a constant value of 0.36 for all doses of alginate. The DR value of control groups varies with age from 0.9 for very young rats to 0.35 for mature ones, though in all cases alginate enhanced physiological discrimination (Waldron-Edward, 1968). The DR values also indicate the variation of effectiveness of alginates from different sources, which was associated with high guluronic acid content.

IV. Conclusions

Three general problems can be recognized in the study of marine biodynamic substances. First, the research that has been done to date has focused attention on marine toxins to an extent that is deleterious to effective progress in the field. It appears that the concept of biodynamic materials has been forgotten or overlooked, and that a broader class of substances that may prove to be more useful than the more spectacular poisons is being overlooked. This is an admonition to the future worker rather than a condemnation of the excellent research that has been accomplished with marine biotoxins. It is encouraging to see that this view has not been neglected, however, and we have endeavored to emphasize it by selection of examples that show specific chemical–physical–cellular correlates.

Second, much research effort has been concerned with isolation of pure compounds (though we recognize that this is a redundancy and should not normally be considered a "problem"). These efforts have been spectacularly rewarding in the instances of saxitoxin, tetrodotoxin, and prostaglandins, to cite only a few examples. There is a danger, even so, that in focusing attention on purity we may have overlooked the obvious fact that mixtures may be significant *in vivo*, and what we gain in model compound correlates, we may lose in ecological significance and even in other useful compounds that comprise the remainder of the mixture.

Third, except in isolated instances, few examples of specific compound screening have been observed. The prevalence of tetrodotoxin in several sources, some remote, has been noted. The same appears to be true of acrylic acid. The general distribution of prostaglandins can only be guessed at, though we are inclined to suspect that the answers would be very significant, from practical and theoretical viewpoints. At present, we can only speculate on the teleological and ecological significance of these and other biodynamic substances.

ACKNOWLEDGMENTS

This work was supported by Grant FD 00120 from the Food and Drug Administration, Consumer Protection and Environmental Health Service, United States Public Health Service to Dr. G. Padilla. One of us (D.F.M.) gratefully acknowledges a PHS Career Award (1K04 GM 4259-03) from the National Institute of General Medical Sciences.

REFERENCES

Abraham, E. (1962). The cephalosporins. *Pharmacol. Rev.* **14,** 473–500.

Albuquerque, E. X. (1972). The mode of action of batrachotoxin. *Fed. Proc., Fed. Amer. Soc. Exp. Biol.* **31,** 1133–1138.

Alender, C., Feigen, G., and Tomita, J. (1965). Isolation and characterization of sea urchin toxin. *Toxicon* **3,** 9–17.

Andersen, N. (1971). Program notes on structure and nomenclature. *Ann. N.Y. Acad. Sci.* **180,** 14–23.

Barnes, W. J., and Horridge, G. A. (1965). A neuropharmacologically active substance from jellyfish ganglia. *J. Exp. Biol.* **42,** 257–267.

Baslow, M. H. (1969). "Marine Pharmacology." Williams & Wilkins, Baltimore, Maryland.

Baslow, M. H. (1971). Marine toxins. *Annu. Rev. Pharmacol.* **11,** 447–454.

Boylan, B. (1966). "The Chemical Nature of the Toxic Secretions of the Boxfish (*Ostracion lentiginosus* Schneider)." Ph.D. Dissertation, University of Hawaii.

Brock, V. E. (1955). Possible production of a substance poisonous to other fish by the boxfish *Ostracion lentiginosus* Schneider. *Copeia* **3,** 195–196.

Buchwald, H. D., Durham, L., Fischer, H. G., Harada, R., Mosher, H. S., Kao, C. Y., and Furhman, F. A. (1964). Identity of tarichatoxin and tetrodotoxin. *Science* **143,** 474–475.

Bull, R. J., and Pringle, B. H. (1968). Saxitoxin as an example of biologically active marine substances. *In* "Drugs from the Sea" (H. D. Freudenthal, ed.), pp. 73–86. Marine Technology Society, Washington, D.C.

Burkholder, P. (1963). Drugs from the sea. *Armed Forces Chem. J.* **17,** 6–16.

Burklew, M. A., and Morton, R. A. (1971). The toxicity of Florida gulf puffers, genus *Sphoeroides*. *Toxicon* **9,** 205–210.

der Marderosian, A. (1968). Current status of drug compounds from marine sources. *In* "Drugs from the Sea" (H. D. Freudenthal, ed.), pp. 19–68. Marine Technology Society, Washington, D.C.

Dettbarn, W. (1971). Mechanism of action of tetrodotoxin (TTX) and saxitoxin (STX). *In* "Neuropoisons" (L. L. Simpson, ed.), Vol. I, pp. 169–186. Plenum, New York.

Dettbarn, W. P., Higman, H., Rosenberg, P., and Nachmansohn, D. (1960). Rapid and reversible block of electrical activity by powerful marine biotoxins. *Science* **32,** 300–301.

Dettbarn, W. P., Higman, H., Bartels, E., and Podleski, T. (1965). Effects of marine toxins on electrical activity and K$^+$ efflux of excitable membranes. *Biochim. Biophys. Acta* **94,** 472–478.

Dewar, E. T. (1956). Sodium laminarin sulphate as a blood anticoagulant. *Int. Seaweed Symp., 2nd, 1955,* pp. 55–61.

Doty, M. S., and Aguilar-Santos, G. (1966). Caulerpicin, a toxic constituent of *Caulerpa*. *Nature (London)* **211,** 990.

Doty, M. S., and Aguilar-Santos, G. (1970). Transfer of toxic algal substances in the marine food chain. *Pac. Sci.* **24,** 351–355.

Fingl, E., and Woodbury, D. M. (1965). Introduction. General principles. *In* "The Pharmacological Basis of Therapeutics" (L. S. Goodman and A. Gilman, eds.), 3rd ed., pp. 1–36. Macmillan, New York.

Gasteiger, E. L., Haake, P. C., and Gergen, J. A. (1960). An investigation of the distribution and function of homarine (*N*-methyl picolinic acid). *Ann. N.Y. Acad. Sci.* **90,** 622–636.

Gennaro, J. F., Jr., and Meszler, J. W. (1968). Research tools from the sea. *In* "Drugs from the Sea" (H. D. Freudenthal, ed.), pp. 151–171. Marine Technology Society Washington, D.C.

Gutknecht, J., and Tosteson, D. C. (1970). Ionic permeability of thin lipid membranes. Effects of *n*-alkyl alcohols, polyvalent cations and a secondary amine. *J. Gen. Physiol.* **55**, 359–374.

Hagiwara, S., and Nakajima, S. (1966). Difference in Na and Ca spikes as examined by application of tetrodotoxin, procaine, and manganese ions. *J. Gen. Physiol.* **49**, 793–806.

Halstead, B. W. (1965). "Poisonous and Venomous Marine Animals of the World," Vol. I. Invertebrates. US Govt. Printing Office, Washington, D.C.

Halstead, B. W. (1967). "Poisonous and Venomous Marine Animals of the World," Vol. II. Vertebrates. US Govt. Printing Office, Washington, D.C.

Halstead, B. W. (1968a). "Poisonous and Venomous Marine Animals of the World," Vol. III. Vertebrates. US Govt. Printing Office, Washington, D.C.

Halstead, B. W. (1968b). Marine biotoxins, new foods, and new drugs from the sea. *In* "Drugs from the Sea" (H. D. Freudenthal, ed.), pp. 229–239. Marine Technology Society, Washington, D.C.

Hartman, W. J., Clark, W. G., Cyr, S. D., Jordon, A. L., and Leibhold, R. A. (1960). Pharmacologically active amines and their biogenesis in the octopus. *Ann. N.Y. Acad. Sci.* **90**, 637–666.

Hashimoto, Y., and Yasumoto, T. (1960). Confirmation of saponin as a toxic principle of starfish. *Bull. Jap. Soc. Sci. Fish.* **26**, 1132–1138.

Haug, A. (1961). The affinity of some divalent metals to different types of alginates. *Acta Chem. Scand.* **15**, 1794–1795.

Jensen, D. (1963). Eptatretin: A potent cardioactive agent from the branchial heart of the Pacific hogfish, *Eptatretus stoutii*. *Comp. Biochem. Physiol.* **10**, 129–151.

Jensen-Holm, J. H., Lausen, H., Milthers, K., and Moller, K. O. (1959). Determination of cholinesterase activity in blood and organs by automatic titration. *Acta Pharmacol. Toxicol.* **15**, 384–394.

Johnson, H. M., and Mulberry, G. (1966). Paralytic shellfish poison: Serological assay by passive haemagglutination and bentonite flocculations. *Nature (London)* **211**, 747–748.

Kao, C. Y. (1966). Tetrodotoxin, saxitoxin and their significance in the study of excitation phenomena. *Pharmacol. Rev.* **18**, 997–1049.

Kao, C. Y. (1967). Comparison of the biological actions of tetrodotoxin and saxitoxin. *In* "Animal Toxins" (F. E. Russell and P. R. Saunders, eds.), pp. 109–114. Pergamon, Oxford.

Kao, C. Y., and Fuhrman, F. A. (1963). Pharmacological studies on tarichatoxin, a potent neurotoxin. *J. Pharmacol.* **140**, 31–40.

Kao, C. Y., and Nishiyama, A. (1965). Actions of saxitoxin on peripheral neuromuscular systems. *J. Physiol. (London)* **180**, 50–66.

Kem, W. R., Abbott, B. C., and Coates, R. M. (1971). Isolation and structure of a hoplonemertine toxin. *Toxicon* **9**, 15–22.

Kuriaki, K., and Nagano, H. (1957). Susceptibility of certain enzymes of the central nervous system to tetrodotoxin. *Brit. J. Pharmacol.* **12**, 393–396.

Lane, C., Coursen, B. W., and Hines, K. (1961). Biologically active peptides in *Physalia* toxin. *Proc. Soc. Exp. Biol. Med.* **107**, 670–672.

Larramendi, L. M. H., Lorente de No, R., and Vidal, F. (1956). Restoration of sodium deficient frog nerve fibers by an isotonic solution of guanidinium chloride. *Nature (London)* **178,** 316–317.

Larsen, J. B., and Lane, C. E. (1966). Some effects of *Physalia physalis* on the heart of the land crab, *Cardisoma guanhumi* (Latreille). *Toxicon* **3,** 69–71.

Li, C. P., Prescott, B., Jahncs, W. C., and Martino, E. C. (1962). Antimicrobial agents from mollusks. *Trans. N.Y. Acad. Sci.* [2] **24,** 504–509.

Li, C. P., Eddy, B., Prescott, B., Caldes, G., Green, W. R., Martino, E. C., and Young, A. M. (1965). Antiviral activities of paolins from clams. *Ann. N.Y. Acad. Sci.* **130,** 374–382.

Li, K. M. (1965). Ciguatera fish poison: A choline esterase inhibitor. *Science* **147,** 714–715.

McCandless, E. L. (1965). Chemical structural requirements of stimulation of connective tissue growth by polysaccharides. *Ann. N.Y. Acad. Sci.* **118,** 867–882.

McCandless, E. L. (1967). Sensitization reaction of carrageenan in the guinea pig. *Proc. Soc. Exp. Biol. Med.* **124,** 1239–1242.

Martin, D. F. (1970). "Marine Chemistry," Vol. II, p. 427. Dekker, New York.

Martin, D. F., and Chatterjee, A. B. (1970). Some chemical and physical properties of two toxins from the red-tide organism, *Gymnodinium breve. U.S. Fish Wildl. Serv. Fish. Bull.* **68,** 433–443.

Martin, D. F., and Padilla, G. M. (1971). Hemolysis induced by *Prymnesium parvum* toxin. Kinetics and binding. *Biochim. Biophys. Acta* **241,** 213–225.

Martin, D. F., Padilla, G. M., and Brown, P. A. (1971). Hemolysis induced by *Prymnesium parvum* toxin. Effect of primaquine treatment. *Biochim. Biophys. Acta* **249,** 69–80.

Martin, E. J. (1966). Anticoagulant from the sea anemone *Rhodactis* howesii. *Proc. Soc. Exp. Biol. Med.* **121,** 1063–1065.

Moore, R. E., and Scheuer, P. J. (1971). Palytoxin: A new marine toxin from a coelenterate. *Science* **172,** 495–496.

Mosher, H., Fuhrman, F., Buchwald, H., and Fischer, H. (1964). Tarichatoxin-tetrodotoxin, a potent neurotoxin. *Science* **144,** 1100–1110.

Mueller, G. P., and Rees, D. A. (1968). Current structural views of red polysaccharides. *In* "Drugs from the Sea" (H. D. Freudenthal, ed.), pp. 214–255. Marine Technology Society, Washington, D.C.

Murakami, S., Takemoto, T., Tei, Z., and Daigo, K. (1955). Effective principles of *Digenea simplex*. VIII. Structure of kainic acid. *J. Pharm. Soc. Jap.* **75,** 866–869.

Murtha, E. F. (1960). Pharmacological study of poisons from shellfish and puffer fish. *Ann. N.Y. Acad. Sci.* **90,** 820–836.

Narahashi, T., Moore, J. W., and Scott, W. R. (1964). Tetrodotoxin blockage of sodium conductance increase in lobster giant axons. *J. Gen. Physiol.* **47,** 965–974.

Narahashi, T., Anderson, N. C., and Moore, J. W. (1966). Tetrodotoxin does not block excitation from inside the nerve membrane. *Science* **153,** 765–767.

Narahashi, T., Moore, J. W., and Poston, R. N. (1967). Tetrodotoxin derivatives: Chemical structure and blockage of nerve membrane conductance. *Science* **156,** 976–979.

Nigrelli, R. F., Jakowska, S., and Calventi, L. (1959). Ectyonin, an antimicrobial agent from the sponge, *Microciona prolifera* Verrill. *Zoologica (New York)*, **44,** 173–176.

Nigrelli, R. F. (1955). The chemical nature of holothurin, a toxic principle from the sea-cucumber (Echinodermata: Holothurioidea). *Zoologica (New York)* **40,** 47–48.

Nigrelli, R. F., and Jakowska, S. (1960). Effects of holothurin, a steroid saponin from the Bahamian sea-cucumber (*Actinopyga agassizi*) on various biological systems. *Ann. N.Y. Acad. Sci.* **90**, 884–892.

Okaichi, T., and Hashimoto, Y. (1962). Physiological activities of nereistoxin. *Bull. Jap. Soc. Sci. Fish.* **28**, 930–935.

Osol, A., Pratt, R., and Altschule, M. D. (1967). "The United States Dispensatory and Physicians Pharmacology." Lippincott, Philadelphia, Pennsylvania.

Padilla, G. M. (1970). Growth and toxigenesis of the chrysomonad *Prymnesium parvum* as a function of salinity. *J. Protozool.* **17**, 456–462.

Parnas, I. (1963). The toxicity of *Prymnesium parvum*. *Isr. J. Zool.* **12**, 15–23.

Paster, Z. (1968). Prymnesin: The toxin of *Prymnesium parvum* Carter. *Rev. Int. Oceanogr. Med.* **10**, 249–258.

Paster, Z., and Abbott, B. C. (1969). Hemolysis of rabbit erythrocytes by *Gymnodinium breve* toxin. *Toxicon* **7**, 245.

Pepler, W. J., and Loubser, E. (1960). Histochemical demonstration of the mode of action of the alkaloid in mussel poisoning. *Nature (London)* **188**, 860.

Percival, E., and McDowell, R. H. (1967). "Chemistry and Enzymology of Marine Algal Polysaccharides," Chapter 5. Academic Press, New York.

Pike, J. E. (1971). Prostaglandins. *Sci. Amer.* **225**, 84–92.

Pratt, R. R., Mautner, H., Gardner, G. M., Sha, Y., and Dufrenoy, J. (1951). Report on antibiotic activity of seaweed extracts. *J. Amer. Pharm. Ass.* **40**, 575–579.

Ramwell, P., and Shaw, J. (1971). The biological significance of the prostaglandins. *Ann. N.Y. Acad. Sci.* **180**, 10–13.

Robertson, W. V. B., and Schwartz, D. (1953). Ascorbic acid and the formation of collagen. *J. Biol. Chem.* **201**, 689–696.

Roos, H. (1957). Untersuchungen über das vorkommen antimikrobieller substanzen in meersalzen. *Kiel. Meeresforsch.* **13**, 41–58.

Russell, F. E., and Emery, J. (1960). Venom of the weevers *Trachinus draco* and *Trachinus vipera*. *Ann. N.Y. Acad. Sci.* **90**, 805–819.

Russell, F. E. (1965). Marine toxins and venomous and poisonous marine animals. *Advan. Mar. Biol.* **3**, 355–384.

Russell, F. E. (1967). Comparative pharmacology of some animal toxins. *Fed. Proc., Fed. Amer. Soc. Exp. Biol.* **26**, 1206–1224.

Schantz, E. J. (1963). Studies on the paralytic poisons found in mussels and clams along the North American Pacific Coast. *In* "Venomous and Poisonous Animals and Noxious Plants of the Pacific Region" (H. L. Keegan and W. V. Macfarlane, eds.), pp. 75–82. Pergamon, Oxford.

Schantz, E. J. (1970). Algal toxins. *In* "Properties and Products of Algae" (J. E. Zajic, ed.), pp. 83–96. Plenum, New York.

Schantz, E. J., Lynch, J. M., Vayvada, G., Matsumoto, K., and Rapoport, H. (1966). The purification and characterization of the poison produced by *Gonyaulax catenella* in axenic culture. *Biochemistry* **5**, 1191–1195.

Scheuer, P., Takahashi, W., Tsutsumi, J., and Yoshida, T. (1967). Ciguatoxin: Isolation and chemical nature. *Science* **155**, 1267–1268.

Schmeer, M. R. (1966). Mercenene: Growth-inhibiting agent of *Mercenaria* extracts further chemical and biological characterization. *Ann. N.Y. Acad. Sci.* **136**, 211–218.

Schweiger, R. G. (1962). Acetylation of alginic acid. II. Reaction of algin acetates with calcium and other divalent metal ions. *J. Org. Chem.* **27**, 1789–1791.

Schwimmer, D., and Schwimmer, M. (1964). Algae and medicine. *In* "Algae and Man," (D. F. Jackson, ed.), pp. 368–412. Plenum, New York.

Shanes, A. M., Freygang, W. H., Grundfest, H., and Amatniek, E. (1959). Anaesthetic and calcium action in the voltage clamped squid giant axon. *J. Gen. Physiol.* **42,** 793–802.

Shilo, M. (1967). Formation and mode of action of algal toxins. *Bacteriol. Rev.* **31,** 180–193.

Starr, J. (1962). Antibacterial and antiviral activities of algal extracts studied by acridine orange staining. *Tex. Rep. Biol. Med.* **20,** 271–279.

Tanaka, K., Ueyanagi, J., Nawa, H., Sanno, Y., Honjo, M., Nakamori, R., Sugawa, T., Uchibayashi, M., Osugi, K., Ueno, Y., and Tatsuoka, T. (1957). The synthesis of L-α-kainic acid. *Proc. Jap. Acad.* **33,** 53–58.

Tasaki, I., Singer, I., and Watanabe, A. (1966). Excitation of squid giant axons in sodium-free external media. *Amer. J. Physiol.* **211,** 746–754.

Thomson, D. A. (1964). Ostracitoxin: An ichthyotoxic stress secretion of the boxfish, *Ostracion lenthiginousus. Science* **146,** 244–245.

Thomson, D. A. (1968). Trunkfish toxins. *In* "Drugs from the Sea" (H. D. Freudenthal, ed.), pp. 203–211. Marine Technology Society, Washington, D.C.

Trieff, N. M., Spikes, J. J., and Ray, S. M. (1970). Isolation and purification of *Gymnodinium breve* toxin. *Toxicon* **8,** 157.

Tsuda, K., Ikuma, S., Kawamura, M., Tachikawa, R., Sakai, K., Tamura, C., and Amakaru, O. (1964). Tetrodotoxin. VII. On structure of tetrodotoxin and its derivatives. *Chem. Pharm. Bull.* **12,** 1357–1374.

Tu, A. T. (1971). Sea snake venom structure probed. *Chem. Eng. News* **49,** 25–26.

Waldron-Edward, D. (1968). The use of alginate in the prevention and treatment of radiostrontium toxicity. *In* "Drugs from the Sea" (H. D. Freudenthal, ed.), pp. 267–275. Marine Technology Society, Washington, D.C.

Weinheimer, A. J., and Spraggins, R. L. (1969). The occurrence of two new prostaglandin derivatives (15-*epi*-PGA$_2$ and its acetate, methyl ester) in the gorgonian *Plexaura homomalla*, chemistry of coelenterates. XV. *Tetrahedron Lett.* No. 59, p. 5185.

Wiberg, G. S., and Stephenson, N. R. (1960). Toxicologic studies on paralytic shellfish poison. *Toxicol. Appl. Pharmacol.* **2,** 607–615.

Wong, J. L., Oesterlin, R., and Rapoport, H. (1971). The structure of saxitoxin. *J. Amer. Chem. Soc.* **93,** 7344–7345.

Yasumoto, T., Watanabe, T., and Hashimoto, Y. (1964). Physiological activities of starfish saponin. *Bull. Jap. Soc. Sci. Fish.* **30,** 357–364.

Youngken, H. W., Jr. (1968). Sources of drugs from the sea and drug screening. *In* "Drugs from the Sea" (H. D. Fruedenthal, ed.), pp. 15–17. Marine Technology Society, Washington, D.C.

Yudkin, W. H. (1944). Tetrodon poisoning. *Bull. Bingham Oceanogr. Coll.* **9,** 1–18.

CHAPTER II

Biochemistry of Nemertine Toxins

WILLIAM R. KEM

I. Introduction

The nemertines (rhynchocoeles) are a small invertebrate phylum containing fewer than 1000 described species. In many ways, these worms resemble the free-living flatworms (from which the nemertines probably evolved), but they are easily distinguished from the turbellarians by the presence of a prominent, eversible proboscis (Fig. 1). The proboscis primarily functions in the capture of prey animals. Nemertine species vary greatly in size (from millimeters to several meters), external coloration, and abundance. Most are marine, but there are also a few land and fresh-water species (Coe, 1943; Hyman, 1951; Gontcharoff, 1961). Nemertines are classified into two subphyla, the Anopla and the Enopla. The mid-region of the enoplan proboscis contains a stylet apparatus for piercing

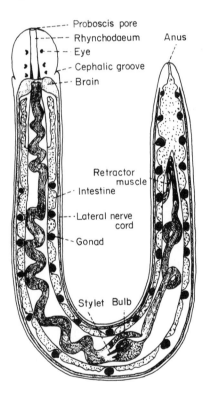

FIG. 1. Drawing of a hoplonemertine, *Prostoma rubrum*, illustrating the anterior, median (stylet-bearing), and posterior regions of the proboscis. (Modified from R. W. Pennak, "Fresh-Water Invertebrates of the United States," Copyright 1953, The Ronald Press Company, New York.)

prey, while the anoplan proboscis lacks this structure. Each subphylum is in turn divided into two orders (Coe, 1943). The Heteronemertinea (Anopla) and the Hoplonemertinea (Enopla) are the two most abundant orders, and most of the research described in this chapter will be concerned with species from these two orders.

Nemertines are carnivorous, feeding mainly upon annelids, crustaceans, mollusks, and even fish. Certain hoplonemertine species are known to immobilize their prey with a viscous venom released from the proboscis (Reisinger, 1926; Gontcharoff, 1948, 1961; Hickman, 1963; Jennings and Gibson, 1969; Roe, 1970). By isolating and observing annelids immediately after they are attacked by *Paranemertes peregrina*, it is possible to observe the time course of prey paralysis separate from the mechanical damage and mucous entanglement that normally also contribute to prey immobilization. During its attack, *Paranemertes* repeatedly jabs the body surface of the annelid with its proboscis stylet, and the segments that come into contact with the proboscis are rapidly paralyzed. If the annelid is not mechanically damaged, it will recover within about 20 minutes. The venom generally does not kill the prey (Roe, 1970).

Several zoologists have suggested that mucous secretions from the body surface of nemertines are toxic. McIntosh (1873) noted that the skin of many heteronemertines gave a marked acid reaction when tested with litmus paper. Wilson (1900) observed with respect to the heteronemertine *Cerebratulus lacteus* that, "If a minute drop of the slime be placed upon the tongue, it will be found so intensely acrid as to parch the whole mouth, and the taste remains for a long time." Hyman (1951) mentioned that the slime secreted by nemertines is obnoxious to other animals and possibly even poisonous.

Bacq (1936, 1937) accidentally discovered the presence of two toxic substances in nemertines during his comparative studies of the distribution of choline esters in various animal phyla. Pharmacological experiments with aqueous extracts of whole nemertines led Bacq to conclude that there are two different toxic substances in this phylum, "amphiporine" and "nemertine" (Table I). Amphiporine extracts (from the hoplonemertines *Amphiporus lactifloreus* and *Drepanophorus crassus*) elicited a nicotinelike contracture of the frog rectus abdominis muscle which was not potentiated by eserine. The contracture reversed more slowly upon washing than was the case after acetylcholine contracture. The *Amphiporus* extract augmented the blood pressure of an atropinized cat anesthetized with chloralose. The cat superior cervical ganglion-nictitating membrane preparation was excited and then blocked by the *Drepanophorus* extract. Both autonomic preparations were blocked subsequent to the initial excitatory effect,

TABLE I

Nemertine Toxins[a]

Amphiporine
1. Produces prolonged contractures in frog rectus abdominis
2. Excites, then blocks cat superior cervical ganglion; lacks negative inotropic effects on Straub heart preparation of frog
3. Induces convulsions in crabs; produced spontaneous action potentials
   in *Carcinus* nerve bundle (one experiment?)
4. Dialyzable; resists boiling 15 minutes at neutral, acid, and alkaline
   (0.5 N NaOH) pH's
5. Soluble in methanol, ethanol, chloroform (alkaline pH; King, 1939);
   slightly soluble in ether; insoluble in acetone
6. Absent in all anoplan nemertines tested
                        Nemertine
1. No contractural effect on frog rectus; negligible effects on frog heart
2. Induces convulsions in crabs; spontaneous action potentials in isolated
   nerve bundles
3. Apparently exists in all nemertine species, at widely variable tissue concentrations
4. Dialyzes slower than amphiporine, resistant to boiling
5. Solubility properties similar to amphiporine

---

[a] Bacq (1936, 1937).

and became insensitive to further applications of the same extracts. The *Amphiporus* extract lacked any negative inotropic actions on the frog heart, unlike what would be expected for a choline ester. The stability of amphiporine to boiling under acid or alkaline conditions and its extraction into chloroform from an alkaline solution unequivocally demonstrated that it is not a choline ester. An *Amphiporus* extract induced repetitive spiking in an isolated crab leg nerve preparation (Bacq, 1936, 1937). Bacq concluded that amphiporine is an alkaloid similar to nicotine.

Heteronemertine extracts failed to contract the frog rectus abdominis, but they did induce repetitive spiking in *Carcinus* nerve bundles. Again, no effect was observed with the frog heart. Nemertine was so named because aqueous extracts of practically all nemertine species stimulated crab nerve or walking leg preparations, at least in high concentrations (Bacq, 1936, 1937). The presence of nemertine in amphiporine-containing species was not ascertained since quantitative bioassays of tissue toxicity were not made. Since only crude extracts were tested, it was not demonstrated that the rectus-contracting, crab nerve-stimulatory, and crab-paralyzing activities in *Amphiporus* are due to the same substance. Amphiporine (by rectus assay) was absent in certain hoplonemertines species and in all the anoplan species tested. All *Amphiporus* tissues were active on the rectus, so it was concluded that amphiporine is not a venom in the usual vertebrate sense of the term (Bacq, 1936, 1937).

King (1939) attempted the purification of the active constituent of *Amphiporus lactifloreus* using the frog rectus contracture for bioassay of the active substance. One thousand worms collected over an 18-month period and kept in 90% ethanol were used. The solvent was removed, and the worms were reextracted with ethanol after being ground with sand. The combined solvent extracts were then evaporated to a small volume under reduced pressure, acidified, and reextracted with chloroform to remove fats and pigments. The solution was made alkaline by adding solid sodium bicarbonate, and was then extracted four times with chloroform. The basic chloroform extract was evaporated to dryness, yielding 44 mg of a brownish varnish that contained most of the rectus-contracting activity. Small amounts of this oil were added to several alkaloidal precipitants in order to find a means of crystallizing the substance. Picric acid, mercuric chloride, flavianic acid, and ammonium reineckate all gave oily or only partially crystalline salts. A chloroplatinate was the only well-defined crystalline salt formed, but it was completely insoluble in boiling water or dilute acid, and could not be decomposed by addition of silver or hydrogen sulfide. Failure to find a sparingly soluble salt of amphiporine suitable for further purification by recrystallization and the difficulties in obtaining sufficient *Amphiporus* extracts apparently caused the termination of this investigation.

The potential of certain neurotoxins as tools for analyzing electrically and chemically excitable membranes is particularly evident from recent pharmacological and electrophysiological studies on tetrodotoxin (Narahashi *et al.*, 1964; Kao, 1966; Moore and Narahashi, 1967) and α-bungarotoxin (Changeux *et al.*, 1970; Miledi *et al.*, 1971). The pharmacological actions of amphiporine and nemertine (particularly their common ability to induce spontaneous, repetitive action potentials in isolated axon preparations) suggested that these compounds might also serve as experimental tools for studying the molecular basis of membrane excitation. The papers of Bacq (1936, 1937) and King (1939) are the only original publications on nemertine toxins prior to 1969, and thus they have served as a foundation for the research presented in this chapter. My initial goal was to collect, purify, and characterize the nemertine toxins prior to carrying out detailed pharmacological and electrophysiological experiments on their mechanisms of action. This was a fortunate strategy since at least five separate toxins have now been isolated from a small number of species, and other toxic compounds will probably be discovered as extracts of other nemertines become available. The present chapter will be concerned with the purification and chemical analysis of several nemertine toxins and their relationships to Bacq's amphiporine and nemertine.

II. Materials and Methods

A. Animals

The major recurring difficulty in investigating nemertine toxins is obtaining sufficient numbers and species for analysis. This chapter is primarily concerned with the toxins present in two of the most abundant North American species. Preliminary experiments (in 1965) on a small ethanolic extract of the Pacific coast hoplonemertine *Paranemertes peregrina* demonstrated the presence of large amounts of amphiporine activity (rectus abdominus contracture) in this species. Two years later, I hand-collected 10,000 (3.70 kg) *Paranemertes* at Friday Harbor Marine Laboratory, San Juan Island, Washington. This species wanders over the exposed sandy mud surface of the intertidal zone as the tide recedes, searching for its annelid prey. Consequently, it is much more readily collected than most nemertines, which generally burrow or hide beneath rocks during low tide.

Approximately 200 living specimens of the East coast heteronemertine *Cerebratulus lacteus* were obtained from the Supply Department, Marine Biological Laboratory, Woods Hole, Massachusetts. *Lineus ruber, Lineus viridis,* and *Amphiporus angulatus* were collected from rocky intertidal areas along the New Hampshire and Maine coasts. Other nemertine species were collected and identified by several generous zoologists (see Acknowledgments).

B. Bioassay of Nemertine Toxins

A quantal bioassay measuring the median effective dose (PD_{50}) necessary to paralyze a 20-g crayfish (*Orconectes virilis* or *Procambarus clarkii*) is used to analyze all nemertine toxin extracts. Crayfish are purchased from commercial suppliers (E. Steinhilber Co., Oshkosh, Wisconsin; Dahl Co., Berkeley, California) and are kept in plastic pans containing about 1 inch of tap water (room temperature) for at least 2 days before use. Animals can be maintained for a month or longer by weekly feedings of shredded pork liver. Crayfish used are of both sexes, and their sizes range from 10 to 30 g (mean of about 20 g). The behavioral end point chosen as a measure of paralysis is righting ability. Before beginning a bioassay, all animals are placed squarely on their backs, and only those individuals that right themselves within 2 minutes and possessing both chelipeds are used. Five randomly selected crayfish are rapidly weighed and injected (dorsal posterior terminus of cephalothorax, 0.06 ml/10 g) within approximately 2 minutes. All toxin samples are prepared in crayfish saline (van Harreveld, 1936), and the final pH is adjusted within the range 6.5–7.5. Fifteen minutes after the first injection, all five crayfish are placed squarely on their backs, and after 2 minutes the number of nonrighting individuals is recorded. In order to minimize bioassay costs (about \$0.50 per crayfish), the intermediate response-producing dose range is routinely estimated with crayfish that had been used in previous bioassays or that lack both chelipeds.

The PD_{50} is estimated by several methods, depending upon the numbers of animals and doses tested. Under optimal conditions, a single bioassay consists of three to four intermediate doses (ten or fifteen animals per dose) prepared by serial twofold dilutions. The PD_{50} is then estimated either by linear regression analysis (Kem, 1971) or by the Spearman-Karber estimation method (Finney, 1964; Brown, 1970). The latter method is recommended when applicable, since it also gives an estimate of the standard error involved in a particular PD_{50} determination. The planning and analysis of bioassays according to the Spearman-Karber method are aptly described in a recent article (Brown, 1970). In the bioassay of numerous chromatographic fractions, it is not possible to use as many doses and animals (see above). In this case, two intermediate doses are usually tested (ten crayfish per dose, same dose interval), and the PD_{50} is graphically estimated by straight-line interpolation. The toxicity of a particular toxin sample is always expressed in crayfish units (1 CU = 1 PD_{50} for a 20-g crayfish).

The advantages of the crayfish paralytic assay are its simplicity, speed, and its responsiveness to a wide variety of neurotoxins. The latter characteristic makes it of general use in monitoring neurotoxin purifications and in exploratory studies of tissue extracts suspected of containing uncharacterized toxic compounds. Since many types of toxin are known to produce spastic or flaccid paralysis of crayfish, this bioassay can usually be expected to ascertain the presence or absence of neurotoxins in a given extract. The low selectivity of this assay was not particularly disadvantageous in the present investigation. When required, selectivity could be be effectively increased by parallel application of the colorimetric assay for *Paranemertes* toxin (Section II,C) or by initial fractionation of a toxic extract by various chromatographic methods. The drawbacks of this bioassay are its cost (about half that for white mice) and the heterogeneity of the commercially supplied crayfish with respect to size, sex, and seasonal status. The relative responsiveness of the two crayfish species to nemertine toxins was not extensively studied, but, at least in their responses to the *Lineus* toxins, they are very similar (W. R. Kem, unpublished). *Orconectes virilis* was used exclusively in the *Paranemertes* toxin studies, while *Procambarus clarkii* was routinely used in the heteronemertine toxin experiments.

C. Colorimetric Determination of Paranemertes Toxin

The first thin-layer separations of *Paranemertes* toxin indicated that it is easily visualized by several spot reagents, the most useful being Dragendorff's (orange spot), ninhydrin–acetic acid (lavender spot), and Ehrlich's reagent (salmon spot). The latter reagent yields a uniquely colored product with the toxin, so the p-dimethylaminobenzaldehyde (DMAB) reaction was adapted for use as a sensitive, specific chemical assay for *Paranemertes* toxin. The colorimetric assay allows a more quantitative analysis of the purification and distribution of this particular nemertine toxin than is possible solely by the bioassay procedure, and it also eliminates much expense.

The standard conditions finally chosen for the colorimetric assay are as follows. The reaction sample consists of 1.0 ml p-dimethylaminobenzaldehyde reagent (1.0 g DMAB, 1.0 ml concentrated HCl, 98.0 ml absolute ethanol), the ethanolic toxin sample, and sufficient ethanol to give a 2.0-ml final sample volume. Absorbance at 490 nm is measured after 3 hours heating at 70°C, since at this time the reaction is nearly complete (Kem, 1971). Absorbance development is independent of hydrogen ion concentration over a thirtyfold range, 2.5×10^{-3}–7.5×10^{-2} N HCl; the acidity under standard conditions is 5.5×10^{-2} N HCl. Absorbance developed is a linear function of *Paranemertes* toxin concentration (Fig. 2). Duplication of sample is recommended since the standard deviation of the mean absorbance of duplicate samples averages 3.7%. Absorbance of refrigerated (5°C) samples is stable for several days, but readings are routinely made within 2 hours. Several dilutions of a toxic sample are usually used for the reaction in order to insure a final 490-nm absorbance of less than 1.0. A 490-nm absorbance of 1.00 is observed with 6 μg of pure toxin in the 2.0-ml sample volume; the molar extinction coefficient of the DMAB-toxin derivative is therefore 5.3×10^4, based on the toxin molecular weight (Section III,B). The linearity of the assay with respect to toxin concentration partly depends upon the presence of a large excess of DMAB (2000-fold excess over toxin, molar basis). Samples containing as much as 60 μg pure toxin also give absorbances expected from Fig. 2, but such amounts are to be avoided in assays of crude toxin extracts in which many other DMAB-reactive substances are present.

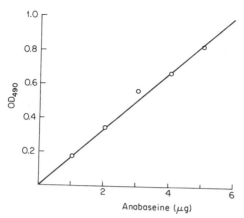

Fig. 2. Standard curve for the colorimetric (*p*-dimethylaminobenzaldehyde) assay of *Paranemertes* toxin (anabaseine). The average slope for four experiments was 6.05 ± 0.18 (SEM) µg per unit absorbance. (Kem, 1971.)

The selectivity of the DMAB method in the determination of the toxin in crude tissue extracts of whole *Paranemertes* was tested. After routine colorimetric assay, an ethanolic sample was flash evaporated, dissolved in aqueous solution, extracted with ethyl acetate under acidic and basic conditions, and then the basic ethyl acetate phase was evaporated and separated on aluminum oxide thin-layers. With ethyl acetate development the DMAB-toxin derivative has R_f 0.4, whereas unreacted DMAB migrates with the solvent front. A similar amount of synthetic toxin (Section III, C) was reacted with DMAB, and purified in parallel with the natural product to correct for losses incurred during the purification process. Over 95% of the initial 490-nm absorbance in the crude extract was accounted for by the toxin (Kem, 1971).

The selectivity of this assay for *Paranemertes* toxin is based on the 488-nm λ_{max} of the product chromophore measured under standard conditions. DMAB also reacts with indoles, amines, amino acids, proteins, etc., but these products generally absorb at shorter wavelengths, or are not formed in appreciable amounts at the moderate acid strength used in the above reaction. However, very concentrated alcoholic tissue extracts lacking anabaseine do contribute a small absorbance of approximately 0.03 OD_{490} units per 10 mg of original tissue extracted, so this interference must be corrected for when dealing with such extracts. The selectivity of the DMAB method for anabaseine in a new nemertine extract must always be established by isolation and identification of the DMAB derivative. The 488-nm λ_{max} and TLC (thin-layer chromatography) R_f of the derivative are good identification criteria. Ultimate identification of small amounts of anabaseine are best accomplished by mass spectrometry of the toxin base (Section III,B) or its DMAB-derivative (Section III,D).

D. Tissue Localization of Nemertine Toxins

Due to the acoelomate body plan and small size, it is difficult to dissect apart various nemertine organs and tissues for separate analysis. An exception is the proboscis, which is easily removed by either of two methods. Some species (*Paranemertes*) evert the proboscis when mechanically irritated with a dissecting needle; the proboscis is then grasped with forceps and pulled until it breaks loose from its anterior and posterior attachments. Examination of *Paranemertes* proboscis obtained in this manner suggests that the entire proboscis plus its posterior rectractor muscle is removed intact. The second method, applicable to all moderately large (diameter >3 mm) nemertines, is to cut through one side of the body wall musculature just behind the cephalic region. Application of pressure to the entire body causes rupture of the proboscis sheath and explosive release of the proboscis through this opening. The proboscis is then removed with forceps as above. The anterior, median, and posterior regions of the hoplonemertine proboscis are easily distinguished with a dissecting microscope, and can be sliced apart with a razor for separate analysis. The median segment contains the entire stylet apparatus, but most of its mass is contributed by adjacent anterior and posterior proboscis tissues. In these experiments, the proboscis parts were separately weighed and homogenized with at least five volumes of methanol–acetic acid (95:5); this material was vacuum filtered through a fine fritted glass disk, and the clear filtrate was flash evaporated, redissolved in ethanol, and then used in the colorimetric assay (Section II,C).

The body wall integument is spatially separated from the proboscis apparatus and digestive tract by several relatively thick muscle layers, making it possible to dissect transverse sections of moderately large nemertines into two portions containing different organs. The "peripheral" portion consists of the integument, its underlying basement membrane, and the external muscle layers, while the "core" portion contains the internal musculature, proboscis sheath, and digestive tract. If a toxin is largely present in only one of these samples, it can be safely concluded that the toxin is absent from the musculature, which contributes considerable mass to both portions. Large nemertines are probosectomized, the bodies are contracted to minimal length by mechanical irritation, and they are then rapidly frozen on pieces of dry ice. The frozen bodies are then transversely sectioned into numerous disks (1–3 mm thick). A disk is placed on a small block of dry ice under a dissecting microscope, and the peripheral tissues are then sliced away with a precooled razor, and are quickly placed in a vial packed in dry ice. The remaining core is then placed in another vial. After numerous repetitions of this procedure, the vial contents are separately freeze-dried, weighed, and then analyzed.

E. Amino Acid Analysis of Cerebratulus Toxins

A Beckman Model 120 amino acid analyzer modified for 2-hour analyses is used (Kem *et al.*, 1972). The two-column system using sodium citrate eluting buffers has been described (Spackman *et al.*, 1958). The CMC-purified toxins (0.3–1.0 mg, in 0.5 ml distilled water) are pipetted into Pyrex hydrolysis tubes containing 0.60 ml 12 N HCl and 0.10 ml 80% phenol. The samples are deaerated (with vortex mixing) and sealed under vacuum. Generally, 24-, 48-, and 72-hour hydrolysates are analyzed, due to the slow release of isoleucine in *Cerebratulus* Toxin III. Serine and threonine are estimated by linear extrapolation to zero hydrolysis time. Other amino acid estimates are mean values for the 24-, 48-, and 72-hour determinations. The calibration constant for carboxymethylcysteine is determined according to the Beckman manual.

The spectrophotometric method of Edelhoch (1967) was used to estimate the tryptophan content of reduced and carboxymethylated *Cerebratulus* Toxin III (RCM-Toxin III), in 6.0 M guanidine hydrochloride, 0.020 M potassium phosphate, pH 6.6. DTNB [5,5'-dithiobis(2-nitrobenzoic acid)] was used for the detection of cysteine (Ellman, 1959). The phenol–sulfuric acid procedure of Dubois (Hirs, 1967) was used to measure carbohydrate in the toxin samples.

F. Reduction and Carboxymethylation of Cerebratulus Toxin III

A procedure similar to that of Crestfield *et al.* (1963) was used. A 100-fold excess of 2-mercaptoethanol and a 90-fold excess of iodoacetate (Baker, recrystallized) are used in the reaction, assuming the presence of four half-cystines and a molecular weight of 4000 (from a preliminary amino acid analysis). The CMC-purified toxin is added to 3.0 ml of a nitrogen-equilibrated solution containing 6.0 M guanidine HCl, 1.0 M tris, and $2 \times 10^{-3} M$ EDTA (pH 8.5). Once the toxin is in solution, 0.07 ml of 2-mercaptoethanol is added, and the vial is closed to exclude air. After 4 hours, 170 mg of iodoacetate in 1.0 ml 1 N NaOH is added with stirring. The pH is immediately adjusted to 8.3, and the vial is closed, wrapped in foil to exclude light, and then maintained at room temperature for 20 minutes. After this period, the pH is 8.15. Ten drops of glacial acetic acid are added to terminate the reaction (final pH below 4), and the entire sample is then immediately applied to a G-25F Sephadex column (1.5 × 81 cm) equilibrated with 30% glacial acetic acid at room temperature. The column is wrapped with aluminum foil, and the separation is carried out in dim light to minimize iodine formation. The RCM-Toxin elutes at the void volume (V_0) and is completely separated from excess reactants and guanidine. The V_0 fractions are pooled and freeze-dried. RCM-Toxin (6.50 mg) is dissolved in 3.25 ml distilled water, and this 2.0-mg/ml standard solution is subsequenly used in the amino acid and molecular weight determinations.

G. Molecular Weight Determinations of Cerebratulus Toxin III

Sedimentation equilibrium ultracentrifugation and 6% agarose gel filtration methods are used to estimate the molecular weight of RCM-Toxin III (Kem *et al.*, 1972). Both experiments are done with the carboxymethylated toxin in buffered 6.0 M guanidine hydrochloride (Heico) solutions to eliminate secondary and tertiary structure. A Beckman Model E ultracentrifuge equipped with a photoelectric scanner is used for the sedimentation equilibrium run. The initial RCM-Toxin concentration is 0.33 mg/ml (OD_{280} = 0.470, in 6.0 M guanidine hydrocholoride, 0.02 M potassium phosphate, pH 6.6). Equilibrium is attained in 30 hours at 30,000 rpm; the final scan is recorded at 45 hours. An additional equilibrium scan is made at 52,000 rpm to check for sample heterogeneity. Log OD_{280} is plotted verses (radius)^2 and the slope, $d \log OD/dr^2$, is then estimated by visually fitting a straight line to the graph, which contains approximately twenty-five data points. Molecular weight is calculated according to Chervenka (1969). The partial specific volume ($\bar{v}$) of RCM-Toxic III is estimated as 0.71 from its amino acid composition, according to Cohn and Edsall (1943).

Insulin, cytochrome c, and α-chymotrypsinogen (all Sigma) are used as markers for the gel filtration determination. Each is separately reduced and carboxymethylated according to Fish *et al.* (1969). Dextran blue and dinitrophenylalanine (DNP-alanine) are used as markers for the void volume (V_0) and interstitial volume (V_e), respectively. A calibrating run with the five marker compounds is first done. The 0.35-ml marker sample applied to the column (1.5 × 85 cm) contains 5.0 mg/ml of each RCM-protein, 0.3% dextran blue, 0.05% DNP-alanine, 6.0 M guanidine HCl, and 0.01 M sodium acetate. Sucrose (110 mg) is added to facilitate layering of the sample on the column. The column flow rate (2.9 g per hour) is controlled by a constant head of pressure, and 0.79-g (mean) fractions are collected on a time basis. Gel filtration is carried out at room temperature (∼25°C). Elution volumes are gravimetrically estimated to increase the accuracy. A single run lasts about 50 hours (∼200 tubes), so it is necessary to remove and weigh eluted fractions (ten tubes at once) at least twice daily to minimize changes in fraction volumes. Absorbance of each marker-containing tube is determined with a Zeiss PMQ-II spectrophotometer at the wavelengths used by Fish *et al.* (1969). The blank is the eluting medium, 6.0 M guanidine hydrochloride, 0.01 M sodium acetate, pH 4.75. The 0.25-ml experimental sample (8.0 mg/ml RCM-Toxin, 0.4% dextran blue, 0.06% DNP-alanine, 6.0 M guanidine HCl, 0.01 M sodium acetate, pH 4.75) is applied and eluted under identical conditions. Molecular weight is estimated from a Porath plot constructed with the K_d estimates for the three marker proteins (Fish *et al.*, 1969).

III. Hoplonemertine Toxins

A. Purification of Paranemertes Toxin

The purification and structure determination of *Paranemertes* toxin have recently been described in some detail (Kem, 1969; Kem *et al.*, 1971). These experiments will now be briefly described, particularly to introduce some of the versatile separatory and analytical techniques now at the disposal of the marine toxinologist or pharmacognosist. A preparative purification of *Paranemertes* toxin is summarized in Fig. 3. The four main steps are (1) tissue homogenization and toxin extraction with 95% ethanol–5% glacial acetic acid, (2) solvent fractionation of the ethanol-soluble materials under acidic and then alkaline conditions, (3) aluminum oxide adsorption chromatography, and (4) crystallization of the toxin picrate. All of these steps are classic separation procedures in alkaloid chemistry, and the first two steps were previously used in the partial purification of amphiporine (King, 1939). The entire procedure was first tested on a small *Paranemertes* extract before scaling it up to extracts containing 500–1000 g fresh weight *Paranemertes*.

Approximately 150-g batches of *Paranemertes* were cleaned, weighed, and then homogenized with 4–5 volumes of 95% ethanol–5% glacial acetic acid. The pH range of these extracts was 3–4; this would most likely protonate a weakly basic toxin, making it more soluble, and would also enhance denaturation and precipitation of proteins in the extract. Acetic acid is very satisfactory for this purpose, since concentration of such extracts to about 10% of their initial volume by rotary evaporation does not lower the pH below 2.8. The concentrates were poured into polyethylene bottles which were then packed in dry ice and transported by car to the University of Illinois for further purification.

Crab paralysis and colorimetric assays of the various solvent phases involved in step (2) show that approximately 70–80% of the initial toxin

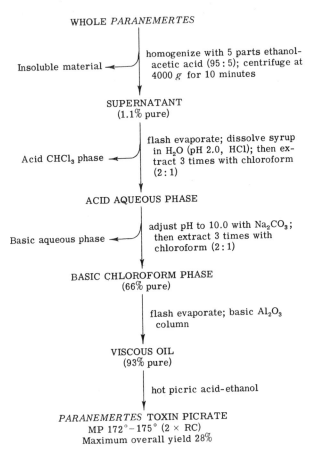

WHOLE *PARANEMERTES*

Insoluble material ←— homogenize with 5 parts ethanol-
acetic acid (95 : 5); centrifuge at
4000 *g* for 10 minutes

SUPERNATANT
(1.1% pure)

Acid CHCl₃ phase ←— flash evaporate; dissolve syrup
in H₂O (pH 2.0, HCl); then ex-
tract 3 times with chloroform
(2 : 1)

ACID AQUEOUS PHASE

Basic aqueous phase ←— adjust pH to 10.0 with Na₂CO₃;
then extract 3 times with
chloroform (2 : 1)

BASIC CHLOROFORM PHASE
(66% pure)

flash evaporate; basic Al₂O₃
column

VISCOUS OIL
(93% pure)

hot picric acid-ethanol

PARANEMERTES TOXIN PICRATE
MP 172°–175° (2 × RC)
Maximum overall yield 28%

FIG. 3. A preparative purification of *Paranemertes* toxin.

is recovered in the basic chloroform phase, and the remainder is largely in the acid chloroform phase. The yield in this step would undoubtedly be increased by using a countercurrent extraction procedure in both the acid and alkaline steps.

Step (3) can be accomplished by either column or preparative layer chromatography. I prefer the latter method because of its simplicity, speed, and better resolution. Collection and analysis of numerous samples are unnecessary. Merck Alox F-254, Type T precoated plates (20 × 20 cm, 0.2-cm thickness, activated 1 hour at 100°C) are capable of separating 300 mg of the oil obtained in step (2). After about 3 hours of development with ethyl acetate, UV-absorbing zones are observed near the origin, at R_f 0.6, and near the solvent front. Crayfish-paralytic and rectus-contracting activities are confined to the R_f-0.6 zone. *Paranemertes* toxin may be readily located on chromatograms by its distinctive spot reaction with the modified Ehrlich's reagent (Section II,C). *Paranemertes* toxin is essentially pure after step (3), as evidenced by its UV absorbance spectrum and vapor phase chromatographic behavior.

The toxin base is unstable over long periods of time, particularly at high concentrations, so a sparingly soluble picric acid salt of the toxin is prepared. The most efficient method for obtaining the toxin picrate is to add 4 g of solid picric acid per gram toxin base (in ethanol). This initially yields a very gummy material, but several minutes of trituration with a spatula finally yields a fine, amorphous precipitate. Two or three recrystallizations from 95% ethanol (75°C) are necessary to obtain a microcrystalline picrate, MP 172°–175°C. To obtain the free base, the picrate salt is dissolved in a saturated lithium hydroxide solution, and the base is recovered by repeated chloroform extraction. Thin-layer chromatography of the recovered base reveals a single DMAB-reactive spot possessing crayfish-paralytic and frog rectus-contracting activities.

B. Elucidation of Paranemertes Toxin Structure

The availability of 400 mg of pure toxin base permitted a complete spectral and chemical analysis of the compound (Kem *et al.*, 1971). The ultraviolet absorption spectrum (ethanol) contains a peak at 229 nm and a prominent shoulder at 265 nm. Both bands obey the Beer-Lambert relation, and thus represent real maxima. Adding a drop of concentrated HCl increases the absorbance at 265 nm by nearly 70%, whereas the 229-nm band is greatly depressed. It was inferred that *Paranemertes* toxin possesses a single double bond conjugated with an aromatic ring; the pH dependence of both absorbance bands indicates that one or more ionizable groups are present in the toxin.

The proton magnetic resonance spectrum of *Paranemertes* toxin (Fig. 4) permitted a tentative structure assignment (Fig. 5). The spectrum of a 10% solution of the toxin base in deuterochloroform consists of seven separate resonances. The four downfield proton resonances possess the chemical shifts and coupling constants expected for a 3-substituted pyridine ring. The $\tau 1.06$ and $\tau 1.45$ peaks are assigned to the 2' and 6' protons of anabaseine. The $\tau 1.9$ resonance must represent the 4' proton since the primary split (due to spin–spin coupling of protons) has $J \sim 8$ Hz, and the secondary split has $J \sim 1.7$ Hz. The $\tau 2.7$ peak is expected for the 5' proton, and it shows the expected primary ($J \sim 8$ Hz) and secondary ($J \sim 5$ Hz) splits. The spin–spin coupling constants for pyridine are

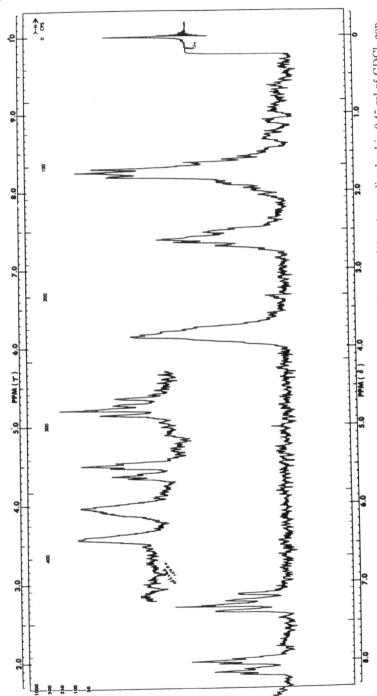

Fig. 4. Proton magnetic resonance spectrum of pure *Paranemertes* toxin. The base (50 mg) was dissolved in 0.45 ml of CDCl₃ containing TMS internal standard, and the spectrum was immediately recorded with a Varian A-60 (60 mHz) spectrometer. The downfield protons were recorded with a 150-Hz offset (two of the resonance peaks are duplicated). (Kem *et al.*, 1971.)

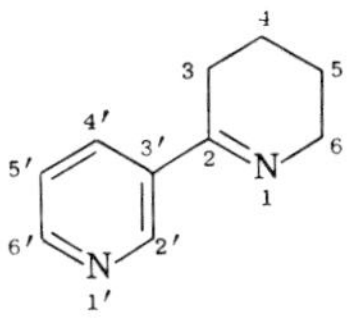

FIG. 5. Structure of *Paranemertes* toxin [anabaseine, or 2-(pyridyl)-3,4,5,6-tetra-hydropyridine].

$J(\alpha,\beta)$, 4.9–5.7 Hz; $J(\alpha,\gamma)$, 1.6–2.6 Hz; $J(\alpha,\gamma)$, 7.2–8.5 Hz (Dyer, 1965). The three remaining upfield peaks are expected for a 2-substituted Δ^1-piperideine ring. The $\tau 6.14$ peak represents the methylene protons adjacent to the nitrogen; the $\tau 7.38$ is characteristic of the allylic methylene protons; and the $\tau 8.25$ resonance is expected for methylene protons in a cyclic hydrocarbon. Electronic integration of the NMR spectrum shows that the relative peak areas are 1:1:1:1:2:2:4, as expected for anabaseine. The NMR spectrum fully agrees with published NMR data for anabaseine (Kamimura and Yamomoto, 1963; Duffield *et al.*, 1965) and for myosmine, the Δ^1-pyrroline analog (Pople *et al.*, 1959).

The mass spectra of both the toxin picrate and the TLC-purified base

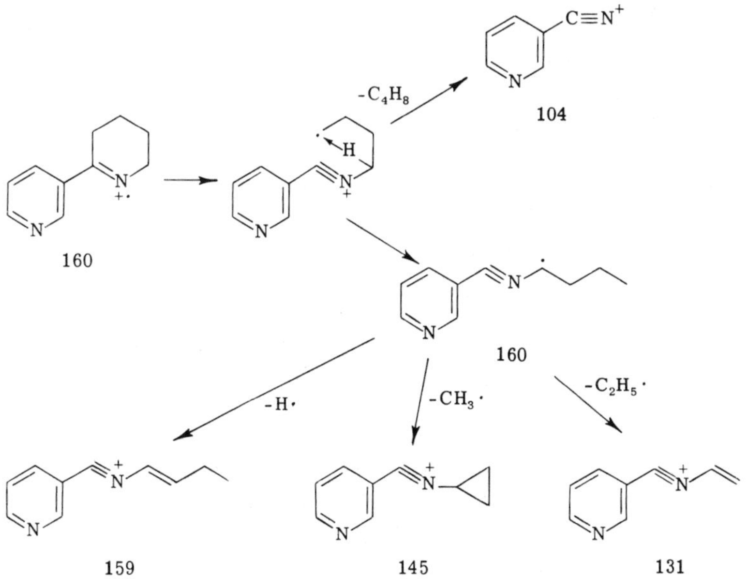

FIG. 6. Proposed mass spectral fragmentation mechanism for *Paranemertes* toxin (anabaseine).

contain a conspicuous molecular ion at m/e 160, as predicted for anabaseine. A plausible fragmentation route is shown in Fig. 6. Initial bond cleavage most likely occurs between carbons 2 and 3, as has also been proposed for myosmine (Duffield *et al.*, 1965). Conjugation of the imine double bond with the π-electron system of the pyridine ring apparently prevents appreciable cleavage at the 2–3′ bond, as evidenced by a small m/e-78 fragment.

Reduction of *Paranemertes* toxin with sodium borohydride would be expected to yield *dl*-anabasine if anabaseine is indeed the correct structure. The toxin reduction product picrate (MP 211–212°C) infrared spectrum is almost identical to the spectrum of *l*-anabasine picrate (Kem *et al.*, 1971). The melting point of *dl*-anabasine has been reported as 214°C (Späth and Mamoli, 1936a).

The elemental composition of *Paranemertes* toxin picrate agrees with the composition calculated for anabaseine dipicrate (found—C, 42.66%; H, 2.98%; N, 18.41%; calculated—C, 42.73%; H, 2.93%, N, 18.12%, $C_{10}H_{14}N_2 \cdot 2 \, C_6H_3N_3O_7$).

C. Anabaseine Synthesis

Interestingly, laboratory synthesis of this compound was reported in the same year that Bacq first reported his discovery of amphiporine. Final verification of the structure proposed for *Paranemertes* toxin was achieved by anabaseine synthesis according to Späth and Mamoli (1936a). Three main steps are involved in this synthesis (Fig. 7): (1) benzoylation of 2-piperidone (δ-valerolactam), yielding N-benzoylpiperidone (I), the precursor of the tetrahydropyridine ring; (2) Claisen ester condensation between (I) and nicotinic acid ethyl ester yielding the β-diketone intermediate α-nicotinoyl-N-benzoyl-2-piperidone (II); and (3) decarboxylation, ring closure, and amide hydrolysis in the presence of concentrated HCl. One such anabaseine synthesis will now be described in detail. All three starting compounds, δ-valerolactam, benzoic anhydride, and nicotinic acid ethyl ester, can be obtained from a single manufacturer (Aldrich).

δ-Valerolactam (29 g, 0.29 mole) and benzoic anhydride (68 g, 0.30 mole) are heated in a boiling flask at 180°C for 3 hours. The reaction mixture is then distilled at 1 mm Hg at temperatures up to 120°C to remove benzoic acid; this is terminated when 34 g of solid have been collected. Benzoic acid (MP 122°C) solidifies in the distillation assembly, so an infrared lamp is used to facilitate collection of the by-product. N-Benzoylpiperidone distills at 120°–180°C, and is recrystallized with ethyl acetate–ether (32.6 g, 55% yield, MP 110°–112°C).

In step (2), sodium ethoxide (15 g, 0.22 moles) is prepared by slowly

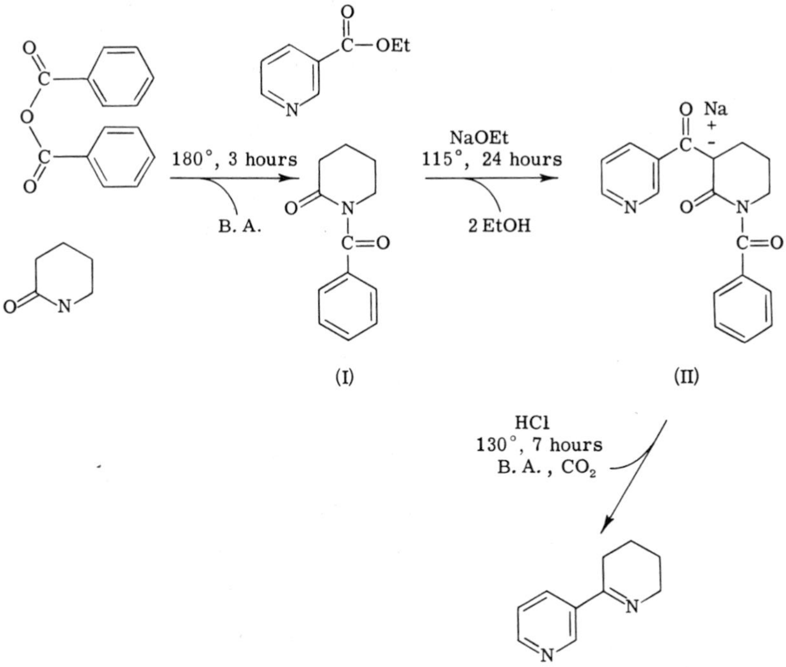

Fig. 7. Synthetic route for anabaseine. (Späth and Mamoli, 1936a.)

adding a total of 5 g of sodium chips to a larger excess of absolute ethanol, keeping the flask near room temperature with ice water. Excess ethanol is then flash evaporated at about 100°C, leaving a white solid. Ethyl nicotinate (24 g, 0.16 mole), *N*-benzoylpiperidone (32.6 g, 0.16 mole), and 65 ml of benzene are then added to the same flask, and the mixture is continuously stirred and refluxed in a 115°C bath under anhydrous conditions. After 20 hours, the solvent is evaporated, and 65 ml of benzene is again added in an attempt to drive the reaction to completion by removal of ethanol.

After a total of 24 hours, the solvent is again evaporated, and step (3) is initiated by slowly adding 460 ml of concentrated HCl. The solution is then poured into several glass (Carius) combustion tubes, which are then sealed and heated at 138°C for 7 hours (intermittent mixing). The tubes are cooled to 5°C before opening to prevent losses due to the considerable pressures generated by carbon dioxide. Slow addition of KOH pellets brings the pH to 11.2. Precipitated KCl is filtered off several times. The 600-ml aqueous solution is extracted three times with 600 ml of ethyl acetate. Rotary evaporation of the solvent yields 4.15 g of crude base which is precipitated with excess picric acid in absolute ethanol. Three recrystallizations yield 7.4 g of anabaseine dipicrate (0.012 moles, 4% overall yield, MP 174°–175°C). Elemental composition is experimentally found to be C, 42.97%; H, 2.98%; N, 18.22% (calculated—C, 42.73%; H, 2.93%; N, 18.12%).

Mixture of equal quantities of the *Paranemertes* toxin dipicrate with anabaseine dipicrate produces no melting point depression. Superimposed IR spectra are identical, as are the NMR spectra of the bases in CDCl₃. The mass spectrum of synthetic anabaseine is identical with the purified toxin. Thin-layer development in parallel gives indistinguishable R_f's. The crayfish paralytic activity of the natural and synthetic products are very similar (W. R. Kem, unpublished).

The 4% overall yield of the present synthesis is disappointing compared with the 24% yield reported by Späth and Mamoli (1936a). Recently, Kamimura and Yamomoto (1963) have reported a 13% yield based on *N*-benzoylpiperidone (I); this is about double the present yield calculated in the same fashion, but the lower melting point of their picrate (167°C) suggests the presence of considerable impurities. No obvious differences in procedure can account for these divergent yields. Since step (1) of the present synthesis gave the same yield as obtained by Späth and Mamoli, the large losses occurred in steps (2) and/or (3). The Claisen ester condensation is the most commonly used synthetic route for such 2-(3-pyridyl) compounds as nicotine, nornicotine, and myosmine, so it would be desirable to determine if the overall yields can be improved beyond the 10–20% yields usually reported. Myosmine dipicrate, the Δ^1-pyrroline analog of anabaseine, was synthesized in 10% yield by the same route, starting with 2-pyrrolidone (Späth and Mamoli, 1936b). A superior means of crystallizing anabaseine would also be helpful since about half of the synthetic product is lost during this step alone.

The synthetic contaminant noted in previous anabaseine syntheses is easily separated from anabaseine using alumina (Merck) thin-layers (Kem, 1969). During ethyl acetate development, the contaminant migrates near the solvent front, compared with R_f 0.6 for anabaseine. It is also more soluble than anabaseine in picric acid–ethanol, and, hence, may be simply removed during the recrystallization process. The TLC-purified contaminant has a peak absorbance at 236 nm in ethanol and a very small "shoulder" near 260 nm, but, upon acidification, one only finds a single, slightly larger peak at 258 nm. The infrared spectrum (neat) contains strong IR bands at 1720, 1280, and 1120 cm⁻¹, as expected for an N-benzoyl moiety (Dyer, 1965). The mass spectrum contains a small molecular ion at m/e 264 and conspicuous fragments at m/e 159, 158, 144, 130, 117, 105 (and 103 and 77). It is proposed that the contaminant is N-benzoyl-2-(3-pyridyl)-2,3-dehydropiperidine, an expected synthetic intermediate.

D. Chemical Basis of the Colorimetric Assay for Anabaseine

Due to the importance of this technique in the analysis of various nemertine extracts, the p-dimethylaminobenzaldehyde–anabaseine reaction product was prepared on a larger scale for structural analysis (Kem, 1971). Synthetic anabaseine was allowed to react with a twofold excess of p-dimethylaminobenzaldehyde for 2.5 hours at 61°C, pH 0.7 (ethanol). The reaction product base was recovered and then separated from unreacted DMAB by preparative layer chromatography, and the pure base was then precipitated with picric acid. The elemental composition of the recrystallized picrate (MP 211°–213°C) was in fair agreement with the composition expected for the reaction of equimolar amounts of the two reactants (found—C, 50.93%; H, 3.96%; N, 16.59%; calculated—C, 49.67%; H, 3.63%; N, 16.82%; for $C_{19}H_{21}N_3 \cdot 2 \ C_6H_3N_3O_7$). The mass spectrum of the product picrate contained a very prominent molecular ion, m/e 291, as expected. The large, conspicuous fragments (m/e 262, 248, 247, and 235) are most easily rationalized as being due to cleavage and fragmentation of the saturated portion of the tetrahydropyridine ring in the proposed structure (Fig. 8). The only other possible structure would be a Schiff base formed by reaction of the DMAB-carbonyl with the tetrahydropyridine nitrogen. This imine could exist under acidic conditions, but it is unlikely to be stable in its neutral form. The DMAB-anabaseine product was quite stable at alkaline pH's, and its intermediate TLC R_f (0.4, aluminum oxide, ethyl acetate development) suggests that it is un-ionized under these conditions.

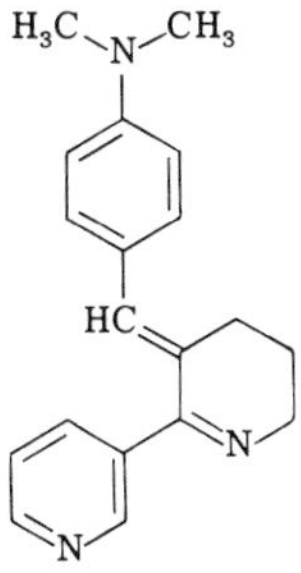

Fig. 8. 3-(N,N-dimethylaminobenzylidene)anabaseine, the product chromophore in the anabaseine colorimetric assay.

The ultraviolet and visible absorbance characteristics of 3-(dimethyl-aminobenzylidene)anabaseine were studied in some detail. In absolute ethanol (pH 1.1) the results were $E_{490nm} = 5.08 \times 10^4$, as expected from the assay standard curve (see Fig. 2). Spectra were also recorded from aqueous solutions (0.10 M potassium phosphate) of the derivative over the pH range 10.4–0.0. The primary λ_{max} for the base occurs at 353 nm; protonation causes the disappearance of this band and the simultaneous appearance of a stronger band at 472 nm. Spectrophotometric estimation (Flett, 1962) of the pK_a of this ionizable group yielded a value of 8.35, which is not surprising for an amidinium-type resonance system. Reducing the pH below about 3 produces two interesting changes in the primary absorbance peak. There is a progressive decline in absorbance, and the λ_{max} shifts from 472 to 490 nm; a new peak occurs at 320 nm. These alterations are probably due to protonation of the two remaining nitrogen base lone electron pairs. It is postulated that the pK_a of the pyridine nitrogen is slightly higher than the pK_a of the remaining nitrogen in the amidinium resonance system; protonation of the pyridine nitrogen would produce the 472–490 nm shift, and would also cause a substantial reduction in the maximal absorbance of this peak. Protonation of the remaining nitrogen would then be responsible for the complete disappearance of the 490-nm peak and the appearance of the 320-nm peak.

The maximum capabilities of the colorimetric procedure for anabaseine have not yet been fully realized. It should be possible to greatly increase the sensitivity of this assay by several changes. Simply reducing the reaction sample volume to 0.50 ml (maintaining the optical path length at 1 cm) would increase the sensitivity fourfold. Although pilot assays run at different pH's showed that maximal absorbance development occurs under standard conditions (Section II,C), spectral measurements on aqueous solutions of pure dimethylaminobenzylidene-anabaseine have recently demonstrated that its absorbance at pH 1.1 is only about 20% of its absorbance in the pH 4–6 range. The pH selected for the standard assay conditions thus appears to be a compromise between two pH optima, one for the rate of reaction, the other for the product chromophore. Considerable improvement in sensitivity should be obtained by raising the pH to the 4–6 region prior to reading the 470-nm absorbance. Incorporation of these two suggested modifications into the assay should make it possible to measure as little as 0.03 μg (0.2 nmoles) of anabaseine per sample. Another possible means of improving the sensitivity would involve the use of p-dimethylaminocinnamaldehyde in place of DMAB. This would be expected to yield a product chromophore with a larger molar extinction coefficient and an absorbance peak at a longer wavelength. With such improvements, it should be possible to analyze very small tissue samples. It may also be possible to adapt this reaction for histochemical localization of anabaseine in tissue sections.

IV. Heteronemertine Toxins

A. Preliminary Experiments with Lineus and Cerebratulus Toxins

Bacq (1936, 1937) stated that nemertine resisted boiling, was soluble in alcohols and chloroform, was barely soluble in ether, was insoluble in acetone, and was probably a small molecule similar to amphiporine. However, initial experiments with a methanol–0.5% concentrated HCl extract of *Lineus ruber* demonstrated that Bacq's nemertine was actually one or more polypeptide neurotoxins (Kem, 1969). Acidic (pH 1.0) and basic (pH 11.7) ethyl acetate extractions of an aqueous solution of the whole animal extract removed only minor amounts of paralytic activity (2.5% of the initial toxicity was found in the pH-1.0 ethyl acetate phase, 0.7% in the pH-11.7 ethyl acetate phase, and 44% of the initial activity remained in the aqueous phase). Approximately 53% of the initial toxicity was destroyed during these extractions. Chloroform extraction of the aqueous phase at pH 7.1 also failed to remove significant paralytic activity. Heating (100°C) aqueous solutions of the original toxin extract caused rapid inactivation of the paralytic activity at extremes of pH, particularly on the alkaline side. Trypsin, α-chymotrypsin, and pronase inactivated the crayfish paralytic activity (Kem, 1969). G-50M Sephadex gel filtration (0.1 M acetic acid) of part of the *L. ruber* extract showed that the paralytic activity eluted in a broad zone, $V_e = 1.6$–2.8 V_0 The peak of crayfish paralytic activity eluted at $V_e = 2.2$ V_0. Since glucagon (MW 3500) also eluted at $V_e = 2.2$ V_0 on the same column, it was concluded that the apparent molecular weight of the main toxin was approximately 3500. A prominent shoulder of activity also occurred near $V_e = 1.8$ V_0, and this suggested that more than one toxin was present.

Recent experiments with acidic methanol extracts of *Lineus ruber* that have been stored below -10°C for nearly 6 months have demonstrated that at least two separate polypeptide toxins are present (Fig. 9). The pharmacological properties of these partially purified toxins have not yet been extensively investigated, but it has been shown that both toxins induce spontaneous spike activity in isolated lobster (*Homarus americanus*) leg nerve preparations. High concentrations of both toxins failed to contract the frog rectus abdominis or to hemolyze human red cells suspended

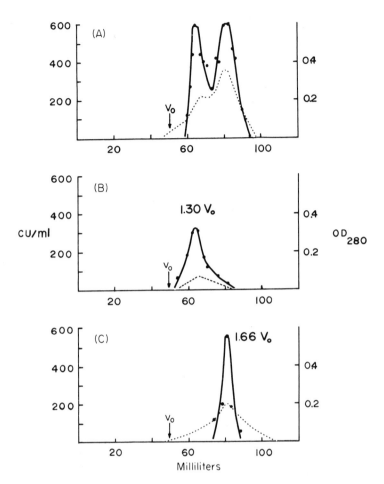

Fig. 9. Partial purification of the "artifact" polypeptide neurotoxins in a 6-month-old acidic methanol extract of the heteronemertine *Lineus ruber*. The G-25F Sephadex gel column (1.5 × 81 cm) was eluted with 0.10 M ammonium acetate–acetic acid (pH 5.0, 5°C). A, the initial separation; B and C show the effluent diagrams obtained by rechromatography of the two partially resolved components obtained in A. Solid lines, crayfish units per ml; dotted lines, OD_{280}.

in isotonic saline. These properties are thus consistent with Bacq's limited description of nemertine.

A milder extraction procedure was required once the paralytic compounds were demonstrated to be polypeptide toxins. Acidic methanol would be expected to denature many polypeptides and proteins, to cause the hydrolysis of certain labile peptide and side-chain amide bonds, and to esterify carboxyl groups. It was suspected that the two observed polypeptides were actually partial degradation products of one or more native toxins of larger molecular size. This was recently demonstrated to be the case, as G-25F Sephadex gel filtration experiments with aqueous extracts of whole *Lineus viridis* and of the body wall mucus of *Cerebratulus lacteus* show that paralytic activity elutes only with the void volume, rather than at 1.3 and 1.7 V_0. Gel filtration of the *Cerebratulus* mucous extract on a G-50F Sephadex column revealed a single toxic peak at $V_e = 1.6\ V_0$. The existence of the G-25 Sephadex 1.3- and 1.7-V_0 components in the *Lineus* and *Cerebratulus* aqueous extracts is extremely doubtful, since biological assays indicate that, if present, they would contribute less than 1% of the total paralytic activity in these extracts. However, storage of toxic *Cerebratulus* mucus in 99% methanol–1% glacial acetic acid for 2 weeks ($< -10°C$) produces an effluent diagram lacking a V_0-eluting toxin, but containing a large toxic peak at $V_e = 1.4\ V_0$ and a minor component near $V_e = 1.7\ V_0$. These resemble the two components present in acidic methanol extracts of *Lineus ruber*. Since it has been shown (Section IV,B) that the *Cerebratulus* $V_e = 1.6\ V_0$ (G-50F) peak actually contains three distinct toxic polypeptides, it is likely that each of the (G-25F) 1.3- and 1.7-V_0 paralytic peaks may also contain more than one active polypeptide. Experiments on the origin and structure of these "artifact" polypeptides are in progress, since an understanding of their structures and pharmacological actions should be very helpful in determining which portions of the "native" toxins are necessary for receptor binding and activity.

B. Purification of the Cerebratulus Toxins

Cerebratulus lacteus is not nearly as toxic as *Lineus ruber* or *L. viridis* (Kem, 1971). However, the large size (3–10 g fresh weight) and abundance of this species make it a choice source for obtaining the polypeptide toxins corresponding to Bacq's nemertine. The most important features of the purification procedure (Fig. 10) will now be discussed. An article concerning the purification and characterization of the most basic *Cerebratulus* toxin (Toxin III) should be consulted for further details (Kem *et al.*, 1972).

Hand dissection of the toxic integumentary tissues from the body proper of *Cerebratulus* is impractical for processing large numbers of *Cerebratulus*. On the other hand, aqueous extraction of whole *Cerebratulus* is also clearly undesirable, since minute amounts of the polypeptide toxins would be diluted with large amounts of various protein contaminants, including proteolytic enzymes from the digestive tract (Jennings, 1960; Jennings and Gibson, 1969). Therefore, a method was devised for obtaining the toxins relatively free of most *Cerebratulus* body constituents. This

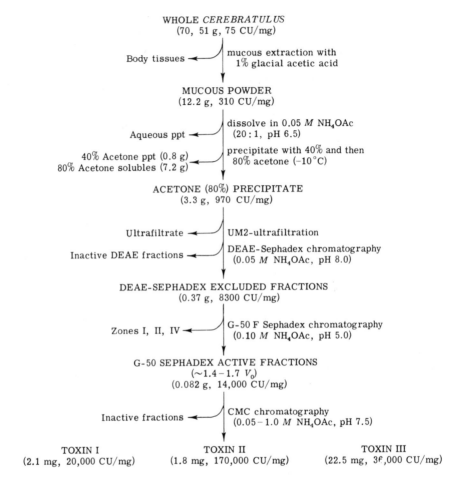

FIG. 10. Purification procedure for *Cerebratulus lacteus* Toxins I–III.

"biological" purification step, based on the observation that *Cerebratulus* secretes a copious, toxic mucus when irritated, should also be useful in the extraction and analysis of other nemertine toxins.

Approximately one dozen (50–80 g fresh weight) *Cerebratulus* are weighed and then placed on a sheet of cheesecloth fitted into the top of a large polyethylene funnel (diameter ∼14 cm). The funnel, in turn, rests in the spout of a 2-liter polyethylene bottle chilled with ice water. The investigator, wearing rubber gloves, sprays 10–30 ml of 1% acetic acid (in distilled water) over the mass of worms, mixes the animals in this medium, closes the gauze sheet over the worms, and firmly squeezes the slimy fluid from the enclosed *Cerebratulus*. The worms vigorously move about and release a copious mucus in response to this combined osmotic, acid (pH 2.8), and mechanical irritation. The clear mucus drains into the chilled container below. This is repeated roughly ten times over a period of about 5 minutes, until the body surfaces of the worms are no longer slippery. In pilot experiments to determine the optimal conditions for collecting the toxin, it was found that mechanical irritation of *Cerebratulus* in artificial seawater is sufficient to release moderate amounts of paralytic activity, but addition of 1% acetic acid doubles the paralytic activity recovered. The hypotonicity of the 1% acetic acid solution appears unnecessary for increasing the toxin yield; it is used to minimize the amounts of inorganic salts in the mucous extract. *Cerebratulus* treated by this procedure are immobile at the end of the 5-minute period, and death ensues shortly thereafter. The volume of a mucous extract collected in this fashion is about seven times the original fresh weight of the *Cerebratulus* used; in the present purification, 2.5 liters were collected from 340 g of *Cerebratulus*. Freeze-drying the mucous extract yielded a tan powder (12.2 g, about 25% of the initial dry weight) whose toxicity was unaffected by 3 months of storage near $-10°C$. The powder contained 3.8×10^6 CU, which corresponds to a tissue toxicity of 1.1×10^4 CU/g fresh weight. Thus, about five times more paralytic activity is observed in the collected mucus than in aqueous homogenates of whole *Cerebratulus* (Section V).

Ammonium acetate was used as a buffering salt in all of the ensuing purification steps due to its volatility during the freeze-drying process routinely used in concentrating toxic fractions. All purification steps except the acetone precipitations were carried out at $2°–5°C$. The entire purification was monitored with the *Procambarus* paralytic assay. Only inactive fractions (less than 200 CU/ml) were discarded. All tubes belonging to an active chromatographic effluent zone were pooled prior to the bioassay. Absorbance at 280 nm was used as a measure of polypeptide concentration at each step. The specific activity of a particular fraction was assessed with respect to dry weight and absorbance (Section IV,B).

The cold acetone, membrane ultrafiltration, and DEAE–Sephadex chromatography steps were successful in removing large quantities of contaminants, particularly inorganic salts. In all three steps, the paralytic activity partitioned as a single component. Ultrafiltration with a UM-2 Diaflo membrane at 5°C was used for desalting, since preliminary experiments had shown that a large proportion of the toxicity of aqueous *Lineus* extracts crossed dialysis tubing. None of the *Cerebratulus* paralytic activity was retained on the DEAE–Sephadex column—bioassays of all subsequent fractions, including those eluted with 0.50 M ammonium acetate, were negative.

The DEAE–Sephadex excluded material (0.366 g) was dissolved in 6.0 ml NH_4OAc –HOAc buffer (pH 5.0), and then 3.0-ml aliquots were separately applied and developed on a G-50F Sephadex column (1.5 × 87 cm). The effluent diagram contained four major OD_{280}-absorbing zones, and the paralytic activity was almost entirely confined to zone III. However, due to the partial overlapping of zones II and III, it was necessary to repeat the G-50F separation twice in order to adequately separate these zones. A considerable loss of paralytic activity was incurred during the molecular sieve step for unknown reasons. Other G-50F column separations of *Cerebratulus* toxins under identical conditions have given excellent (>90%) yields of paralytic activity. It is suspected that storage of the DEAE-excluded material at pH 8.0 near 0°C for several days prior to gel filtration may have caused these unusual losses.

The final purification step involved cation exchange separation with a carboxymethylcellulose (CMC) column. After equilibration with 0.05 M ammonium acetate (pH 7.5) and "fines" removal, Whatman preswollen

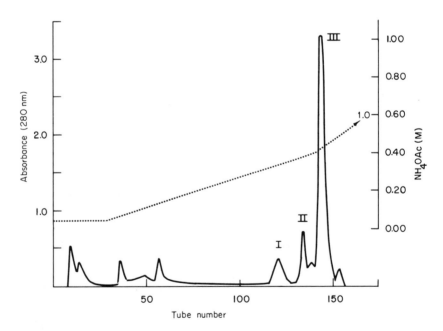

Fig. 11. Carboxymethylcellulose column separation of *Cerebratulus* Toxins I–III. Solid line, OD_{280}; dotted line, estimated ammonium acetate gradient (pH 7.5, 0.05– 0.40 M, then 0.40–1.00 M). (Kem *et al.*, 1972.)

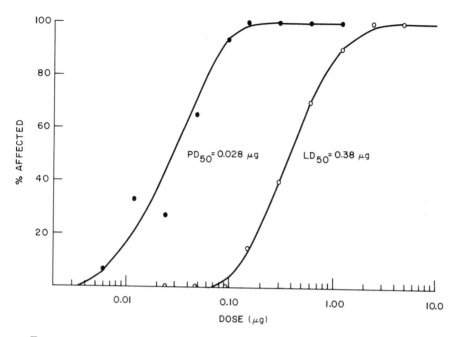

Fig. 12. Paralytic and lethal dose-response relations for carboxymethylcellulose-purified *Cerebratulus* Toxin III injected into crayfish, *Procambarus clarkii*. PD_{50} and LD_{50} estimates were numerically estimated by the Spearman-Karber method. Paralysis was determined 15 minutes after injection, death at 24 hours. (Kem *et al.*, 1972.)

CMC (CM 52) was packed with increasing pressure (maximum pressure 5 pounds/square inch), yielding a 1.5 × 24 cm column. The sample (.082 g) was applied in 2.0 ml of 0.05 *M* ammonium acetate (pH 7.5). Ten different zones of OD_{280}-absorbing material were obtained, and at least four of these zones are toxic (Fig. 11). The first paralytic zone (tubes 8–12) appeared near the exclusion volume of the column and contained very little activity, so its status as a separate toxin is questionable. The remaining three paralytic zones will hereafter be specified as *Cerebratulus* Toxins I, II, and III, in their order of elution from the CMC column. Toxin III was the major toxin both in terms of dry weight and in total paralytic activity. Evidence for the homogeneity of the Toxin III peak was obtained from the amino acid and molecular weight analyses (Section IV,C), and by Edman N-terminal analysis (Kem *et al.*, 1972).

A bioassay of Toxin III is illustrated in Fig. 12. The LD_{50} is about ten times the PD_{50}. Crayfish paralysis by the three *Cerebratulus* toxins is indistinguishable from that due to anabaseine, except for the slower onset.

TABLE II

ANALYSIS OF THE FIRST PREPARATIVE PURIFICATION OF *Cerebratulus lacteus*
TOXINS I–III [a]

Material	Dry weight (g)	OD_{280}/ml [b]	Specific toxicity (CU/mg)	Specific toxicity $(CU/OD_{280}/ml)$	Toxicity $(CU \times 10^{-6})$	% Initial toxicity
Mucous extract	12.20	5,200	310	—	3.83	100.0
Acetone phases						
40% Precipitate	0.80	—	60	—	0.048	1.2
80% Soluble	7.20	—	3×10^{-8}	—	0.020	0.5
80% Precipitate	3.30	750	970	4,300	3.20	84.0
DEAE–Sephadex excluded fractions	0.366	260	8,300	—	3.0	78.0
G-50 Sephadex active fractions	0.0821	67.4	14,000	17,000	1.1	29.0
CMC active fractions						
Excluded fractions	—	5.20	—	<250	—	<0.03
Toxin I	0.0021 [c]	5.56	20,000 [d]	7,700	0.04	1.0
Toxin II	0.0018 [c]	4.73	170,000 [d]	64,000	0.30	7.8
Toxin III	0.0225	33.05	36,000	24,000	0.80	21.0

[a] Kem *et al.* (1972).
[b] Measured in van Harreveld's saline (pH 7.2), except the CMC column fractions, which were dissolved in ammonium acetate solution (pH 7.5).
[c] Dry weight estimated by amino acid analysis, assuming MW 6000.
[d] Based on dry weight estimated by amino acid analysis.

Crayfish injected with a median paralytic dose of anabaseine are all rapidly paralyzed (in terms of righting ability) within 5 minutes after injection, but, at 15 minutes, 50% have recovered. A median paralytic dose of one of the three *Cerebratulus* toxins has its maximal effects at about 15 minutes, the normal testing time. Although Toxin II is present in much smaller amounts than Toxin III, it is approximately three times as toxic, on a molar basis (Table II). Efforts are presently being made to improve this *Cerebratulus* toxin purification procedure, particularly to increase the yields of these three purified toxins.

C. Amino Acid Composition and Molecular Weight of Cerebratulus Toxin III

Results from three separate analyses of Toxin III are tabulated in Table III. Each value represents the mean of the 24-, 48-, and 72-hour hydrolysates, except serine, threonine, and isoleucine. Serine and threonine are estimated by linear extrapolation to zero hydrolysis time. Isoleucine is slowly liberated during hydrolysis, and so it is estimated from samples hydrolyzed for at least 72 hours. The agreement between the three analyses is generally quite good. The CMC-purified toxin contains small amounts of valine and proline impurities which are absent in the reduced and carboxymethylated (RCM) derivative. For this reason, a small portion of the CMC-purified Toxin III was separated once more on a G-50F Sephadex

TABLE III

AMINO ACID COMPOSITION OF *Cerebratulus lacteus* TOXIN III [a]

| | CMC-purified toxin | | Residues/mole | | |
Amino acid	1[b]	2[c]	RCM-toxin	Mean	Nearest interger
Lysine	9.97	10.39	10.00	10.12	10
Histidine	1.21	0.99	0.98	1.06	1
Arginine	2.93	2.96	2.88	2.92	3
Aspartic acid	4.46	5.22	4.78	4.82	5
Threonine[d]	0.92	0.98	1.01	0.97	1
Serine[d]	1.09	1.05	1.00	1.05	1
Glutamic acid	3.38	4.15	3.73	3.75	4
Proline	0.59	0.37	0.15	0.37	0
Glycine	4.59	5.26	4.88	4.91	5
Alanine	6.92	8.10	6.94	7.32	7
Half-cysteine	>5	>5	7.99[e]	—	8
Valine	0.18	0.00	0.00	0.06	0
Methionine	0.00	0.00	0.00	0.00	0
Isoleucine	2.37	2.77[f]	2.56	2.57	3
Leucine	0.99	0.98	1.00	0.99	1
Tyrosine	1.57	1.86	1.83	1.75	2
Phenylalanine	0.00	0.00	0.00	0.00	0
Tryptophan[g]	—	—	2.11	—	2
Total residues					53
Formula weight					5940

[a] Kem *et al.* (1972).

[b] Original carboxymethylcellulose-purified toxin sample.

[c] CMC-purified toxin subsequently eluted through a G-50F Sephadex column with 1.0 M acetic acid–ammonium acetate, pH 3.2.

[d] By linear extrapolation to zero hydrolysis time.

[e] Measured as carboxymethyl cysteine.

[f] Estimated from a 102-hour hydrolysate.

[g] Spectrophotometric method of Edelhoch (1967).

column (1.5 × 87 cm, equilibrated with 1.0 *M* acetic acid–ammonium acetate, pH 3.2). The effluent diagram contained a single, sharp absorbance peak. Amino acid analysis of the hydrolysate indicate that valine was now absent, and the apparent proline content was reduced by 40% There is considerable doubt that the "proline" peak is entirely due to proline, since the ninhydrin product absorbances measured at 440 and 570 nm were nearly equal. Amino acid standards run immediately before and after the toxin hydrolysates yielded proline 440-nm absorbances that were consistently about five times the 570-nm absorbance.

The composition of RCM-Toxin III indicates a very high degree of purity, since four amino acids (proline, valine, methionine, and phenylalnine) are absent, and the other residues are present in nearly integral amounts. Edman N-terminal analysis of RCM-Toxin III also yielded only alanylphenylthiohydantoin (Kem *et al.*, 1972). The carboxymethylation procedure (Section II,F) appears satisfactory, as there is complete carboxymethylation of the half-cystines, but no reaction with lysyl and histidyl amino groups. CMC-purified Toxin III does not significantly react with Ellman's reagent, so it may be concluded that there are four

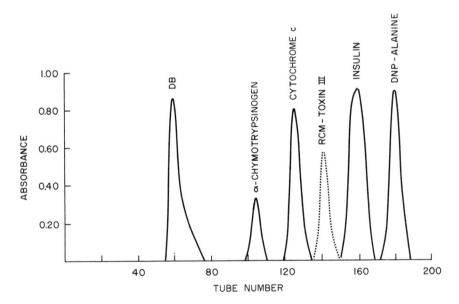

Fig. 13. Elution behavior of reduced and carboxymethylated *Cerebratulus* Toxin III and molecular marker polypeptides on a 6% agarose gel filtration column (1.5 × 85 cm) eluted with buffered 6 *M* guanidine hydrochloride. Absorbance wavelengths: dextran blue, 630 nm; α-chymotrypsinogen, 280 nm; cytochrome c, 405 nm; Toxin III, 280 nm; insulin, 280 nm; DNP-alanine, 360 nm. (Kem *et al.*, 1972.)

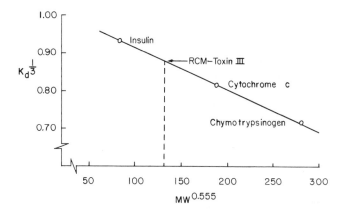

Fig. 14. Porath plot of the molecular marker distribution coefficients (K_d) estimated from the agarose column experiment. Placing $K_I = 0.681$ (RCM-*Cerebratulus* Toxin III) on this linear plot yields $MW^{0.555} = 132$ or $MW = 6620$. (Kem *et al.*, 1972.)

disulfide bonds in Toxin III. The Dubois carbohydrate test was negative.

The molecular weight of RCM-Toxin III is estimated as 6700 ± 200 (1 SD) by the sedimentation equilibrium method. There is a small departure from linearity in the OD_{280} versus (radius)^2 plot near the botton of the ultra-centrifuge cell in the 30,000-rpm run suggesting the presence of some higher molecular weight contaminants or some self-association. However, such components contribute only about 2% of the total absorbance and can be neglected. The agarose gel filtration estimate was made with the same RCM-Toxin III solution used in the ultracentrifugation experiment. The effluent diagram (Fig. 13) for RCM-Toxin III is sharp, and there is no indication of the heterogeneity implied by the first ultracentrifuge run. The molecular size estimated from a Porath plot (Fig. 14) is 6650; if we assume that eight carboxymethylcysteines are present in RCM-Toxin III (see Table III), the molecular weight estimate for Toxin III is 6200, which is slightly higher than the 5900 estimate from the amino acid analysis. This disparity of approximately 6% is not alarming since the amino acid analyzer and the molecular weight methods normally contain errors in the 2–5% range.

Preliminary amino acid analyses of *Cerebratulus* Toxins I and II show that they have approximately the same molecular size as Toxin III, as expected from their coelution behavior on G-50F Sephadex. Their amino acid compositions are also similar to Toxin III, but fewer basic residues are present. This seems reasonable in view of their order of elution from the CMC column. Their different compositions indicate that they are not degradation products of *Cerebratulus* Toxin III (W. R. Kem, unpublished).

V. Tissue and Species Distributions of Nemertine Toxins

The most extensive tissue localization experiments have been done on the proboscis, longitudinal, and transverse distributions of anabaseine in *Paranemertes* using the colorimetric method (Section II,C). The results of three identical experiments are tabulated in Table IV. The anterior proboscis contains a very high concentration of anabaseine, about 7% of the tissue dry weight. Although the median posterior proboscis determinations show considerable variation due to their small size and to varying amounts of adjacent proboscis regions, it is clear that their anabaseine concentrations are lower than the anterior portion. This roughly corresponds to the lower density of basophilic (hematoxylin-staining) gland cells observed in histological section of these regions of the *Paranemertes* proboscis (W. R. Kem, unpublished). The anabaseine concentration along the length of a probosectomized *Paranemertes* remains constant (Kem, 1971).

Transverse localization of the toxins is accomplished by dissection of the integumentary and external muscle layers from the rest of the body (Section II,D). In view of the difficulties in completely separating the integumentary tissues from the internal viscera and musculature, the sixteenfold greater concentration of anabaseine in the *Paranemertes* peripheral sample indicates that this toxin is solely confined to the integument (Kem, 1971). The small quantities present in the core sample are almost certainly due to incomplete dissection, as small patches of the black integumentary pigment

TABLE IV

ANABASEINE DISTRIBUTION IN *Paranemertes peregrina*
MEASURED BY THE COLORIMETRIC ASSAY[a]

Body part	Anabaseine concentration (mg/g fresh weight)	% Total anabaseine
Whole body	3.17 ± 0.66	100.00
Body minus proboscis	2.42 ± 0.48	69.30 ± 3.80
Anterior proboscis	10.83 ± 1.05	27.30 ± 3.50
Median proboscis	7.28 ± 2.65	0.76 ± 0.46
Posterior proboscis	2.21 ± 1.58	0.25 ± 0.12
Peripheral part of body wall	2.72	—
Body core tissues	0.18	—

[a] Each value represents the mean ± 1 SEM for three experiments, except the body wall and body core estimates, which were obtained from a single experiment (Kem, 1971).

are observed on some core blocks. The same dissection procedure applied to frozen transverse disks of similarly sized *Lineus viridis* yields a similar partition of toxicity between the peripheral and core samples, whereas dissection and analysis of the much wider *Cerebratulus* transverse section yields a sixtyfold greater activity in the peripheral sample than in the core sample. This suggests that the ratios obtained for *Paranemertes* and *Lineus* are due to limitations in the dissection technique for that particular size of worm. It is concluded that in these three species the toxins are localized within the body wall integument and the proboscis.

Aqueous or acidic methanol extracts of several species were made in order to determine the generality of occurrence of anabaseine in the nemertine phylum. Due to its sensitivity and selectivity, the colorimetric method for measuring anabaseine was invaluable in these experiments. Crayfish paralytic assays were done in parallel to test for the presence of other toxins besides anabaseine (Kem, 1971). Toxicities of these extracts are found in Table V.

Several tentative conclusions can be made from these experiments if one keeps in mind that less than 2% of the described species in this phylum have been sampled, and many nemertine families are not represented in this initial comparative survey. Anabaseine was found in four of the eight hoplonemertine species tested, including *Amphiporus lactifloreus*, the species in which Bacq discovered amphiporine. Identification of anabaseine in these four species was accomplished by isolating the *p*-dimethylamino-benzaldehyde derivatives, which showed identical visible spectra and TLC R_f's with the synthetic derivative (Section III,D). *Paranemertes peregrina* contains much larger concentrations of anabaseine than the other three species, so it was a fortunate choice for the toxin purification experiments described above. The absence of anabaseine in certain hoplonemertines and in all anoplans parallels Bacq's observations on the distribution of amphiporine.

Two hoplonemertines have been shown to contain one or more toxic compounds different from anabaseine. Unfortunately, due to difficulties in obtaining adequate extracts of these species, the investigation of their paralytic constituents has lagged behind that of the other toxins described in this article. Anabaseine contributes only about 5% of the total paralytic activity in acidic methanol extracts of *Amphiporus angulatus*. Most of the toxicity is due to a compound that migrates just ahead of anabaseine on alumina thin-layers. The two compounds normally overlap during ethyl acetate development, but resolution can be improved by doubling the activation time at 100°C or by use of a less polar solvent for development. The toxic compound does not produce a chromophore with the Dragendorff, ninhydrin–acetic acid, or Ehrlich sprays, but it does have two absorbance

TABLE V

ANABASEINE CONTENT AND TOXICITY OF SEVERAL NEMERTINE SPECIES[a]

Species[b]	Anabaseine		Crayfish paralytic activity	
	mg/g Fresh weight	Detection limit[c]	CU/g Fresh weight	Species used[d]
Anopla				
Paleonemertinea				
Procephalothrix spiralis (Coe)	Absent	(0.06)	80	P
Carinoma sp.	—	—	<130	P
Heteronertinea				
Cerebratulus lacteus (Leidy)	Absent	(0.20)	1,600	P
			11,000[e]	P
Lineus bicolar Verrill	—	—	>10,000[f]	P
Lineus dubius Verrill	—	—	2,900	P
Lineus ruber (Müller)	Absent	(0.05)	26,000	P
Lineus socialis (Leidy)	Absent	(0.30)	>30,000[f]	O
Lineus viridis Verrill	Absent	(0.05)	55,000	P
Micrura leidyi (Verrill)	Absent	(0.50)	160[e]	P
Enopla				
Hoplonemertinea				
Amphiporus angulatus (Fabricius)	13	—	80	O
Amphiporus lactifloreus (John-stone)[g]	>60	—	>90[f]	P
Amphiporus ochreceus (Verrill)	Absent	(2.7)	>150	O
Paranemertes peregrina (Coe)	3,200	—	1,200	O
Prostoma rubrum (Leidy)	Absent?	(20)	700	P
Tetrastemma workii (Corrêa, 1961)	>200	—	—	—
Zygonemertes virescens (Verrill)	Absent?	(20)	—	—
Bdellonemertinea				
Malacobdella grossa (Müller)	Absent	(2.0)	>100[f]	O

[a] Updated from Kem (1971).

[b] Coe (1943).

[c] $OD_{490} = 0.050$ was arbitrarily taken as the limit of spectrophotometric measurement.

[d] Crayfish species used: O, *Orconectes virilis*, P, *Procambarus clarkii*.

[e] Estimated by bioassay of 1% HOAc–distilled H_2O mucous extracts.

[f] These bioassay estimates are minimum values since acidic methanol extracts were used.

[g] Anabaseine assay was done on a 9-month-old acidic methanol extract of this species, whereas the bioassay acidic methanol extract was 3 weeks old.

peaks of nearly equal intensity at 238 and 272 nm (ethanol); acidification shifts the λ_{max} values to 220 and 277 nm, respectively. The PD_{50} (*Procambarus*) of the partially purified compound is less than 7 μg (<350 μg/kg). The purification, chemistry, and distribution of this interesting compound are presently being investigated. The small freshwater hoplonermertine *Prostoma rubrum* probably lacks anabaseine, although it is toxic (see Table V).

The hoplonemertine *Amphiporous ochraceus* illustrates the perils of uncritical application of the colorimetric assay for anabaseine. Fresh acidic methanol extracts of this small nemertine (collected by dredging near Woods Hole) contain an unstable compound with solvent extraction and TLC behavior practically identical with anabaseine. It gives an orange spot with Dragendorff's reagent, but the ninhydrin–acetic acid spot is yellow. The eluted DMAB derivative has λ_{max} at 477 nm in the standard assay solution, rather than at 488 nm, as expected for DMAB-anabaseine. Unlike DMAB-anabaseine, the DMAB derivative base of this compound remains at the origin of Brinkmann alumina thin-layers developed with ethyl acetate. The same TLC run demonstrated that anabaseine is absent in this species. The toxicity of this unstable compound, which is probably an imine, has not yet been established.

The most toxic nemertines yet studied belong to the heteronemertine family Lineidae. Six of the seven species tested are toxic (see Table V). The marginal toxicity of *Micrura leidyi* may perhaps be due to minute amounts of one or more polypeptide toxins, but this point has not yet been experimentally resolved. Analysis of acidic methanol extracts of *Cerebratulus lacteus* have shown that both anabaseine and the *Amphiporus angulatus* paralytic compound are absent in this heteronemertine. It was possible to exclude the presence of anabaseine in all the anoplan species tested. In view of the instability of the polypeptide toxins in acidic methanol (at least in their native forms), it is not yet possible to exclude the possible presence of these polypeptide neurotoxins in the enoplan species studied. The mucous extraction method (Section IV,B) should be applied to *Paranemertes* and other hoplonemertines to determine whether any polypeptide toxins are present in this nemertine order.

VI. Discussion

A. Chemical and Pharmacological Properties of Nemertine Toxins

It is rather surprising that a nicotinelike compound such as anabaseine should be found in a marine animal, rather than in the tobacco plant.

Anabaseine was synthesized in the laboratory (Späth and Mamoli, 1936a) several decades before it was identified as a natural product (Kem *et al.*, 1971). It was also recently isolated from the leaves of tobacco plants (*Nicotiana tabacum*) that had been fed large amounts of anabasine, 2-(3-pyridyl)piperidine. Anabaseine was not found in control plants. Myosmine, the Δ^1-pyrroline analog of anabaseine, was also isolated from plants that were fed nornicotine, 2-(3-pyridyl)pyrrolidine (Kisaki and Tamaki, 1966). These experiments indicate that oxidative enzymes capable of synthesizing the two imines from their piperidine and pyrrolidine ring precursors are present in *Nicotiana*, but it is still uncertain whether these cyclic imines are normally present in fresh tobacco tissues. Due to its sensitivity and selectivity, the colorimetric assay for anabaseine should be useful in screening extracts of various tobacco species for the presence of anabaseine (and perhaps myosmine).

Although the pharmacological properties of anabaseine have not yet been extensively investigated, it has been shown that 2.5×10^{-6} M anabaseine produces a half-maximal contracture of the frog rectus abdominis, which is antagonized by d-tubocurarine. Anabaseine contractures relax very slowly—a maximal contracture elicited by 2.5×10^{-5} M anabaseine had not completely subsided after 2 hours of washing with frog Ringer (W. R. Kem, unpublished). Further experiments on several cholinergic and noncholinergic synaptic preparations are planned in order to determine whether anabaseine possesses any pharmacological properties that differ from those of nicotine. Parallel experiments with anabasine will be done to ascertain the pharmacological importance of the potentially reactive imine bond in anabaseine. In aqueous solutions it is quite possible that the open chain amino ketone form of anabaseine (produced by the reaction of a water molecule or OH^- with the Δ^1-imine group and a subsequent tautomeric shift) may exist in equilibrium with the cyclic imine form. Evidence for such an equilibrium has been obtained for myosmine (Witkop, 1954). It would be desirable to know the pharmacologically active forms of anabaseine in aqueous solution; this interconversion between the cyclic and open chain forms of anabaseine is currently being investigated with titrimetric and spectral (UV, NMR) techniques.

Although the nicotinelike effects of anabaseine on the frog rectus are comparable with Bacq's amphiporine, anabaseine has no effect on the resting and action potentials of the crayfish median giant axon (concentrations up to 2.8×10^{-3} M) or the compound action potential of the lobster walking leg nerve bundle (10^{-2} M). Furthermore, acidic methanol extracts of *Amphiporus lactifloreus*, *A. angulatus*, and *A. ochraceus* containing at least 10 CU/ml have no effect on the lobster nerve preparation

(W. R. Kem, unpublished). Bacq (1936, 1937) mentions only a single experiment in which a concentrated aqueous extract of two *Amphiporus lactifloreus* (in 2.0 ml seawater) elicited repetitive spiking in a walking leg nerve bundle of the crab *Carcinus maenas*. This activity partially subsided within 2–3 minutes. Although the tissue concentration of this extract was unfortunately not specified, it is likely to have been about 100 mg/ml; such a solution would contain approximately twice the potassium ion concentration of normal seawater. This may have depolarized certain fibers sufficiently to elicit a brief train of action potentials. Due to the difficulty in obtaining live specimens of *A. lactifloreus*, this contradiction has not been unequivocally settled, but it is possible to conclude that the three *Amphiporus* species tested contain negligible amounts of axonal toxins, if any are present at all. Neither anabaseine nor the *A. angulatus* toxin affects isolated crustacean axon preparations, in contrast with Bacq's amphiporine extract. Since there are at least two distinct toxic compounds in the genus *Amphiporus* which do not completely correspond with Bacq's amphiporine, the latter term no longer seems appropriate and should be abandoned.

The toxic heteronemertines so far examined contain one or more polypeptide toxins that apparently correspond with Bacq's nemertine (Kem, 1969; Kem *et al.*, 1972). Three different paralytic polypeptides have been purified from *Cerebratulus lacteus*. All three toxins are active in very minute amounts (see Table II). If one assumes that the injected toxins equilibrate only with the crayfish extracellular space (about 25% body weight; Prosser and Weinstein, 1950), the concentrations of Toxins I–III in animals injected with 1 CU are estimated as $16 \times 10^{-10} M$, $2 \times 10^{-10} M$, and $8 \times 10^{-10} M$, respectively. The pharmacology of these three toxins will be investigated on several axonal and synaptic membrane preparations to determine whether there are major differences in the mechanisms of action of these polypeptides. Microelectrode and voltage clamp experiments on crayfish and squid giant axons are planned. Initial experiments with the "artifact" polypeptides of *Lineus ruber* have shown that these toxins prolong the falling phase of the action potential and induce spontaneous action potentials. The irreversibility of these actions suggests that it may be feasible to use radioisotope-labeled heteronemertine toxins as "affinity labels" for their axolemmal receptor sites, in a fashion similar to recent successful experiments where the curarelike polypeptide α-bungarotoxin was used to label and isolate the cholinergic receptor protein (Changeux *et al.*, 1970; Miledi *et al.*, 1971).

Cerebratulus Toxins I–III share several features in common with other polypeptide neurotoxins recently isolated from scorpion (Rochat *et al.*, 1967; Miranda *et al.*, 1970) and snake (Karlsson *et al.*, 1966; Tamiya and

Arai, 1966) venoms. All of these toxins consist of a single polypeptide chain containing 50–65 amino acid residues, with a high proportion of basic (lysyl, histidyl, and arginyl) residues and disulfide bonds (4–5). Methionine and cysteine are lacking in most of these toxins. This fascinating similarity in general molecular characteristics will require explanation. Since certain of these toxins are curarelike synaptic blockers, while others affect action potential generating systems, these features alone are not sufficient to explain the great differences in the pharmacological properties of these toxins. Delineation of the tertiary as well as primary structures of these polypeptides will be necessary to understand the relationships between polypeptide structure and activity in this important group of membrane toxins.

Further investigation of a variety of nemertine species, particularly those belonging to the paleonemertine and hoplonemertine orders, is likely to unearth other neurotoxic compounds which may be useful to the pharmacologist. At least five paralytic compounds are now known to occur in this phylum, whereas only two were previously suspected. It seems obvious that the time and effort expended in purifying crude toxic extracts prior to extensive pharmacological experimentation is most worthwhile, since it greatly simplifies the interpretation of such data and eliminates the need to repeat many experiments when the pure compounds become available.

B. Biological Function of Nemertine Toxins

It is likely that most plant and animal toxins confer adaptive advantages upon the organisms producing them. Many secondary plant substances are animal attractants or repellents (Fraenkel, 1959; Whittaker and Feeney, 1971). The biological importance of chemical communication between different species has only recently gained considerable attention (Sondheimer and Simeone, 1970). I now wish to discuss the probable biological roles of the nemertine toxins in the light of our present knowledge of their biochemistry, pharmacology, and distribution.

Behavioral observations have demonstrated that at least certain hoplonemertines paralyze their annelid of arthropod prey with their proboscis secretions (Reisinger, 1962; Gontcharoff, 1948, 1961; Hickman, 1963; Roe, 1970; Jennings and Gibson, 1969). Now there is experimental evidence that prey paralysis by *Paranemertes peregrina* is due to anabaseine. It has been demonstrated that the *Paranemertes* proboscis contains much more anabaseine than is needed to paralyze an annelid as large as the nemertine. Although the proboscis contributes only 6% of the *Paranemertes* body weight, it contains 30% of the total anabaseine. The toxicity of aqueous extracts of *Paranemertes* probosces can be accounted for by the anabaseine present. Mucus collected from intact everted proboscis of irritated *Paranemertes* contains at least 50 mg of anabaseine per gram dry weight. Subepidermal injection of 50–100 μg of synthetic anabaseine rapidly paralyzes body movements in 8- to 10-g specimens of the annelid *Amphitrite ornata*. On this basis, it is estimated that a 300-mg *Paranemertes* would be able to paralyze an annelid its own size by introducing into the prey about 3 μg of anabaseine, or 2% of the proboscis anabaseine (Kem, 1971).

In *Paranemertes*, the anterior proboscis contains a much higher concentration of anabaseine than is found in the median and posterior regions (see Table IV). This portion contributes 95% of the total proboscis weight and 99% of its anabaseine. Therefore, it can be concluded that in this species anabaseine is chiefly synthesized and stored in the anterior proboscis region. This was somewhat unexpected, since morphological observations on the hoplonemertine proboscis have suggested that the most efficient means of envenomating prey would involve ejaculation of a paralyzing sectetion from the median and posterior proboscis chambers at the time that the stylet punctures the skin of the annelid (Bürger, 1904; Reisinger, 1926; Pawlowksy, 1927; Jennings and Gibson, 1969; Gibson, 1970). The small duct that connects the poststylet chambers with the anterior proboscis chamber bypasses the stylet apparatus, so this means of envenomation would not be strictly identical with a "needle syringe" mechanism (used by certain snakes and arthropods) in which the venom is directly introduced through the puncturing device. Anabaseine released directly from the everted anterior proboscis surface would probably be diluted in the seawater, and, therefore, only small amounts would enter the stylet wounds (Gibson, 1970). The discrepancy between the proboscis anabaseine measurements and these a priori considerations may only be apparent, since some of the anabaseine synthesized and stored in the anterior region may be released and then transferred (by contraction of the proboscis wall musculature) to the poststylet chambers prior to prey attack. Roe (1970) reports that the anterior half of a *Paranemertes* recoils from the annelid immediately before the attack, so perhaps it is during this time that such a transfer would occur. Since the anabaseine measurements were made on proboscis sections that had been soaked in cold seawater for several minutes, they probably would not include anabaseine that had been released into the various proboscis chambers. It is obvious that much remains to be learned about the mechanisms of biosynthesis, storage, and release of anabaseine. Several types of gland cell are abundant in the proboscis epithelium, but their biological functions are not well understood (McIntosh, 1873; Bürger, 1890; Gontcharoff and Léchenault, 1966; Jennings and Gibson, 1969; Gibson, 1970; Ling, 1971).

Observations on the feeding behavior of the heteronemertines *Cerebratulus lacteus* (Wilson, 1900), *Lineus ruber* (Gontcharoff, 1948; Jennings, 1960; Jennings and Gibson, 1969), and *Lineus viridis* (W. R. Kem, unpublished) have failed to provide any evidence for an initial chemical paralysis of prye during capture by nemertines of this order. Annelid prey often violently thrash about for several minutes while they are being seized and injested by *Lineus*. Paralysis does not occur when the common prey annelid *Nereis virens* is subepidermally injected with several thousand CU's of crude *Lineus* or *Cerebratulus* toxin extracts (W. R. Kem, unpublished). Histological studies have demonstrated the absence of a stylet apparatus and of a dense papillalike arrangement of epithelial glands in the heteronemertine proboscis. The behavioral, pharmacological, and anatomical data together indicate that the proboscis toxins of *Lineus* and *Cerebratulus* are not used in prey capture.

Hoplonemertine (*Paranemertes*) and heteronemertine (*Lineus, Cerebratulus*) toxins have been localized within the body wall integument (see Section V). The same toxins are also probably localized in the proboscis integument, since this layer is homologous with the body wall integument (Hyman, 1951). The general body surface of these nemertines does not make intimate contact with prey animals during capture, so the body wall toxins must function as a chemical defence against predators. Behavioral observations support this hypothesis. It has already been demonstrated (Section IV,B) that either mechanical or chemical irritation of *Cerebratulus* causes the secretion of large amounts of a highly toxic mucus. While at Woods Hole, I made several observations on the "palatability" of two heteronemertine species to potential predators. *Cerebratulus lacteus* was rapidly seized by either the lobster (*Homarus americanus*) or the spider crab (*Libinia emarginata*), and pieces of this nemertine were then torn loose and moved toward the mouth for ingestion. However, the pieces were rejected soon after chewing commenced. No convulsions were observed in these crustaceans, but they showed no further interest in eating *Cerebratulus*. Similarly, the crab *Carcinus maenas* refused to eat *Lineus viridis*, even after several days of starvation. Small sea bass (*Centriopristes strictus*) also refused to eat *L. viridis* over a 3-day period of starvation, although they then readily fed on similarly sized *Nereis* placed in the same aquarium with the *Lineus*. Another littoral fish, *Paranenophrys bubalis*, also consistently refuses to eat lineids, even when starved and eager to accept other artificial and natural foods (Gibson, 1970). At this time, almost nothing is known about predation on nemertines under natural conditions, so the function of nemertine toxins as chemical repellents can only be surmised. Feeding experiments with a wide variety of potential predators and nemertines should provide an answer to this question.

The unpalatability of these heteronemertines probably results from one or more substances present in the body surface secretions. These substances are probably the polypeptide toxins described in Section IV. Repellent substances could affect certain chemoreceptors (Case and Gwilliam, 1961; Kleerekoper, 1969) or could act directly on nerve endings in the oral cavity (Beidler, 1965). Since the crustaceans rapidly rejected the toxic lineids, it seems highly improbable that the toxins would pass across the gastrointestinal wall and equilibrate with the hemolymph in order to exert their actions. A direct action on nerve endings in the oral cavity of crustaceans seems most likely, since the *Lineus ruber* toxins have already been shown to cause repetitive spiking in isolated lobster nerve bundles (see Section IV,A). Electrophysiological experiments on crustacean and fish chemoreceptor–nerve preparations should provide information on the cellular basis of this phenomenon. Experiments with the purified nemertine toxins will obviously be necessary to determine whether they do act as repellent substances.

VII. Conclusions

Five neurotoxic compounds were isolated and partially characterized from the primitive animal phylum Nemertinea (Rhynchocoela). Methods for biological and chemical assay, purification, and structural analysis of these toxins were described. The pharmacology and distribution of these toxins were investigated in order to determine their affinities with Bacq's amphiporine and nemertine, their usefulness as research tools in the analysis of excitable membranes, and their biological functions.

The toxin of a hoplonemertine, *Paranemertes peregrina*, was purified by solvent extraction, aluminum oxide chromatography, and crystallization of the toxin picrate. UV, IR, NMR, and mass spectral measurements indicated that the toxin is anabaseine, 2-(3-pyridyl)-3,4,5,6-tetrahydropyridine. This proposed structure was confirmed by selective reduction with sodium borohydride [yielding anabasine, 2-(3-pyridyl)piperidine] and by comparison of the natural product with synthetic anabaseine. Anabaseine possesses the arthropodicidal ($PD_{50} = 0.8$ μmoles/kg) and nicotinoid properties of Bacq's amphiporine, but it has no effect on crustacean nerve action potentials.

Reaction of *p*-dimethylaminobenzaldehyde with anabaseine yields an intense chromophore, 3-(N,N-dimethylaminobenzylidene) anabaseine;

standardization of this reaction provided a sensitive colorimetric method for measuring microgram amounts of anabaseine in crude tissue extracts. Colorimetric determinations demonstrated that anabaseine is confined to the body wall integument and proboscis in *Paranemertes peregrina*. The anterior proboscis contains about 99% of the total proboscis anabaseine in *Paranemertes*. Since anabaseine constitutes 7% of the anterior proboscis dry weight, it must be stored at very high local concentrations ($>0.1\ M$). Anabaseine was observed in four of eight hoplonemertine species, but was absent in all anoplan species tested. Another crayfish-paralyzing compound ($PD_{50} < 350\ \mu g/kg$) was discovered in extracts of the hoplonemertine *Amphiporus angulatus;* its structure and pharmacological actions are being investigated. It also has no effect on the lobster nerve preparation. Since at least two toxic compounds lacking axonal actions have now been isolated from the genus *Amphiporus*, the generic term amphiporine should be abandoned.

Three toxic polypeptides were isolated from body wall mucous extracts of the heteronemertine *Cerebratulus lacteus*. *Cerebratulus* Toxin III was completely purified by acetone precipitation, ultrafiltration, DEAE–Sephadex cation exclusion chromatography, G-50F Sephadex column chromatography, and ammonium acetate gradient elution from a carboxymethylcellulose column. The median paralytic doses of carboxymethylcellulose-purified Toxins I–III are 0.4, 0.05, and 0.2 nmoles/kg, respectively. Toxin III consists of a single polypeptide chain (N-terminal alanine) with an unusually high proportion of lysyl and cystinyl residues. Amino acid, sedimentation equilibrium, and gel filtration determinations provided a mean molecular weight estimate of 6100 for *Cerebratulus* Toxin III. Two smaller polypeptide neurotoxic fractions have been partially purified from acidic methanol extracts of *Lineus ruber*. It was demonstrated that these toxins are partially degraded forms of one or more larger polypeptide toxins. These "artifact" polypeptides induce repetitive spiking in crustacean nerves and irreversibly prolong the repolarization phase of the action potential. The native polypeptide neurotoxins isolated from *Lineus* and *Cerebratulus* correspond with Bacq's nemertine.

Nemertine toxins appear to be used both in food capture and as chemical defences against predators. The hoplonemertine *Paranemertes* uses its proboscis anabaseine to paralyze its annelid prey. However, behavioral and pharmacological observations indicate that the heteronemertines *Lineus* and *Cerebratulus* do not use their polypeptide toxins for prey capture. The localization of nemertine toxins in the body wall integument strongly suggests a defensive role for these toxins. The copious secretion of a highly toxic mucus by irritated *Cerebratulus* is strong evidence for this hypothesis. It is suggested that nemertine toxins act as repellents to potential predators.

The cellular and molecular mechanisms of synthesis, storage, release, and membrane action of these recently purified toxins are being investigated. Since a large number of nemertine species appear to have developed offensive and/or defensive toxic mechanisms, it is likely that future investigations of a wider variety of nemertine species will reveal other natural compounds of interest to the pharmacologist.

ACKNOWLEDGMENTS

I am particularly grateful to Doctors B. C. Abbott (University of Southern California), R. M. Coates (University of Illinois, Urbana), R. E. Fellows (Duke University), and T. Narahashi (Duke University) for providing advice, encouragement, and laboratory facilities during various phases of this research. Dr. N. A. Meinkoth (Swarthmore College) initially interested me in the nemertines and has also generously provided extracts of several nemertine species. I am indebted to two marine laboratories for providing personal and laboratory accommodations: University of Washington, Friday Harbor Laboratories (summer, 1967) and Marine Biological Laboratory, Woods Hole, Massachussets (summers, 1969, 1970). Doctors M. Apley, A. Kirby, E. Kirsteuer, P. Roe, and J. Ropes provided samples of various nemertine species. C. Kem assisted in numerous collecting trips. Elemental (J. Nemeth), NMR spectral (R. Thrift), and mass spectral (R. Wrona) analyses were done by personnel in the School of Chemical Sciences, University of Illinois (Urbana). Doctors R. Painter and J. Huston (both of Duke University) generously assisted in the molecular weight determinations of *Cerebratulus* Toxin III. A. Mudge and J. Martin provided assistance in the initial amino acid analyses. Miss D. Whaley typed the final manuscript. This research was supported in part by NIH pre- and postdoctoral fellowships, a Duke University Research Council grant (T. Narahashi), and a Pharmaceuticais Manufacturers Association Foundation Research Starter Grant.

I am also indebted to Pergamon Press for permission to include Figs. 2, 4, and 5 and Tables IV and V.

REFERENCES

Bacq, Z. M. (1936). Les poisons des némertiens. *Bull. Cl. Sci., Acad. Roy. Belg.* [S] **22,** 1072–1079.

Bacq, Z. M. (1937). L'"Amphiporine" et la "nemertine," poisons des vers némertiens. *Arch. Int. Physiol.* **44,** 109–204.

Beidler, L. M. (1965). Comparison of gustatory receptors, olfactory receptors, and free nerve endings. *Cold Spring Harbor Symp. Quant. Biol.* **30,** 191–200.

Brown, B. W. (1970). Quantal-response assays. *In* "Statistics in Endocrinology" (J. W. McArthur and T. Colton, eds.), p. 129. MIT Press, Cambridge, Massachusetts.

Bürger, O. (1890). Untersuchungen über die Anatomie and Histologie der Nemertinen nebst Beitragen zur Systematik. *Z. Wiss. Zool.* **50,** 1–277.

Bürger, O. (1904). Nemertini. *Tierreich* **20**, 1–151.

Case, J., and Gwilliam, G. F. (1961). Amino acid sensitivity of the dactyl chemoreceptors of *Carcinides maenas. Biol. Bull.* **121**, 449–455.

Changeux, J-P., Kasai, M., and Lee, C-Y. (1970). Use of a snake venom toxin to characterize the cholinergic receptor protein. *Proc. Nat. Acad. Sci. U.S.* **67**, 1241–1247.

Chervenka, C. H. (1969). "A Manual of Methods for the Analytical Ultracentrifuge." Spinco Division of Beckmann Instruments, Inc., Palo Alto, California.

Coe, W. R. (1943). Biology of the nemerteans of the Atlantic Coast of North America. *Trans. Conn. Acad. Arts Sci.* **35**, 129–328.

Cohn, E., and Edsall, J. T. (1943). "Proteins, Amino Acids, and Peptides." Van Nostrand-Reinhold, Princeton, New Jersey.

Crestfield, A. M., Moore, S., and Stein, W. H. (1963). The preparation and enzymatic hydrolysis of reduced and *S*-carboxymethylated proteins. *J. Biol. Chem.* **238**, 622–627.

Duffield, A. M., Budzikiewicz, H., and Djerassi, C. (1965). Mass spectrometry in structural and chemical problems. LXXII. A study of the fragmentation processes of some tobacco alkaloids. *J. Amer. Chem. Soc.* **87**, 2926–2932.

Dyer, J. R. (1965). "Applications of Absorption Spectroscopy of Organic Compounds." Prentice-Hall, Englewood Cliffs, New Jersey.

Edelhoch, H. (1967). Spectrophotometric determination of tryptophane and tyrosine in proteins. *Biochemistry* **6**, 1948–1954.

Ellman, G. L. (1959). Tissue sulfhydryl groups. *Arch. Biochem. Biophys.* **82**, 70.

Finney, D. J. (1964). "Statistical Method in Biological Assay," 2nd ed. Hafner, New York.

Fish, W. W., Mann, K. G., and Tanford, C. (1969). The estimation of polypeptide chain molecular weights by gel filtration in 6 M guanidine hydrochloride. *J. Biol. Chem.* **244**, 4989–4994.

Flett, M. (1962). "Physical Aids to the Organic Chemist." Elsevier, Amsterdam.

Fraenkel, G. S. (1959). The raison d'être of secondary plant substances. *Science* **129**, 1466–1470.

Gibson, R. (1970). The nutrition of *Paranemertes peregrina* (Rhynchocoela: Hoplonemertea). II. Observations on the structure of the gut and proboscis, site and sequence of digestion, and food reserves. *Biol. Bull.* **139**, 92–106.

Gontcharoff, M. (1948). Note sur l'alimentation de quelques Némertes. *Ann. Sci. Natr.* (Paris) **10**, 75–78.

Gontcharoff, M. (1961). Embranchement des némertiens. *In* "Traité de Zoologie" (P. P. Grassé, ed.), Vol. 4, pp. 783–886. Masson, Paris.

Gontcharoff, M., and Léchenault, H. (1966). Ultrastructure et histochimie des glandes sous épidermiques chez *Lineus ruber* et *L. viridis. Histochemie* **6**, 320–335.

Hickman, V. V. (1963). The occurrence in Tasmania of the land nemertine *Geonemertes australiensis* Dendy, with some account of its distribution, habits, variations, and development. *Pap. Proc. Roy. Soc. Tasmania* **97**, 63–75.

Hirs, C. H. W. (1967). Glycopeptides. *In* "Methods in Enzymology" (C. H. W. Hirs, ed.), Vol. II, pp. 411–413. Academic Press, New York.

Hyman, L. H. (1951). The acoelomate Bilateria. *In* "The Invertebrates," Vol. 2, p. 459. McGraw-Hill, New York.

Jennings, J. B. (1960). Observations on the nutrition of the rhynchocoelan *Lineus ruber. Biol. Bull.* **119**, 189–196.

Jennings, J. B., and Gibson, R. (1969). Observations on the nutrition of seven species of rhynchocoelan worms. *Biol. Bull.* **136**, 405–433.

Kamimura, H., and Yamomoto, I. (1963). Studies on nicotinoids as insecticides. III. Structure of anabaseine. *Agr. Biol. Chem.* **27**, 450–453.

Kao, C. Y. (1966). Tetrodotoxin, saxitoxin, and their significance in the study of excitation phenomena. *Pharmacol. Rev.* **18**, 997–1049.

Karlsson, E., Eaker, D. L., and Porath, J. (1966). Purification of a neurotoxin from the venom of *Naja nigricollis. Biochim. Biophys. Acta* **127**, 505–520.

Kem, W. R. (1969). "A Chemical Investigation of Nemertine Toxins." Ph.D. Thesis, University of Illinois, Urbana.

Kem, W. R. (1971). A study of the occurrence of anabaseine in *Paranemertes* and other nemertines. *Toxicon* **9**, 23–32.

Kem, W. R., Abbott, B. C., and Coates, R. M. (1971). Isolation and structure of a hoplonemertine toxin. *Toxicon* **9**, 15–22.

Kem, W. R., Narahashi, T., and Fellows, R. E. (1972). In preparation.

King, H. (1939). Amphiporine, an active base from the marine worm *Amphiporus lactifloreus. J. Chem. Soc. London*, p. 1365.

Kisaki, T., and Tamaki, E., (1966). Phytochemical studies on the tobacco alkaloids. X. Degradation of the tobacco alkaloids and their optical rotatory changes in plants. *Phytochemistry* **5**, 293–300.

Kleerekoper, H. (1969). "Olfaction in Fishes." Indiana Univ. Press, Bloomington.

Ling, E. A. (1971). The probascis apparatus of the nemertine *Lineus ruber. Phil. Trans. Roy. Soc. London, Ser. B* **262**, 1–22.

McIntosh, W. C. (1873). A monograph of the British Annelids. Pt. 1. The Nemerteans. *Ray Soc. Publ.* **22**, 1–218.

Miledi, R., Molinoff, P., and Potter, L. T. (1971). Isolation of the cholinergic receptor protein of *Torpedo* electric tissue. *Nature (London)* **229**, 554–557.

Miranda, F., Kupeyan, C., Rochat, H., Rochat, C., and Lissitzky, S. (1970). Purification of animal neurotoxins. Isolation and characterization of eleven neurotoxins from the venoms of the scorpions *Androctonus australis* Hector, *Buthus occitanus tunetanus*, and *Leiurus guinguestriatus guinguestiratus. Eur. J. Biochem.* **16**, 514–523.

Moore, J. W., and Narahashi, T. (1967). Tetrodotoxin's highly selective blockage of an ionic channel. *Fed. Proc. Fed. Amer. Soc. Exp. Biol.* **26**, 1655–1663.

Narahashi, T., Moore, J. W., and Scott, W. R. (1964). Tetrodotoxin blockage of sodium conductance increase in lobster giant axons. *J. Gen. Physiol.* **47**, 965–974.

Pawlowsky, E. N. (1927). "Giftiere Und Ihre Giftigkeit." Fischer, Jena.

Pennak, R. W. (1953). "Fresh-Water Invertebrates of the United States," Chapter 6. Ronald Press, New York.

Pople, J. A., Schneider, W. G., and Bernstein, H. J. (1959). "High Resolution Nuclear Magnetic Resonance." McGraw-Hill, New York.

Prosser, C. L., and Weinstein, S. J. F. (1950). Blood volume of the crayfish. *Physiol. Zool.* **23**, 113.

Reisinger, E. (1926). Nemertini. *Biol. Tiere Deutschl.* **1**, 1–24.

Rochat, C., Rochat, H., Miranda, F., and Lissitzky, S. (1967). Purification and some properties of the neurotoxins of *Androctonus australis* Hector. *Biochemistry* **6**, 578–585.

Roe, P. (1970). The nutrition of *Paranemertes peregrina* (Rhynchocoela: Hoplonemertea). I. Studies on food and feeding behavior. *Biol. Bull.* **139**, 80–91.

Sondheimer, E., and Simeone, J. B., eds. (1970). "Chemical Ecology." Academic Press, New York.

Spackman, D. H., Stein, W. H., and Moore, S. (1958). Automatic recording apparatus for use in the chromatography of amino acids. *Anal. Chem.* **30**, 1190-1206.

Späth, E., and Mamoli, L. (1936a). Eine neue Synthese des *d,l*-Anabasins. *Chem. Ber.* **69**, 1082–1085.

Späth, E., and Mamoli, L. (1936b). Syntheses des Myosmins. *Chem. Ber.* **69**, 757–760.

Tamiya, N., and Arai, H. (1966). Studies on sea-snake venoms. Crystallization of erabutoxins a and b from *Laticauda semifasciata* venom. *Biochem J.* **99**, 624–630.

van Harreveld, A. (1936). A physiological solution for freshwater crustaceans. *Proc. Soc. Exp. Biol. Med.* **34**, 428–432.

Whittaker, R. H., and Feeney, P. P. (1971). Allelochemics: Chemical interactions between species. *Science* **171**, 757–770.

Wilson, C. B. (1900). Habits and early development of *Cerebratulus*. *Quart. J. Microsc. Sci.* **43**, 97–198.

Witkop, B. (1954). Infrared diagnosis of the hydrochlorides of organic bases. II. The structure of myosmine. *J. Amer. Chem. Soc.* **76**, 5597–5599.

CHAPTER III

Effects of Toxin from the Blue-Ringed Octopus (Hapalochlaena maculosa)

PETER W. GAGE and ANGELA F. DULHUNTY

I. Introduction

Many marine species contain powerful toxins that they use both as offensive and defensive weapons. The value of some of these toxins as pharmacological tools in research laboratories is becoming increasingly recognized. One outstanding example is tetrodotoxin (TTX), which is extracted from the ovaries of puffer fish (genus *Fugu*) and is now widely used by physiologists throughout the world because of its selective inhibition of action potentials.

It has been known for some time that many octopuses secrete substances that kill crustacea, but in general these toxins were not thought to be lethal to humans. In 1954, however, Mabbet reported a death from an octopus bite. A skin-diver who was collecting small octopuses was attracted by one with particularly bright coloring. For a while he allowed it to crawl over his arms and shoulders. Soon afterward he complained of a dry mouth and difficulty in swallowing. Then he began to vomit, showed signs of extreme respiratory distress, and, despite being placed in an artificial respirator, died 2 hours after being bitten. No positive identification of the octopus was made, but it was thought to be a blue-ringed octopus (*Hapalochlaena maculosa*).

The next year, Flecker and Cotton (1955) reported the death of two soldiers who both died of respiratory failure after bites from an octopus. The octopuses responsible were positively identified as *Hapalochlaena maculosa*. Another death, from respiratory failure caused by an octopus bite, was reported by Lane and Sutherland in 1967. Attracted by its bright colors, a soldier picked up a small octopus to show it to his companions and was bitten while it rested on the back of his hand. He died shortly afterward, and positive identification of the blue-ringed octopus was reported.

The bite of this octopus is not invariably fatal, and there are documented reports of several people having survived (McMichael, 1956; Cleland and Southcott, 1965; Sutherland and Lane, 1969). The symptoms in all cases were characteristic: respiratory distress, numbness of the mouth and tongue, blurring of vision, difficulty in speech and swallowing, loss of tactile sensation, ataxia, and muscular paralysis.

The toxic effects of the saliva from the blue-ringed octopus indicate that its salivary secretions contain a component not present in the saliva of other octopuses. On the other hand, some of the substances normally found in the saliva of other octopuses (see Ghiretti, 1960) are present also in the saliva of *Hapalochlaena maculosa*. Tyramine and octopamine have been identified by Simon *et al.* (1964), and histaminelike pharmacological reactions to the saliva have been described (Trethewie, 1965; Freeman and Turner, 1970

Hapalochlaena maculosa is commonly known in Australia as the blue-ringed octopus (Fig. 1). The origin of this name becomes obvious when an octopus is approached or frightened. Its dusty brown appearance changes dramatically. Dark blue rings and bands appear on its body and tentacles, but the coloring is not maintained for more than a minute or so, either be-

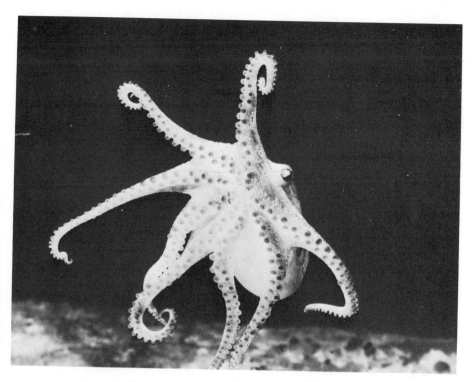

Fig. 1. A female blue-ringed octopus (*Hapalochlaena maculosa*).

cause the octopus adapts to the situation or because the coloring cannot be maintained. The octopus is quite small and measures 3–6 cm across its body. Its total spread rarely exceeds 20 cm. The octopus is found in the shallow coastal waters of Australia, India, and the Indo-Pacific.

The blue-ringed octopus is not naturally aggressive. Its human victims have generally been attracted by its bright unusual markings. It is only when it has been picked up and played with that it has bitten and ejected its toxin, probably in self-defense. The normal behavior of the octopus has been studied by Sutherland and Lane (1969) using live specimens collected from Port Phillip Bay and confined in an aquarium. In particular, the way in which it immobilizes its prey was observed when small live crabs were placed in the aquarium. The octopus would glide through the water and squirt saliva from its beak into the water above the crab; then it would move away and wait for the crab to die. Within 2 minutes, the crab became very excited and ataxic in its gait, and was finally incapable of movement.

When the crab was completely paralyzed, the octopus moved in again and tore the meat from the shell with its beak. If the octopus had been starved for several days, the behavior was somewhat different. It became more daring and aggressive, darted at the crab, and did not wait for paralysis to set in before tearing at the shell. When an octopus was placed on a rabbit that had been shaved and immobilized in a restraining box, the first reaction of the octopus was to try to slide off and get away, but, if it was replaced again and again, it would eventually settle on the rabbit's back for a few seconds. Several puncture marks were then found on the areas where it had settled, and these bled freely for some time, suggesting that the saliva contained an anticoagulant as is commonly found in the salivary secretions of other octopuses. The rabbit went into convulsions shortly after the bite, and then became completely paralyzed. The same octopus could kill a second rabbit in the same way less than 1 hour after the first.

II. Methods

A. Isolation and Chemistry of the Toxin

The toxin is contained in the large posterior salivary glands. The posterior gland is the primary source of toxin in all octopuses, but the anterior gland can also be a source of toxin in some species (Fleig and De Rouville, 1910), but not in the blue-ringed octopus. Sections of this gland show ducts of many sizes lined with large glandular cells grouped closely together into tightly packed acini. The cells are packed so full of secretory granules that the large nuclei appear compressed. In fact, the salivary gland closely resembles the mucous glands of vertebrates (Halstead, 1965; Sutherland and Lane, 1969).

Ghiretti (1960) has described elegant experiments in which the common salivary duct of an octopus was cannulated and secretion of toxin induced by electrical stimulation of the gland. Sutherland and Lane (1969) had no success with this method in attempts to obtain toxin from the blue-ringed octopus, apparently because the trauma of the operation stimulated secretion of the toxin before the duct could be cannulated. The final saliva collection was minute and low in toxicity. Because the octopus could not be induced to bite through a rubber membrane, the toxin could not be obtained by milking, and it was necessary to extract the toxin from whole glands. The glands can be frozen and stored with no apparent loss of toxicity.

The following method for the isolation of maculotoxin (MTX) was developed by Croft (1971). Posterior salivary glands are dissected from dead octopuses and homogenized in methanol. Proteins and cell debris are removed by filtration making any further deproteination unnecessary. The crude extract is purified by adsorption chromatography on a silica gel column, and the toxin is eluted from the column with 50% methanol in chloroform. A second toxic fraction can be eluted from the column with 5% acetic acid in methanol. This second fraction is contaminated with ninhydrin-positive compounds. Neither thin-layer chromatography nor infrared spectroscopy has revealed any difference between the two toxic fractions (Croft, 1971). Possibly, the second fraction is lightly complexed to a larger ninhydrin-positive molecule. Sutherland and Lane (1969) and Simon *et al.* (1964) have reported the presence of more than one toxic fraction also, but Freeman and Turner (1970) found only one toxic component.

B. Physical and Chemical Properties

These have been described in full by Croft (1971). Fractions collected from the column can be dried to a white powder that is readily soluble in water and methanol, but insoluble in acetone or chloroform. MTX is stable at room temperature for more than 3 months and can be kept indefinitely at 2°C. Exposure to 1 M HCl or heating to 60°C for 2 hours does not result in a loss of toxicity. However, in alkaline solutions (pH greater than 8), toxicity is lost completely.

MTX has a relatively low molecular weight. Experiments using ultrafiltration membranes show that it is probably considerably less than 540 (Sutherland *et al.*, 1970). The toxin behaves as a cation. Strong cation exchange resins (Dowex-50W–sulfonic acid) retain the toxin from aqueous solution, whereas anion exchange resins do not. Thin-layer electrophoresis on silica gel or cellulose MN300 at pH 1.9 also shows the cationic property of maculotoxin; it moves toward the cathode because of a net positive charge. Tetrodotoxin and saxitoxin, which are also retained by cation exchangers, possess basic nitrogen atoms. It is possible that the cation exchange properties of maculotoxin may also be due to the presence of a basic nitrogen atom.

Eluents of MTX from cation exchange systems contain sodium, but no small anions, suggesting that the molecule can complex sodium. The sodium can be separated out using MN300 cellulose thin-layer chromatography, and the sodium-free maculotoxin is no less toxic than its sodium-bound counterpart. The ability of MTX to complex with sodium may be fundamental to its toxicity.

Freeman and Turner (1970) have reported that maculotoxin is probably identical chemically to the marine toxins tetrodotoxin and saxitoxin. However, when tetrodotoxin and maculotoxin are compared using thin-layer chromatography (Croft, 1971), the two can be readily distinguished. The

TABLE I

THIN-LAYER CHROMATOGRAPHY COMPARISON OF TETRODOTOXIN
AND MACULOTOXIN

Absorbent	Solvent	R_f TTX	R_f MTX
Silica gel	i-PrOH–HOAc–H$_2$O (70–5–25)	0.6	0.1–0.2
Cellulose MN300	n-BuOH–HOAc–H$_2$O (2:1:1)	0.55	0.3–0.4
Cellulose MN300	t-BuOH–HOAc–H$_2$O (2:1:1)	0.65	0.3–0.4

results of some thin-layer chromatographic studies are summarized in Table I.

Tetrodotoxin and maculotoxin can be distinguished also with color reagents. Tetrodotoxin gives a positive color reaction with ninhydrin and other reagents used for the detection of amines, whereas MTX gives negative reactions. Jaffe, Sakaguchi, Voges-Proskauer, Fearon, and nitroprusside–hexacyanoferrate reagents all fail to give a color with MTX, but give strong color reactions with TTX. The nontoxic, ninhydrin-positive substance that moves just ahead of MTX on a silica gel column gives a strong color reaction with Jaffe reagent. The presence of a ninhydrin-positive contaminant may explain why MTX has been considered chemically similar to TTX.

Spectral studies and microanalysis have yielded little information about the molecular configuration of MTX. No UV absorption bands were found (Simon et al., 1964; Croft, 1971), and potassium ferricyanide–ferric sulfate reagent for phenols did not react with the toxin. These negative tests for catecholamines distinguish MTX from the salivary toxins of many other octopuses (Ghiretti, 1960).

Infrared spectra give peaks indicative of several groups; namely hydrogen-bonded OH groups, a secondary amine or hydroxyl group, and possibly a carboxyl group. NMR spectral analysis has given only negative results. Microanalysis shows the presence of the following elements: Na, 14.3%; K, 6.4%; C, 9.7%; H, 1.98%; N, 3.52%. No evidence of phosphate has been found. Oxygen is present in significant quantities, but the exact percentage was not calculated.

From these results, it is clear that there is little positive information about the chemistry of the toxin. The white powder obtained from the silica gel column is probably a mixture of toxic and nontoxic substances, so that the concentrations of MTX cited in this paper can be regarded only as upper limits. For this reason, the quantitative experiments of Dulhunty and Gage (1971) were done with one extract of MTX so that the percentage of purity was constant. There are some useful statements that can be made about the nature of the toxin, however. It is not a protein, probably does not contain amino groups, and has a molecular weight less than 540. It is positively charged and can form complexes with sodium ions. Finally, it is clearly different in structure from TTX or STX.

C. Immunologic Properties of the Toxin

Several attempts have been made to prepare an antibody to maculotoxin (Sutherland and Lane, 1969; Sutherland et al., 1970). Immunization of rabbits with whole gland extracts produced antibodies to nontoxic components of high molecular weight, but these afforded no protection against MTX. Much of the high molecular weight protein present in the whole muscle extract is hyaluronidase, which can be removed by dialysis. Immunization with the dialyzed extract, containing no protein, produced neither neutralizing nor precipitating antibodies. Toxin further purified by thin-layer chromatography was dried and absorbed onto finely pulverized carbon, which had been twice activated with concentrated hydrochloric acid. The intrasplenic and intrainguinal lymph nodes of six rabbits were injected with the carbon–toxin mixed with Freunds complete adjuvant to stimulate antigenic responses: ten days later, all the rabbits were given intramuscular injections of carbon–toxin twice weekly for 6 weeks. After this time, the rabbits had developed no immunity and did not survive an injection of MTX.

III. Results

A. Experiments on Whole Animals

The systemic effects of the toxin have been tested in anesthetized and unanesthetized animals with similar results. Croft (1971) used unanesthetized mice to determine which of his fractions, obtained from columns, were toxic. When MTX was injected intraperitoneally, the mice became restless and ataxic, their breathing was labored, and death was preceded by spasmodic convulsions. In cats, rabbits, and rats, similar toxic signs have been recorded (Simon et al., 1964; Trethewie, 1965; Freeman and Turner, 1970). A fall in blood pressure has been reported by some investigators, but is probably secondary to the respiratory failure that is a striking feature. Electrical activity recorded from the phrenic nerve in intact animals injected with MTX increases progressively whereas electromyogram activity decreases. The former is probably due to a central feedback response to respiratory insufficiency. It is noteworthy that the increased activity of the phrenic nerve is insignificant in comparison to the effect of neuromuscular blocking agents.

The curve relating "time until death" to dose is very steep (Croft, 1971). One-half of the minimum lethal dose produced no toxic symptoms. Intravenous and intraperitoneal injections were equally effective, but the toxin was much less potent when administered orally. The toxin has a cumulative effect. When a sublethal dose is administered, recovery may appear to be complete in 30 minutes. A second identical dose leads to respiratory failure within 5 minutes. This additive effect is not surprising in view of the steep dose-response curve.

B. Isolated Preparations

When the isolated heart of a guinea pig or cat is exposed to MTX, a transient change in heart rate is observed (bradycardia in the cat and tachycardia in the guinea pig), but this disappears within 5 minutes. Trethewie (1965) could not record any reduction in the amplitude of cardiac contraction during observation periods up to 90 minutes after injection of MTX. These results suggest that the maintained bradycardia in the intact animal is due either to neural or to hormonal influences, which do not operate in the isolated preparation.

The most striking features in the whole animal are muscular paralysis and respiratory insufficiency. Isolated nerve–muscle preparations have proven very useful for investigating the paralysis caused by MTX. In the rat phrenic nerve–diaphragm preparation and the frog sciatic nerve–sartorius muscle preparation, the toxin rapidly abolished twitches in response to stimulation of the nerve (Trethewie, 1965; Freeman and Turner, 1970). When neuromuscular transmission has stopped, the muscle can still be made to contract with direct stimulation, though it is necessary to use a stronger stimulus than before. Compound action potentials can also be recorded from the sciatic nerves of toads after neuromuscular transmission has been blocked by MTX. It has been suggested, therefore, that MTX is a neuromuscular blocking agent (Simon et al., 1964; Freeman and Turner, 1970).

In more recent experiments, Dulhunty and Gage (1971) have found that MTX is not a neuromuscular blocker; that is, it does not inhibit the secretion of transmitter or the postsynaptic effects of acetylcholine. In these experiments, intracellular recording techniques were used, and these will be described in some detail.

A sciatic nerve and innervated satorius muscle were dissected from a toad (*Bufo marinus*) and placed in a bath milled from Lucite. In one chamber, the muscle was immersed in a Ringer solution containing (mmoles/liter) NaCl, 115; KCl, 2.5; CaCl₂, 1.8; sodium phosphate buffer, 3 (pH = 7.2). The nerve was laid across five platinum wires in a second narrower chamber at right angles to the first, and immersed in Ringer also. The distal two wires were connected to a stimulator, the middle one to ground, and the proximal two to the input of a preamplifier. The bath that contained the preparation was transilluminated from below with light reflected from a concave focusing mirror. To stimulate the nerve, an isolated stimulator (Devices, Type 2533) was used. Compound action potentials were recorded differentially from the proximal two wires connected to a preamplifier (Tektronix 122) and displayed on an oscilloscope (Tektronix 502) where they were photographed.

When compound action potentials had been recorded with a supramaximal stimulus, the solution in the bath was replaced with a solution containing MTX (5 × 10⁻⁶ g/ml). Results obtained in one of these experiments are illustrated in Fig. 2. Although muscle twitches in response to nerve stimulation stopped within 10 minutes in this experiment, it took more than 2 hours for the compound action potential to disappear (Fig. 2). However, if the sciatic nerve is desheathed, MTX blocks action potentials

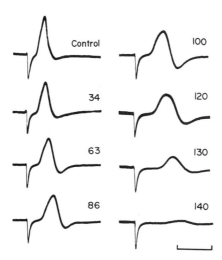

Fig. 2. Compound action potentials recorded extracellularly from a toad sciatic nerve. The upper left record shows the control compound action potential. The subsequent records were obtained at the times indicated in minutes after exposure of the nerve to 5 × 10⁻⁶ g/ml MTX. Calibration 10 mseconds.

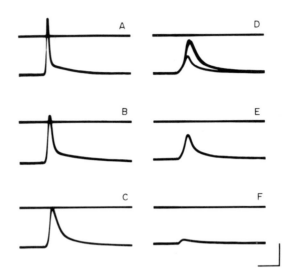

Fig. 3. The effect of maculotoxin (4×10^{-6} g/ml) on action potentials in glycerol-treated toad sartorius muscle fibers. Each frame, A to F, contains five superimposed traces of responses to stimuli at ten per second. In A are shown action potentials before exposure to MTX; B, C, D, E, and F were recorded after 6, 10, 16, 18, and 20 seconds' stimulation in MTX. Calibration: vertical, 50 mV; horizontal, 10 mseconds. (Dulhunty and Gage, 1971.)

within 15 minutes (Simon *et al.*, 1964), and it can be concluded that the sheath acts as an effective diffusion barrier to the toxin.

Muscle fibers have no sheath, but have action potentials very similar to those of nerve cells. The effects of MTX on action potentials in individual muscle cells were investigated using intracellular microelectrodes filled with 2.5 *M* KCl (Dulhunty and Gage, 1971). These electrodes have resistances of 5–50 megohms, so that it is necessary to use an impedance matching device to display signals without attenuation or distortion on oscilloscopes. A convenient and inexpensive way of doing this is to connect the electrode to the positive input of an operational amplifier with a high input resistance (10^{11}–10^{12} ohms). A variable capacitator (0–10 pF) connected between the output and the positive input can be used to compensate for unavoidable stray capacitances that may slow signals of interest (capacity neutralization).Commercial versions are available, but are more than ten times the cost. The operational amplifier used for this purpose was a Philbrick 1009, but there are many others that would be suitable.

Normally, an action potential causes contraction in a skeletal muscle fiber, but it is possible to prevent this by glycerol treating the fiber (Howell and Jenden, 1967; Gage and Eisenberg, 1967, 1969b). Toad sartorius muscles were soaked for 1 hour in a Ringer solution containing 400 mM glycerol in addition to the normal constituents. When these muscles were returned to the Ringer solution, action potentials could be elicited, but there was no contraction (Gage and Eisenberg, 1969b; Dulhunty and Gage, 1969).

Two microelectrodes were inserted in a fiber, one for passing a current pulse to depolarize the surface membrane and the other to record the resting membrane potential and action potentials. Recordings obtained in one of these experiments are shown in Fig 3. The resting potential and five superimposed action potentials elicited at ten per second are shown in each frame, A to F. The preparation was exposed to MTX (4 $\times$ 10^{-6} g/ml) after frame A had been recorded as a control, and frames B, C, D, E, and F were recorded 6, 10, 16, 18, and 20 seconds later. After MTX was added, the action potential disappeared rapidly, but there was no change in membrane potential. This distinguishes MTX from other agents or procedures that block action potentials by depolarizing the membrane. If the microelectrodes were inserted in a neighboring muscle fiber after one had been blocked by stimulation, the same sequence of events could be recorded again. If a concentration greater than 10^{-5} g/ml was used, no action potentials could be elicited (see below). Action potentials quickly returned when the toxin was washed out of the bath.

It soon became clear that MTX at low concentrations was not effective in blocking action potentials until a certain number had occurred. In fact, the total number of action potentials that could be elicited before the nerve was blocked was related exponentially to the concentration of MTX used. This is illustrated in Fig. 4. By extrapolation, it is evident that only one action potential at most would be expected when MTX at a concentration of 10^{-5} g/ml is used, and this, in fact, was found to be true. The blockage of action potentials at lower concentrations depended on the total number of action potentials, not on the duration of the stimulation. When a muscle was stimulated at different rates (0.1–10 per second), block occurred after a certain number of action potentials, irrespective of the time taken to elicit them.

The number of action potentials obtained with a given concentration of MTX was reasonably constant from fiber to fiber and from preparation to preparation. For example, in 110 muscle fibers in five sartorius muscles, the mean number of action potentials before block occurred in 4.5 $\times$ 10^{-6} g/ml MTX was 46.2 with a standard error of 3.2. The number of action potentials before block is obviously well defined for a given concentration of MTX, and should be a very useful standard for assaying the relative concentrations of MTX in different extracts of the toxin.

Because MTX blocks action potentials rapidly, yet causes no change in resting membrane potential, it must block the depolarization-activated sodium conductance that normally leads to an action potential. When an excitable membrane is depolarized, the permeability to sodium ions increases. Because the electrochemical gradient for sodium is inward, sodium ions enter the cell and depolarize the membrane further, leading to an even greater sodium permeability. The process is thus self-regenerative, and the membrane potential moves rapidly toward the sodium equilibrium potential, where there is no net movement of sodium ions. The increase in sodium permeability is accompanied by an increase in potassium permeability, which is lower in magnitude and has a slower time course. Some drugs that block action potentials are nonspecific and inhibit both the sodium and potassium conductance increases in response to membrane depolarization. An example of this type is the group of local anesthetics including procaine (Shanes *et al.*, 1959; Taylor, 1959). Some marine toxins (tetrodotoxin and saxitoxin) block the depolarization-activated sodium conductance change specifically, and do not affect the slower developing potassium conductance increase (Narahashi *et al.*, 1964; Kao, 1964). For convenience, we have called these agents "natrotoxins," and MTX probably belongs in this category. The relative immunity of the depolarization-activated potassium conductance is revealed by the persistence of "delayed rectification" in muscle fibers in which action potentials have been blocked by MTX. If a constant depolarizing current is passed across an excitable

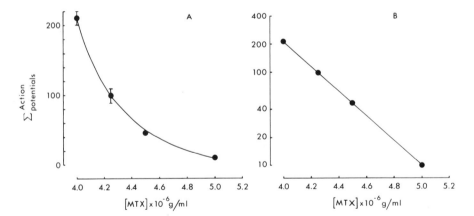

FIG. 4. The relationship between the number of action potentials before block ($\sum$ Action potentials) and MTX concentration. The graphs show averages obtained in 365 glycerol-treated fibers in 25 preparations. The vertical bars in A denote 1 SEM, where this is large enough to extend beyond the symbol. A, Linear plot; B, semilogarithmic plot. (Dulhunty and Gage, 1971.)

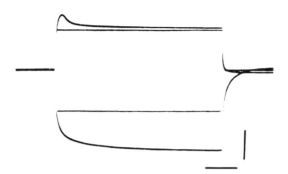

Fig. 5. Delayed rectification in a glycerol-treated muscle fiber in which action potentials have been blocked by MTX, 5×10^{-6} g/ml. The inner rectangular pulses show the current and the outer traces the voltage: depolarization, upward; hyperpolarization, downward. Calibration: vertical, 10^{-7} A for current, 25 mV for voltage; horizontal, 20 mseconds. (Dulhunty and Gage, 1971.)

membrane in which the depolarization-activated sodium conductance channel has been selectively inhibited, the resultant membrane depolarization falls after an initial peak to a steady level (Fig. 5). Because the depolarizing current is constant, a decrease in membrane depolarization must represent an increase in membrane conductance, and this is due to the increase in potassium conductance. MTX seems, therefore, to act selectively on the depolarization-activated sodium conductance. These experiments do not exclude the possibility that MTX might have a small effect on the potassium conductance, and this will have to be determined with voltage clamp techniques.

C. Resting Membrane Conductance

By recording the magnitude and time course of the displacement of membrane potential as a function of the distance from the site of injection of current in nerve or muscle fibers, it is possible to determine the specific resistance and capacitance of the cell membrane (Hodgkin and Rushton, 1946; Katz, 1948; Fatt and Katz, 1951; Gage and Eisenberg, 1969a). In toad sartorius fibers, neither of these parameters is changed significantly by MTX.

The resting membrane conductance in skeletal muscle consists essentially of the sum of the resting chloride and potassium conductances. The toxin, therefore, affects neither of these conductances, nor does it increase the resting sodium conductance. The latter would cause a decrease in resting membrane potential and resistance, neither of which occurs.

D. Inhibition by Sodium Ions

The activity of MTX is influenced by the concentration of sodium ions in the solution: the higher the sodium concentration, the less effective is MTX in blocking action potentials. This effect is illustrated in Fig. 6, which shows results obtained from 1395 fibers in 42 sartorius muscles. Whether or not sucrose was added to maintain a constant osmotic pressure when the sodium concentration was changed made no difference to the results. It is not known whether sodium directly inactivate the toxin. There is evidence that the toxin forms complexes with sodium ions and that the toxin is still active when sodium ions are removed (Croft, 1971), but there is no evidence to suggest that sodium ions reduce the potency of the toxin by binding to it. Another possible explanation for the interaction between sodium ions and MTX is that they both compete for negatively charged sites on the membrane. MTX binds strongly to cation exchangers (Croft, 1971) and migrates to the cathode during electrophoresis. It is possible that during an action potential, sodium ions are bound to a negatively charged group that is exposed by membrane depolarization. MTX might gain access to these sites more readily during an action potential, which would, hence, potentiate the effect. At present, however, there is hardly sufficient evidence to support further speculation.

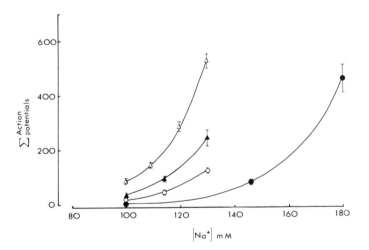

FIG. 6. The influence of extracellular sodium ion concentration on the activity of MTX in blocking action potentials in glycerol-treated muscle fibers. Four concentrations of MTX were used: 4.0×10^{-6} g/ml, open triangles; 4.25×10^{-6} g/ml, filled triangles; 4.5×10^{-6} g/ml, open circles; 5.0×10^{-6} g/ml, closed circles. Each point shows an average obtained in 50–100 fibers in three or four preparations. The vertical bars show ± 1 SEM if this extends beyond the symbol. (Dulhunty and Gage, 1971.)

E. Neuromuscular Transmission

MTX blocks neuromuscular transmission in the rat diaphragm and toad sartorius muscle (Simon *et al.*, 1964; Trethewie, 1965; Freeman and Turner, 1970). With extracellular recording techniques, it has generally been found that transmission is blocked by MTX before the compound action potential in the nerve or the twitch response in the whole muscle (induced by direct stimulation) has disappeared. For this reason, MTX has been said to have a direct neuromuscular blocking action (Simon *et al.*, 1964; Freeman and Turner, 1970). In order to determine whether this is so, the effect of MTX on synaptic transmission has been investigated using microelectrodes.

The sequence of events that occur between stimulation of the nerve and contraction of the muscle may be listed as follows:

1. An action potential in the nerve propagates to the nerve terminal.

2. The membrane depolarization causes the release of a burst of quanta of transmitter (excitation–secretion coupling; see Gage, 1967).

3. The transmitter diffuses to the postsynaptic membrane and complexes with the postsynaptic receptors.

4. The permeability of the subsynaptic membrane increases to both sodium and potassium ions, leading to a current flow that depolarizes the postsynaptic membrane.

5. This depolarization, the end plate potential, leads to an action potential in the muscle membrane.

6. The action potential propagates rapidly along the muscle and causes contraction (excitation–contraction coupling).

When the muscle twitch in response to nerve stimulation (indirect stimulation)is observed as the indicator of neuromuscular efficiency, a drug that stops twitches could act at any one of these steps. If end plate potentials (epp's) and miniature end plate potentials (mepp's) are recorded from the end plate region of a muscle fiber exposed to a drug, it is possible to be much more specific about its site of action.

At neuromuscular junctions, there is a spontaneous, slow, random leakage of discrete, uniform packets or quanta of transmitter from the presynaptic terminals. It is these quanta that cause the miniature end plate potentials that can be recorded in the muscle fiber. In general, the frequency of mepp's is determined by events occurring in the presynaptic nerve terminal, whereas their amplitude is determined by the properties of the postsynaptic cell (Katz, 1962). The presynaptic terminal can be regarded as a supplier of uniform squirts of transmitter, which otherwise might have to be delivered by iontophoretic or cruder techniques. In the presence of drugs like curare, which compete with acetylcholine for the postsynaptic receptors, mepps cannot be recorded. If a drug does not change the amplitude of miniature end plate potentials, it cannot have affected any of steps (3–5) above.

MTX does not have any effect on the amplitude of mepps. Therefore, it cannot have any effect on the interaction between acetylcholine and the postsynaptic receptors, nor on the sodium and potassium conductance changes caused by acetylcholine (Takeuchi and Takeuchi, 1959), nor on the resistance and capacitance of the postsynaptic cell (P.W. Gage and R. N. McBurney, unpublished).

When an action potential reaches a nerve terminal, there is a transient increase in the rate of release of quanta of transmitter as a result of depolarization of the membrane (Bloedel *et al.*, 1966a,b; Katz and Miledi, 1966, 1967; Gage, 1967). The sequence of events that occur in the process of excitation–secretion coupling is not well understood but calcium ions are involved (Katz, 1969). If the release of transmitter is decreased by a drug or toxin, the cause may be either a decrease in the amplitude of presynaptic action potentials or an alteration of the secretory response of the presynaptic terminal to an action potential. An example of a toxin with the latter action is botulinum toxin, which probably blocks synaptic transmission by inhibiting excitation–secretion coupling (see Drachmann, 1971). (See also Chapter IV, Section III,C,D.)

MTX causes a rapid fall in transmitter release from sciatic nerve terminals in response to nerve stimulation. Recordings of end plate potentials in a curarized (*d*-tubocurarine chloride, 2×10^{-6} g/ml) preparation are shown in Fig. 7. As MTX does not change the response of the postsynaptic membrane to a quantum of transmitter, the fall in the amplitude of end plate potentials must be due to a decrease in the amount of transmitter released by an action potential. To find out whether MTX causes any change in excitation–secretion coupling, nerve terminals were depolarized by raising the extracellular potassium ion concentration (Liley, 1956; Gage and Quastel, 1965). This procedure increases the frequency of mepp's, presumably by depolarizing the presynaptic membrane. The increase in the frequency of mepp's caused by raising the potassium concentration to 20 m*M* was not significantly different when action potentials had been inhibited by MTX. Therefore, MTX can have no significant effect on excitation–secretion coupling. Another, though more difficult, technique that could have been used to show that MTX does not block excitation–secretion coupling would have been to record the effect of MTX on end plate potentials elicited by subthreshold depolarization of presynaptic terminals. It is possible to position a microelectrode close to nerve terminals and to elicit end plate potentials by depolarizing the nerve terminals directly

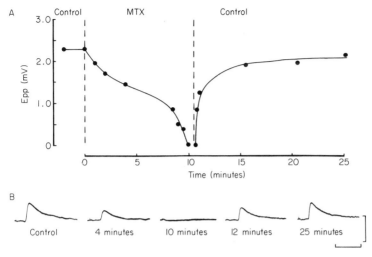

FIG. 7. The effect of MTX (5×10^{-6} g/ml) on end plate potentials in a sartorius muscle fiber. The preparation was curarized (tubocurarine, 2×10^{-6} g/ml) to prevent twitches. (A) Amplitude of end plate potentials against time. The first vertical broken line denotes the introduction of MTX. The second vertical line denotes the return to control solution. (B) The amplitude and time course of end plate potentials recorded at the indicated times. Vertical calibration, 3 mV; horizontal calibration, 10 mseconds. (Dulhunty and Gage, 1971.)

with current pulses passed through the electrode (Hubbard and Schmidt, 1963; Katz and Miledi, 1965). If MTX does not affect excitation–secretion coupling, there should be no change in the amplitude of these current-evoked epp's.

By exclusion, MTX must block neuromuscular transmission by inhibiting action potentials in presynaptic terminals and muscle fibers. It has no effect on the other steps involved in neuromuscular transmission, and, therefore, is not a specific neuromuscular blocking agent.

F. Comparison of the Cellular Effects of MTX and TTX

So far, the biological effects of TTX and MTX would seem to be identical. However, there are some differences. Sodium ions depress the effect of MTX, but this is not found with TTX. It was found that at low concentrations TTX (like MTX) does not block action potentials immediately. For example, in 56 muscle fibers from six toad sartorius muscles exposed to 10^{-8} g/ml TTX, the mean number of action potentials before block was 597 ± 37 (mean $\pm$ SE), whereas in 48 fibers from five other muscles exposed to 2×10^{-8} g/ml TTX, the mean number of action potentials was 81 ± 9.2. However, when the sodium concentration of toad Ringer con-

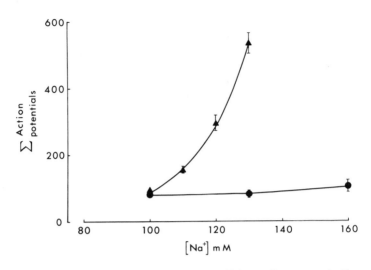

FIG. 8. A comparison of the influence of extracellular sodium concentration on the activity of MTX (4×10^{-6} g/ml, filled triangles) and TTX (2×10^{-8} g/ml, filled circles). The points show average results ± 1 SEM. (Dulhunty and Gage, 1971.)

taining TTX (2×10^{-8} g/ml) was varied from 100 to 180 mM, there was no change in the effectiveness of the toxin. This is shown in Fig. 8 in which a comparison is made between the effect of sodium ion concentration on the potency of MTX and of TTX. In the concentration range used, sodium ions reduced the effectiveness of MTX but not TTX.

IV. Discussion

Maculotoxin is a new toxin extracted from the salivary glands of an octopus, and has pharmacological effects similar to those of tetrodotoxin and saxitoxin, which are also derived from marine species. Because of these similarities, it has been suggested that MTX and TTX are identical compounds (Freeman and Turner, 1970), but the evidence for this is not strong. The pharmacological effects of the toxins are indeed very similar, as might be expected from their selective mode of action. Another point of similarity is that MTX and TTX appear in roughly the same fraction when eluted from a Sephadex G-25 column (Freeman and Turner, 1970).

There are, however, some definite pharmacological differences between the three toxins and some even more striking chemical differences (Croft, 1971). A clear differentiation between TTX and the toxic fraction of MTX can be made on silica gel plates using a mixture of isopropanol and acetic acid as solvent. Ninhydrin gives four red spots with MTX, the toxic fraction appearing at R_f 0.15. In contrast, on the same plate, TTX is located as a yellow spot at R_f 0.6 (Croft, 1971). In view of observations such as these, it is difficult to support the hypothesis of identity between TTX and MTX. The lack of a positive test for guanidine with MTX also argues against structural identity, as clear positive reactions are obtained with TTX and STX. Therefore, it would appear that MTX is a new, distinct toxin with cellular effects similar to those of TTX and STX.

Although the structure of TTX has been determined, the structural basis of its activity has not (see, however, Chapter I, Section III,B). It would appear that the presence of a guanidinium group is not an essential prerequisite for a toxin to block depolarization-activated sodium channels. When the structure of MTX is known, it is possible that the group responsible for its activity will be discovered and, perhaps, will be found to be common to the natrotoxins. Information such as this could provide valuable insight into the nature and structure of the sodium channel itself.

Because MTX has not been extracted pure and since its molecular weight has not been defined precisely, it is difficult to estimate its potency relative to that of TTX and STX. A concentration of crude MTX between 10^{-5} and 10^{-6} g/ml is equivalent in potency to TTX at a concentration of 10^{-7}–10^{-8} g/ml in toad sartorius fibers. If we assume a molecular weight of 200–500, MTX would have a potency equivalent to TTX if the crude extract contained approximately 1% MTX.

It is rather striking that three marine organisms have produced highly specific toxins of low molecular weight. The animals themselves are immune to these toxins. The puffer fish is not affected by TTX, although its nerves carry action potentials that depend on sodium conductance changes. Injections of MTX into a blue-ringed octopus at concentrations that would kill a mouse ten times its weight appeared merely to annoy the creature without otherwise affecting it (A. F. Dulhunty and P. W. Gage, unpublished).

The discovery of these three toxins in the last decade makes it seem likely that more marine toxins with specific pharmacological actions will be discovered in the near future (see Chapter I). The species to examine are those that are already known to be noxious. Interest in naturally occurring toxins and venoms is increasing as it becomes apparent that evolutionary processes have preserved those species that have elaborated chemicals affecting vital tissues such as nerve cells in foe, prey, or predator. An interesting question, as yet unanswered, is what are the mechanisms that protect the possessor of a toxin from its own toxin? Slight modification of an excitable membrane may be all that is needed to protect a depolarization-activated sodium channel from blockage by natrotoxins, and recognition of the modification could help identify the channel and, perhaps, lead to the discovery of antidotes.

The natrotoxins may also have therapeutic uses. Elucidation of the structural basis of the activity of MTX could lead to the synthesis of new, more powerful, anesthetic agents. Consciousness and sensation depend basically on the transfer of information by action potentials, and must cease when these are inhibited. The natrotoxins do not appear to have marked effects on the cardiovascular system; respiratory failure is probably due to the disappearance of action potentials. It is not clear yet whether the effects of the toxin on the central nervous system would preclude their use as general anesthetics. The convulsions that follow administration of the drugs are probably due to the respiratory effects of the drugs. However, it might be preferable if anesthetic agents such as these did not cross the blood–brain barrier. It should not be impossible to synthesize analogs that would not act centrally.

The dependence of the effect of the toxins on action potential activity would be a very useful characteristic. For example, painful procedures are recognized as painful by the victim only because the afferent pain fibers carry volleys of action potentials signaling the presence of noxious stimuli. These fibers carry a large number of action potentials, and therefore, should be highly susceptible to block by MTX. An added advantage of this toxin as a local anesthetic would be that its effects are rapidly reversible. Perhaps more use would be made of the natrotoxins as local or general anesthetics if an active subgroup is identified and can be synthetized inexpensively. Only further research will tell if this is possible.

When the structure of MTX is known, it may be possible to find an antidote to counteract its effects. None of the pharmacological antidotes tested has been found effective. The general assumption that the toxin is a neuromuscular blocking agent led Sutherland and Lane (1969) to test neostigmine as an antidote, since this anticholinesterase antagonizes the effects of many other neuromuscular blocking agents. Simon *et al.* (1964) also tested the effects of neostigmine on isolated nerve–muscle preparations, but could not reverse the effects of MTX. The latter investigators also injected a respiratory center stimulant, tetrahydroaminoacridine, in the hope of improving respiration. There was a temporary improvement in respiratory rate and depth, but this was not maintained. Freeman and Turner (1970) used catecholamines to relieve the severe hypotension that accompanies the respiratory failure. Epinephrine raised the blood pressure transiently, as did nonepinephrine, but neither of these could prevent the dramatic fall in arterial pressure after respiratory failure.

Death is caused by respiratory paralysis. If a victim is artificially ventilated, his chances of survival should be considerably enhanced, and, in fact, this method has been used successfully in one patient who survived. Presumably, the toxin is complexed or quickly eliminated *in vivo*, and, if the affected systems are supported, paralysis should disappear, and the victim should fully recover.

REFERENCES

Bloedel, J., Gage, P. W., Llinas, R., and Quastel, D. M. J. (1966a). Transmitter release at the squid giant synapse in the presence of tetrodotoxin. *Nature (London)* **212,** 49–50.

Bloedel, J. R., Gage, P. W., Llinas, R., and Quastel, D. M. J. (1966b). Transmission across the squid giant synapse in the presence of tetrodotoxin. *J. Physiol. (London)* **118,** 52P–53P.

Cleland, J. B., and Southcott, R. V. (1965). Injuries to man from marine invertebrates in the Australian region. *Nat. Health Med. Res. Counc., Rep.* No. 12.

Croft, J. (1971)."Chemistry of Marine Natural Products" M.Sc. Thesis, Macquarie University, Sydney, Australia.

Drachmann, D. B. (1971). *In* "Neuropoisons" (L. L. Simpson, ed.), Vol. I, p. 187. Plenum, New York.

Dulhunty, A. F., and Gage, P. W. (1969). Neuromuscular transmission in toad sartorius muscles without transverse tubules. *Aust. J. Exp. Biol. Med. Sci.* **47,** 8P.

Dulhunty, A. F., and Gage, P. W. (1971). Selective effects of an octopus toxin on action potentials. *J. Physiol. (London)* **218,** 433–445.

Fatt, P., and Katz, B. (1951). An analysis of the endplate potential recorded with an intracellular electrode. *J. Physiol. (London)* **155,** 320–370.

Flecker, H., and Cotton, B. G. (1955). Fatal bite from octopus. *Med. J. Aust.* **2,** 329–331.

Fleig, C., and De Rouville, E. (1910). Origine intra-glandulaire des produits toxiques des cephalopodes pour les crustaces. Toxicite comparée du sang, des extraits de glandes salivaires et d'extraits de foie des cephalopodes. *C. R. Soc. Biol.* **69,** 502–504.

Freeman, S. E., and Turner, R. J. (1970). Maculotoxin, a potent toxin secreted by octopus maculosus Hoyle. *Toxicol. Appl. Pharmacol.* **16,** 681–690.

Gage, P. W. (1967). Depolarization and excitation–secretion coupling in presynaptic terminals. *Fed. Proc., Fed. Amer. Soc. Exp. Biol.* **26,** 1627–1632.

Gage, P. W., and Eisenberg, R. S. (1967). Action potentials without contraction in frog skeletal muscle fibers with disrupted transverse tubules. *Science* **158,** 1702–1703.

Gage, P. W., and Eisenberg, R. S. (1969a). Capacitance of the surface and transverse tubular membrane of frog sartorius muscle fibers. *J. Gen. Physiol.* **53,** 265–278.

Gage, P. W., and Eisenberg, R. S. (1969b). Action potentials, after potentials and excitation contraction coupling in frog sartorius fibers without transverse tubules. *J. Gen. Physiol.* **53,** 298–312.

Gage, P. W., and Quastel, D. M. J. (1965). Dual effect of potassium on transmitter release. *Nature (London)* **206,** 625–626.

Ghiretti, F. (1960). Toxicity of octopus saliva against crustacea. *Ann. N.Y. Acad. Sci.* **90,** 726–741.

Halstead, B. W. (1965). "Poisonous and Venomous Marine Animals of the World,"
    Vol. I. Invertebrates, pp. 731–769. U.S. Govt. Printing Office, Washington, D.C.
Hodgkin, A. L., and Rushton, W. A. H. (1946). The electrical properties of a crustacean
    nerve fibre. *Proc. Roy. Soc., Ser. B* **133**, 444–479.
Howell, J. N., and Jenden, D. J. (1967). T-tubules of skeletal muscle: Morphological
    alterations which interrupt excitation–contraction coupling. *Fed. Proc., Fed. Amer.
    Soc. Exp. Biol.* **26**, 553P.
Hubbard, J. I., and Schmidt, R. D. (1963). An electrophysiological investigation of
    mammalian motor nerve terminals. *J. Physiol. (London)* **166**, 145–167.
Kao, C. Y. (1964). Tetrodotoxin, saxitoxin and their significance in the study of excit-
    ation phenomena. *Pharmacol. Rev.* **18**, 997–1048.
Katz, B. (1948). The electrical properties of the muscle fibre membrane. *Proc. Roy. Soc.,
    Ser. B* **135**, 506–534.
Katz, B. (1962). The transmission of impulses from nerve to muscle and the subcellular
    unit of synaptic action. *Proc. Roy. Soc., Ser B.* **155**, 455–477.
Katz, B. (1969). "The Release of Neural Transmitter Substances." Liverpool Univ.
    Press, Liverpool.
Katz, B., and Miledi, R. (1965). Release of acetylcholine from a nerve terminal by
    electric pulses of variable strength and duration. *Nature (London)* **207**, 1097–1098.
Katz, B., and Miledi, R. (1966). Input–output relation of a single synapse. *Nature
    (London)* **212**, 1242–1245.
Katz, B., and Miledi, R. (1967). A study of synaptic transmission in the absence of
    nerve impulses. *J. Physiol. (London)* **192**, 407–436.
Lane, W. R., and Sutherland, S. K. (1967). The ringed octopus bite. A unique medical
    emergency. *Med. J. Aust.* **2**, 475–476.
Liley, A. W. (1956). The effects of presynaptic polarization on the spontaneous activity
    at the mammalian neuromuscular junction. *J. Physiol. (London)* **134**, 427–443.
Mabbet, H. (1954). Death of a skindiver. *Aust. Skin Diving Spear Fish. Dig.* **17** [Dec.],
    13.
McMichael, D. F. (1956). Poisonous bites by octopus. *Proc. Roy. Zool. Soc. N.S.W.* **92**,
    110–111.
Narahashi, T., Moore, J. W., and Scott, W. (1964). Tetrodotoxin blockage of sodium
    conductance increase in lobster giant axons. *J. Gen. Physiol.* **47**, 965–974.
Shanes, A. M., Freygang, W. H., Grundfest, H., and Amatniek, E. (1959). Anesthetic
    and calcium action in the voltage clamped squid giant axon. *J. Gen. Physiol.* **42**,
    793–801.
Simon, S. E., Cairncross, K. D., Satchell, D. G., Gay, W. S.,´and Edwards, S. (1964).
    The toxicity of octopus maculosus Hoyle venom. *Arch. Int. Pharmacodyn. Ther.*
    194, 318–329.
Sutherland, S. K., and Lane, W. R. (1969). Toxins and mode of envenomation of the
    common ringed or blue-banded octopus. *Med. J. Aust.* **1**, 893–898.
Sutherland, S. K., Broad, A. J., and Lane, W. R. (1970). Octopus neurotoxins: Low
    molecular weight non-immunogenic toxins present in the saliva of the blue-ringed
    octopus. *Toxicon* **8**, 249–250.
Takeuchi, A., and Takeuchi, N. (1959). Active phase of frogs' end-plate potential.
    J. Neurophysiol. **22**, 395–411.
Taylor, R. E. (1959). Effect of procaine on electrical properties of squid axon membrane.
    Amer. J. Physiol. **196**, 1071–1078.
Trethewie, E. R. (1965). Pharmacological effects of the venom of the common octopus,
    Hapalochlaena maculosa. Toxicon **3**, 55–59.

CHAPTER IV

Mode of Action of Nereistoxin on Excitable Tissues

TOSHIO NARAHASHI

I. Introduction

Among the many known toxins and venoms from marine sources, only a small number have been studied for their chemical structures and pharmacological actions. Nereistoxin (NTX) is the toxic principle from the marine annelid, *Lumbriconereis heteropoda* Marenz, and is one of the best examples of one which has been developed into a useful chemical. A number of NTX derivatives have been synthesized and tested for their insecticidal activity and mammalian toxicity, and one of them called "cartap" is now being used as a commercial insecticide in Japan. In this chapter, the historical background of the study of NTX is reviewed, and recent studies on the mode of action of NTX on the neuromuscular junction are discussed.

A. Initial Study

It has long been known among anglers that flies and ants are paralyzed upon contact with the body of *Lumbriconereis*, which is commonly used as a bait. However, it was not until 1934 that the toxin from this annelid was subjected to scientific research. Nitta (1934) succeeded in isolating a toxic substance from the annelid and named it nereistoxin. He postulated an empirical formula of $C_5H_9NS_2$ as a result of analyses of its picrate and hydrogen oxalate salts. An extensive survey of pharmacological actions of the toxin was then performed using about ten species of animals ranging from the fly to the monkey, and it was concluded that NTX was a potent cholinergic drug (Nitta, 1941).

B. Recent Progress in the Chemistry of Nereistoxin

No progress was made in the study of NTX during the 20 years subsequent to Nitta's pioneering work. The presence of one nitrogen and two sulfurs in the NTX molecule deserves much attention from the biochemical point of view, since a number of biochemically active compounds found in living tissues contain sulfur, e.g., vitamin B_1, methionine, and cystine. Drs. Y. Hashimoto and T. Okaichi of the University of Tokyo did indeed notice such a unique property of NTX, and began an extensive study of the chemical structure of NTX. In 1960, they proposed $C_5H_{11}NS_2$ as the empirical formula, which was slightly different from that originally proposed by Nitta (1934), and reported N,N-dimethylamino-1,2-dithiolanes as the possible structures (Hashimoto and Okaichi, 1960). Shortly thereafter, the structure of NTX was identified as 4-N,N-dimethylamino-1,2-dithiolane (Okaichi and Hashimoto, 1962a).

$$
\begin{array}{cc}
\text{H}_2\text{C} - \text{S} & \text{H}_2\text{C} - \text{SCONH}_2 \\
(\text{CH}_3)_2\text{N} - \text{CH} \quad | & (\text{CH}_3)_2\text{N} - \text{CH} \qquad \text{HCl} \\
\text{H}_2\text{C} - \text{S} & \text{H}_2\text{C} - \text{SCONH}_2 \\
\text{Nereistoxin} & \text{Cartap}
\end{array}
$$

The amount of NTX contained in a worm varies with the size of the animal. It ranged from 60 to 100 mg toxin per 100 g of worm and was inversely related to the body weight (Okaichi and Hashimoto, 1962b). This relationship probably reflects the fact that the toxin is mainly contained in the skin (Hirayama *et al.*, 1960).

Investigators in Takeda Chemical Industries, one of the leading pharmaceutical companies in Japan, were attracted by the unique yet rather simple chemical structure of NTX and by its insecticidal activity, and started extensive research on the synthesis and insecticidal properties of NTX and its derivatives. In 1965, they were successful in synthesizing NTX from 1,3-bis(benzylthio)-2-propanol (Hagiwara *et al.*, 1965). However, the yield of NTX by this method was so poor that they explored several other methods of synthesis (Numata and Hagiwara, 1968; Konishi, 1968a,b, 1970a,b). During the course of these studies, a number of derivatives of NTX were prepared and tested for insecticidal activity and mammalian toxicity. It was found that 4-alkylamino-1,2-dithiolanes and 2-dimethylamino-1,3-propane dithiols were generally effective as insecticides, whereas 1-alkylamino-2,3-propane dithiols and nonsulfurated aminopropanes were not insecticidally active (Sakai, 1969). After extensive experiments in both laboratory and field (Sakai, 1964; Sakai *et al.*, 1967), 1,3-bis(carbamoylthio)-2-(N,N-dimethylamino)propane hydrochloride (cartap, Padan) was selected and developed into a commercial product. Cartap was chosen because it had a potent insecticidal activity, relatively low mammalian toxicity and ichthyocidal activity, and was easy to synthesize. Particular emphasis was placed on the insecticidal activity against the rice stem borer, *Chilo suppressalis*, one of the most serious insect pests in Japan and other Asian countries.

C. Historical Background on the Mode of Action of Nereistoxin

Studies on the mode of action of NTX and its derivatives were also performed along with the chemical studies outlined above. The values for LD_{50} were estimated to be 38 mg/kg (mice, subcutaneous), 1.8 mg/kg (rabbits, subcutaneous), and 0.8 mg/kg (rabbits, intravenous) by Nitta (1941). More recently, the values for LD_{50} were estimated to be 30–33.6 mg/kg (mice, intravenous) and 118–130 mg/kg (mice, oral) (Okaichi and Hashimoto, 1962b; Chiba *et al.*, 1967; Sakai *et al.*, 1967). Cartap exhibited lower toxicity, the LD_{50} values being 59 mg/kg (mice, intravenous) and 165 mg/kg (mice, oral) (Chiba *et al.*, 1967; Sakai *et al.*, 1967). The LD_{50} values of NTX and cartap are listed in Table I together with those of parathion and DDT for comparison. It can be said that the mammalian toxicity of NTX and cartap is rather moderate, especially when compared

TABLE I

Toxicity of Nereistoxin, Cartap, Parathion, and DDT[a]

Animal and route of administration	Chemicals			
	Nereistoxin	Cartap	Parathion	DDT
Mouse				
Intravenous	33.6[b], 30[c]	59[c]		
Oral	130[d], 118[e]	165[d]	6[f]	
Rat				
Intravenous	0.8[g]			50[h]
Oral			3[i]	400[h]
Rabbit				
Intravenous				50[h]
Oral		250[d]		300[h]

[a] LD_{50} in mg/kg.
[b] Okaichi and Hashimoto (1962b).
[c] Chiba *et al.* (1967).
[d] Sakai *et al.* (1967).
[e] Konishi (1968a).
[f] Yamamoto (1968).
[g] Nitta (1941).
[h] O'Brien (1967).
[i] Albert (1968).

with that of parathion, one of the most effective yet dangerous insecticides. Various cholinomimetic effects were observed after injection of NTX, i.e., increased motility of the gastrointestinal tract and uterus, increased secretion of the salivary and lachrymal glands, and constriction of the pupil (Nitta, 1941). Since these effects are antagonized by atropine, NTX appears to have the cholinomimetic action on the muscarinic receptors. In addition, NTX exerts cholinergic blocking action on neuromuscular junctions. The muscle contraction produced by nerve stimulation was suppressed, while that produced by direct stimulation remained unimpaired (Nitta, 1941). This observation suggests that NTX blocks the nicotinic receptors.

Several derivatives of NTX were compared for their effects on the peripheral neuromuscular junctions and on the central nervous system (Chiba *et al.*, 1967; Chiba and Nagawa, 1971). At low doses, they all suppressed neuromuscular transmission, whereas at higher doses they stimulated the central nervous system to produce seizure discharges. They seem to be able to penetrate the brain. NTX resembles *d*-tubocurarine in its peripheral action in that the block is antagonized by anticholinesterases, such as physostigmine and neostigmine, or by agents that increase the release of transmitter substance from the nerve terminals, i.e., calcium and tetraethylammonium (Chiba *et al.*, 1967; Nagawa *et al.*, 1971).

In view of the unique chemical structure of NTX, it is very significant that certain sulfhydryl compounds were effective in antagonizing the neuromuscular block caused by NTX. They include *l*-cysteine, cysteamine, *d*-penicillamine, and dimercaprol (BAL) (Nagawa *et al.*, 1971). This observation may indicate that the disulfide bond of the NTX molecule plays an important role in exerting the cholinergic blocking action.

The mechanisms of action of NTX in insects were further explored by Sakai (1966a). The motor discharge in the German cockroach, *Blattella germanica*, and the housefly, *Musca domestica*, was stimulated after direct application of NTX onto the ganglia, the frequency of discharge being increased. This initial stage of NTX poisoning was followed by a decrease in the frequency of discharges. These effects on the nervous system were considered to be related to convulsions and prostration of NTX-poisoned insects. There is some evidence to support the notion that certain synapses in insect ganglia are cholinergic (Yamasaki and Narahashi, 1960; Callec and Boistel, 1967; Kerkut *et al.*, 1969). Although the nature of the cholinergic receptors in insect synapses remains to be seen, these effects of NTX are compatible with the observed stimulating action of NTX on mammalian muscarinic receptors.

The contraction of the rectus abdominis muscle of the frog produced by acetylcholine (ACh) was effectively suppressed by NTX at concentrations of 10^{-4}–10^{-6} M. The suppressive action of NTX was overcome by an increase in ACh concentration, and was antagonized by eserine. However, NTX had no effect on the contraction produced by direct muscle stimulation (Sakai, 1966b). These observations indicate that the sensitivity of the cholinergic receptor to ACh is competitively suppressed by NTX.

The synaptic transmission across the last (sixth) abdominal ganglion of the American cockroach, *Periplaneta americana*, was blocked by direct application of NTX (2×10^{-6} to $5 \times 10^{-4} M$) (Sakai, 1967). However, the conduction of the presynaptic (the cercal nerve) and postsynaptic (the abdominal nerve cord) nerves was not impaired. The excitatory postsynaptic potential (epsp) as recorded by the external electrodes from the ganglion was suppressed in amplitude after application of NTX. The amplitude of the epsp increased with increasing stimulus intensity, and eventually the action potentials were produced when appropriate concentrations of NTX were used. This suggests that NTX competes with ACh for the site in the postsynaptic membrane.

Nereistoxin was found to be a weak cholinesterase inhibitor (Sakai, 1966c). The value of I_{50} for fly head cholinesterase was estimated to be $1\text{--}2 \times 10^{-3}$ M. The inhibition was of a reversible type and was exerted in a competitive manner. It was concluded that the anticholinesterase activity of NTX plays little or no role in the development of poisoning symptoms unless the dose is extremely high.

To summarize the experimental observations mentioned above, NTX stimulates the muscarinic receptor and suppresses the nicotinic receptor. These two effects may be exerted at different dose levels. However, no further mechanism can be deduced from the available literature. Therefore, the blocking action of NTX on the postsynaptic membrane of the frog skeletal muscle has been analyzed in detail by means of microelectrode and voltage clamp techniques.

II. Methods

A. Materials

The sartorius muscle of the frog, *Rana pipiens*, is isolated with a short segment of the nerve attached. The muscle is mounted in a chamber and perfused with Ringer solution. The adhering connective tissues are carefully removed with a fine forceps and scissors to facilitate the penetration of microelectrodes. The attached nerve is mounted in a small compartment adjacent to the main compartment holding the muscle. This small nerve compartment contains a pair of silver wire electrodes for electrical stimulation and is kept moist to prevent the nerve from drying. Alternatively, the end of the nerve can be sucked into a glass capillary containing Ringer solution, and electrical stimulation is applied between the capillary and the bathing solution which is grounded (suction electrode).

For experiments in which the contraction of muscle is produced and dislodges intracellular electrodes, the muscle is treated with glycerol to block the excitation–contraction coupling (Gage and Eisenberg, 1967; R. S. Eisenberg and Gage, 1967). The muscle is soaked in a Ringer solution containing 400 mM glycerol for a period of 1–2 hours or, occasionally, overnight at about 5°C, and it is then transferred back to normal Ringer solution. The excitation–contraction coupling is inhibited by disrupting the transverse tubular system (B. Eisenberg and Eisenberg, 1968), but the electrical activity remains unimpaired. However, the resting potential usually starts decreasing after the muscle is brought back to normal Ringer solution, and continues decreasing over a period of a few hours. The rate of depolarization can be slowed by having 5 mM calcium ion and

5 mM magnesium ion present in Ringer solution (R. S. Eisenberg *et al.*, 1971), but this method is not always successful in our laboratory. Since the muscle fibers located deep in the preparation are affected slowly, the whole muscle might still contract even after the surface fibers become immobile. Therefore, good results can usually be obtained with small muscle preparations isolated from small frogs.

B. Microelectrodes

A variety of methods have been developed by many investigators for filling microelectrodes with a solution. It is possible to fill an electrode to the tip with a solution simply by tapping the half-filled electrode. However, it takes about 10–15 minutes to fill one electrode. This method would be especially convenient when the filling solution is available only in a small amount, or when an electrode is urgently needed.

The so-called alcohol method originally developed by Tasaki *et al.* (1954) has been used in our laboratory quite successfully. Several (five to eight) capillary electrodes, drawn in a machine, are tied on a microscopic glass slide by means of cotton threads. Several of these glass plates holding capillaries are placed in a staining jar containing methanol. The jar is then placed in a desiccator, and negative pressure is applied at room temperature. Methanol is boiled, and the capillaries are filled with the methanol. Methanol in the jar is then replaced with distilled water, and the capillaries are now filled with water by simple diffusion in about 1 hour. The water-filled capillaries can be kept in a refrigerator for at least several months. One or two days before experiments, the glass slides holding capillaries are transferred into a staining jar containing 3 M KCl. It takes at least 1 night for the water in the capillaries to be replaced with 3 M KCl by diffusion at room temperature. The KCl-filled electrodes can be kept in a refrigerator up to 1 week. After that, the tip potential will start increasing, and electrodes will no longer be suitable for use.

C. Measurements of Resting Potential, Action Potential, and End Plate Potential

An end plate area can easily be located by observation of miniature end plate potentials (mepp's). A recording microelectrode is inserted in a muscle fiber very close to fine nerve branches. If the mepp's of about 0.5–1 mV amplitude are observed and the rising phase is brief, the electrode is located very close to the end plate. The frequency of the mepp's is usually on the order of one per second, but sometimes it reaches as high as 100 per second or more.

When an electrical stimulus is applied to the nerve, an action potential is recorded from the end plate region. The action potential recorded here is slightly different in amplitude and shape from that recorded from an area other than the end plate; the former has small humps during the rising and falling phases and is smaller in amplitude by about 20 mV than the latter (Fatt and Katz, 1951).

The end plate potential can be observed when it fails to reach the threshold for the production of action potential. This occurs in the glycerol-treated muscle, when the resting potential decreases beyond a certain critical level, or in the muscle treated with the Ringer solution containing 10 mM Mg^{2+} or other nondepolarizing blocking agents such as d-tubocurarine and nereistoxin.

D. Iontophoretic Application of Acetylcholine

The sensitivity of the end plate membrane to acetylcholine (ACh) can be examined by recording a transient depolarization produced by an iontophoretic application of ACh (Nastuk, 1951; del Castillo and Katz, 1955). A glass capillary microelectrode filled with 1 M ACh is brought very close to the outside of the end plate, and a positive pulse of current is applied to the ACh electrode. A small amount of ACh ions ejected from the tip of the electrode depolarizes the end plate. The ACh depolarization is recorded by means of an intracellular electrode filled with 3 M KCl. The time course of the ACh depolarization is much slower than that of the epp because the tip of the ACh pipette cannot be brought as close to the end plate as the nerve terminals. The location of the ACh pipette relative to the end plate is very critical, and a very small movement of the electrode causes a great change in ACh depolarization. Despite such technical difficulty, this method is extremely useful to study the sensitivity of the end plate membrane to ACh without being disturbed by any possible change in the activity of the nerve terminals.

E. Measurements of End Plate Conductances by Voltage Clamp Techniques

Voltage clamp techniques were first applied to squid giant axons by Cole (1949) and Marmont (1949). Hodgkin, Huxley, and Katz extensively used the techniques to analyze the behavior of nerve membrane in terms of ionic conductances (Hodgkin *et al.*, 1952; Hodgkin and Huxley, 1952a–d). In short, a wire electrode is inserted into the squid giant axon longitudinally to short-circuit the axoplasm. This makes the membrane potential and membrane current density uniform over the entire length of the axon inserted with the wire, establishing a space clamp condition. Then the membrane potential is suddenly displaced to a new level and held there by means of an electronic feedback circuit, and the membrane current necessary for such voltage clamping is measured. Since the time course of each component of the membrane current is different, it is possible to measure the capacitive current, transient sodium current, and steady state potassium current separately. The sodium and potassium conductances can then be measured from the currents and the membrane potentials. The voltage clamp techniques are widely being used for various giant axons and nerve cells.

Takeuchi and Takeuchi (1959) applied a voltage clamp technique to the end plate membrane for the first time. They concluded that sodium and potassium currents are the major carriers of the end plate current produced by the transmitter action (Takeuchi and Takeuchi, 1960). The voltage clamp method used in our study of nereistoxin action is essentially the same as that used by them, although a number of minor modifications are made in the circuit.

The rationale of voltage clamping of the end plate membrane is as follows: the end plate area is generally very small compared with the space constant of the muscle fiber. In the case of the frog sartorius muscle, an end plate extends from 100 to 200 μm along the muscle fiber having a space constant of 2.4 mm (Fatt and Katz, 1951). Therefore, if two glass capillary microelectrodes, one for potential recording and the other for current delivery, are transversely inserted into the muscle fiber at the end plate region, a space clamp condition is established with respect to the end plate. Now, when the nerve is stimulated, the transmitter substance released from the nerve terminal will increase the end plate conductances to sodium and potassium ions, and the resultant ionic current, instead of membrane potential change, can be recorded. This current is called the "end plate current" (epc).

Unlike the membrane current recorded from the voltage clamped axon, the epc cannot easily be separated into sodium and potassium components because they have very similar time courses. However, since the equilibrium potentials for potassium and sodium (E_K and E_{Na}) of the frog muscle are calculated to be -100 mV and $+50$ mV, respectively, it is possible to record each component of the epc at those potentials (Gage and Armstrong, 1968; Deguchi and Narahashi, 1971). That is, only the sodium epc flows at E_K, and only the potassium epc flows at E_{Na}. In order to make such measurements, one would have to eliminate the contraction of the muscle accompanied with strong depolarization. The glycerol treatment described before is used for this purpose.

The diagram of the voltage clamp circuit used in the present experiment is shown in Fig. 1. Before penetrating microelectrodes in the end plate region, switch 1 (SW1) is kept on, and switch 2 (SW2) is off as shown in the diagram. The potential microelectrode filled with 3 M KCl and having a resistance of about 5 megohms is inserted in the end plate region. If the electrode is properly located, the mepp's can be observed at terminal Vm. Then the current microelectrode also filled with 3 M KCl and with a resistance of 1–5 megohms is inserted in the same region at a distance of less than 50 μm from the potential electrode. When a weak square pulse of current is applied to the current electrode, an electronic membrane potential is observed at the Vm terminal. Such an electrotonic potential cannot be observed if the current electrode is not penetrating the muscle fiber. This mode of stimulation is often called "current clamp," because constant current pulses are applied.

After locating both electrodes in the end plate region, we are ready for voltage clamping. Switch 1 is turned off, and switch 2 is turned on, and the voltage clamp potentiometer is turned clockwise (CW) to the end as is shown in the diagram. Now the control amplifier 2 attains the maximum gain, and the current microelectrode is short-circuited with the output of

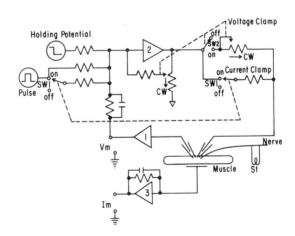

Fig. 1. Circuit diagram for voltage clamp of end plate membranes. See text for explanation. (Deguchi and Narahashi, *J. Pharmacol. Exp. Ther.*, © 1971, The Williams and Wilkins Co., Baltimore, Md.)

the control amplifier 2. The end plate membrane is voltage clamped, and its membrane potential can be changed by applying holding potential. When the nerve is stimulated, an epc is recorded at terminal Im.

F. Solutions and Drugs

The Ringer solution used as the bathing medium contains 115 mM Na$^+$, 2.5 mM K$^+$, 1.8 mM Ca^{2+}, 121.1 mM Cl$^-$, 2.15 mM Na$_2$HPO$_4$, and 0.85 mM NaH$_2$PO$_4$·2 H$_2$O, and the final pH is adjusted to 7.2. The glycerol-Ringer is prepared by addition of 400 mM glycerol to normal Ringer solution. Nereistoxin hydrogen oxalate, supplied by Dr. Y. Hashimoto of the University of Tokyo, is used.

III. Results

Detailed experimental results have already been published elsewhere (Deguchi *et al.*, 1971). Only the highlights of the results directly pertinent to the interpretation of the mode of action of NTX will be discussed here.

A. Effect on Neuromuscular Transmission

When the recording microelectrode was impaled in the end plate region, an action potential was recorded upon nerve stimulation (Fig. 2, Control). The action potential thus recorded was somewhat different in shape and amplitude from that recorded from an area of the muscle other than the end plate. The action potential recorded from the end plate showed a hump during its rising phase, attained a smaller peak, and was more prolonged in its falling phase showing another hump. This is due to the short-circuit effect of the epp exerted on the action potential (Fatt and Katz, 1951).

Nereistoxin blocked the neuromuscular transmission at a concentration of 1–3 × 10^{-4} M. About 10–20 minutes after application of NTX, nerve stimulation evoked only an epp at the end plate, and no action potential was produced (Fig. 2, NTX). The action potential generated at the end of the record of Fig. 2 originated from the other end plate of the same muscle fiber, which was not yet blocked at the time of recording. The amplitude of the epp ranged from 5 mV to 25 mV, depending on the concentration of NTX and on the time of exposure to NTX. The whole muscle preparation still contracted in response to nerve stimulation at the initial stage of NTX poisoning, because muscle fibers located in deeper layers of the preparation were not yet blocked. As these fibers were blocked with the advance of time, the whole muscle became quiescent even with repetitive nerve

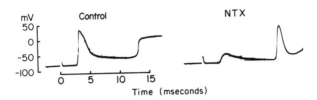

FIG. 2. Records of action potential and end plate potential before and during application of nereistoxin (NTX) at a concentration of 1×10^{-4} M. Control, an action potential evoked by nerve stimulation at the end plate. Depolarization at the end of the record shows that the intracellular electrode was withdrawn due to muscle contraction after the action potential. NTX, an end plate potential recorded from another end plate 18 minutes after beginning of NTX perfusion. The end plate potential was too small to evoke an action potential. The action potential that appeared after the end plate potential originated from the other end plate on the same muscle fiber, which turned out to be unimpaired at the time when the recording was made. (Deguchi *et al.*, 1971.)

stimuli. These effects of NTX were partially reversed upon washing with NTX-free Ringer solution.

B. Effect on Muscle Membrane

Despite such a potent blocking action on the neuromuscular transmission, the muscle fiber itself remained unimpaired under the influence of NTX. The resting potential as measured either at the end plate region or at another region was unaffected by NTX. The action potential was elicited by an intracellular stimulating microelectrode and recorded by another microelectrode inserted nearby. No change was observed in the shape and amplitude of the action potential after application of NTX. The threshold membrane potential for firing also remained unaltered. Thus it can be concluded that the electrical excitability of the muscle membrane is unaffected by NTX. It was also observed that NTX had no effect on the nerve conduction (Sakai, 1967). Therefore, NTX affects either the mechanism of transmitter synthesis in the nerve terminals or its release, or the end plate membrane, or both.

C. Effect on Miniature End Plate Potentials

The frequency of spontaneous mepp's is a measure of the mechanism by which the transmitter substance is released. This parameter is entirely independent of any effect of drugs on the postsynaptic element. After application of NTX at a concentration of $0.6-3 \times 10^{-4}$ M, the frequency of the mepp's gradually decreased, and eventually attained a very low value. The frequency usually varied widely from 0.5 to 100 per second, so that the data could not be expressed in terms of the absolute frequency. It suffices to mention that the frequency, regardless of the initial control value, steadily decreased after introduction of NTX into the chamber. Very low frequencies toward the end of experiment should be considered with some reservation, because the amplitude of the mepp's also decreased together with the frequency, and eventually became indistinguishable from noise. Therefore, it was concluded that NTX suppressed the transmitter release mechanism to some extent.

Under normal conditions, ACh molecules are spontaneously released from the nerve terminal in quanta, thereby producing mepp's. Each quantum contains a few thousand molecules of ACh. When a nerve action potential arrives at the nerve terminal, large numbers ACh quanta are suddenly released producing an epp, which in turn initiates an action potential and contraction. The number of ACh quanta released by a nerve action potential is called "quantum content," and is taken as a measure of the ability of the nerve terminal to release ACh in response to the nerve action potential. One of the methods of estimating the quantum content is to divide the mean amplitude of the epp's by the mean amplitude of the mepp's (del Castillo and Katz, 1954) (see also Chapter III).

In order to use this method for the measurements of the quantum content, the amplitude of the epp's must be kept small to avoid errors. This was achieved by addition of Mg^{2+} ions at a concentration of 10 mM in Ringer solution. Magnesium suppresses the transmitter release from the nerve terminal, thereby reducing the amplitude of the epp. NTX tended to decrease the quantum content to some extent.

D. Effect on the Sensitivity of End Plate Membrane to Acetylcholine

The observed decrease in quantum content by NTX was too small to account for a drastic decrease in the amplitude of the epp's and mepp's. Therefore, either the quantum size, which is an indication of the number of ACh molecules contained in one quantum, or the sensitivity of the end plate membrane to ACh, or both, are decreased by application of NTX. The sensitivity of the end plate membrane can be estimated by application of ACh directly to the end plate membrane. A small amount of ACh is iontophoretically ejected from the tip of the microelectrode containing ACh. If the tip of the ACh pipette is brought very close to the end plate membrane, the resultant end plate depolarization can be recorded by another microelectrode inserted in the end plate region. The end plate sensitivity to ACh was indeed suppressed very effectively by application of NTX at a concentration of 6×10^{-5} M. Thus it is concluded that the decrease in ACh sensitivity of the end plate membrane is one of the major factors responsible for the decrease in the epp and mepp. However, it remains to be seen whether the quantum size is affected by NTX. There is no easy way of measuring this parameter when the end plate sensitivity is reduced.

E. Effects on End Plate Membrane Conductances

The observed decrease in ACh sensitivity of the end plate membrane is presumably due to changes in ionic conductances. As described earlier, the transmitter ACh causes both sodium and potassium conductances to increase (Takeuchi and Takeuchi, 1960). The resting potential is about -90 mV, which is very close to E_K (-100 mV), but far from E_{Na} ($+50$ mV). Therefore, a large amount of inward sodium flux occurs during the transmitter action, which in turn produces an epp.

The contribution of sodium and potassium currents to the epc observed at the resting potential of -90 mV can be calculated. Sodium current (I_{Na}) and potassium current (I_K) are related to conductances and membrane potentials by the following equations.

$$I_{Na} = g_{Na}(E - E_{Na}) \qquad (1)$$

$$I_K = g_K(E - E_K) \qquad (2)$$

The terms g_{Na} and g_K refer to sodium and potassium conductances, and E refers to the membrane potential. From Eqs. (1) and (2) one obtains

$$\frac{I_{Na}}{I_K} = \frac{g_{Na}(E - E_{Na})}{g_K(E - E_K)} \qquad (3)$$

The ratio of the peak amplitude of epc measured at -100 mV to that measured at $+50$ mV is estimated to be 1.8 (Deguchi and Narahashi, 1971). This ratio I_{Na}/I_K is equal to the ratio of g_{Na} measured at -100 mV to g_K measured at $+50$ mV. If one assumes that the ratio g_{Na}/g_K remains constant over the entire membrane potential ranging from -100 mV to $+50$ mV, the ratio I_{Na}/I_K at -90 mV can be calculated to be 25.2 from Eq. (3). This means that only about 4% of the epc at -90 mV is carried by potassium ions.

This calculation indicates that it is impossible to conclude whether both I_{Na} and I_K are suppressed or whether I_{Na} alone is suppressed when the epp is reduced at the resting potential. Any suppression of I_K does not significantly affect the observed epp at the resting potential. It is therefore necessary to perform voltage clamp experiments with NTX-poisoned preparations whereby one can examine the effects on I_{Na} and I_K separately.

The experimental procedure used in this study was as follows: the epc's were recorded when the membrane potential of the end plate was changed in 10-mV steps from −100 mV to +50 mV. A family of epc's at various membrane potentials was thus obtained. NTX was applied, and, after 10–20 minutes, another family of epc's was recorded (Fig. 3). The peak amplitudes of the epc's recorded were then plotted as a function of the membrane potential (Fig. 4). The measured values fell on a straight line in most cases, and the line intersected the abscissa near zero membrane potential. This point represents the equilibrium potential for the epc, and the slope of the line represents the overall conductance of the end plate membrane. The sodium conductance at E_K (−100 mV) is given by Eq. (1), and graphically obtained by connecting the epc at −100 mV with the zero current abscissa at +50 mV. The potassium conductance at E_{Na} (+50 mV) is given by Eq. (2), and obtained by connecting the epc at +50 mV with the zero current abscissa at −100 mV. There is no easy way of calculating each

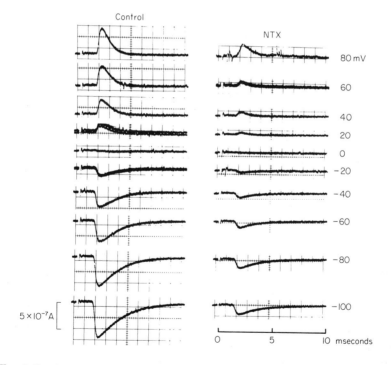

Fig. 3. Families of end plate currents recorded at various holding membrane potentials before and 12 minutes after application of NTX at a concentration of 4×10^{-5} *M* Downward deflections indicate inward end plate currents. (Deguchi *et al.*, 1971.)

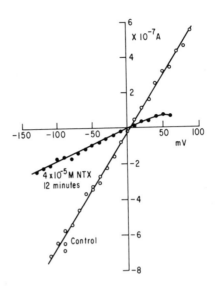

FIG. 4. Relationship between the peak amplitude of the end plate current and the membrane potential before and 12 minutes after application of NTX at a concentration of $4 \times 10^{-5}\ M$. Positive currents indicate outward currents. (Deguchi *et al.*, 1971.)

component of the membrane conductance at the membrane potential other than E_K and E_{Na}, because I_{Na} and I_K have a similar time course and cannot be separated (Deguchi and Narahashi, 1971).

The results shown in Figs. 3 and 4 are straightforward. NTX suppresses both sodium and potassium conductances of the end plate membrane to almost the same extent. The average values indicate that I_K is suppressed slightly more than I_{Na}; the percentage of suppression was estimated to be 72% for I_K as opposed to 52% for I_{Na} by $2 \times 10^{-5}\ M$ NTX, and 81% for I_K as compared with 70% for I_{Na} by $4 \times 10^{-5}\ M$ NTX.

The kinetics of the epc were affected by NTX only to a small extent. The time for I_{Na} to reach its peak was not affected at all either by $2 \times 10^{-5}\ M$ or $4 \times 10^{-5}\ M$ NTX. The time to peak I_K was not affected by $2 \times 10^{-5}\ M$ NTX, but was shortened by 18% by $4 \times 10^{-5}\ M$ NTX. The falling phase of the epc was slightly affected also. The time for I_{Na} to decay to half amplitude was accelerated by 8% by $2 \times 10^{-5}\ M$ NTX and by 21% by $4 \times 10^{-5}\ M$ NTX. The half decay time for I_K was not affected by $2 \times 10^{-5}\ M$ NTX, but was accelerated by 23% by $4 \times 10^{-5}\ M$ NTX.

It can be concluded that the observed decrease in the sensitivity of the end plate membrane to ACh by application of NTX is due to the suppression of both sodium and potassium conductances, the former being affected slightly more than the latter. There is no marked preferential action of NTX on either sodium or potassium components of the end plate conductance.

IV. Discussion

Nereistoxin suppresses the sensitivity of the end plate membrane to ACh very effectively without causing depolarization. This is the major factor responsible for neuromuscular blockage caused by NTX. The decrease in the end plate sensitivity to ACh is due to the inhibition of the mechanisms by which sodium and potassium conductances undergo an increase upon transmitter stimulation. In addition, NTX partially inhibits the mechanism underlying the release of transmitter substance. This action also contributes to the observed neuromuscular blockage to some extent.

In view of the potent end plate suppressive action, NTX may be categorized as a curare-type, nondepolarizing neuromuscular blocking agent. The results of experiments described here are also in agreement with those of Sakai (1966b) who used the rectus abdominis muscle of the frog. Such an inhibitory effect of NTX on cholinergic receptors appears to be responsible for the blockage of synaptic transmission of the cockroach nerve cord observed by Sakai (1967). Some synapses in insect ganglia seem to be cholinergic in nature (Yamasaki and Narahashi, 1960; Callec and Boistel, 1967; Kerkut *et al.*, 1969).

However, stimulating effects of NTX on certain tissues cannot be ac-accounted for on the basis of the cholinergic blocking action. At concentrations greater than $1 \times 10^{-4} M$, NTX stimulates the cockroach ganglia to produce a burst of spontaneous discharges (Sakai, 1967). In mammals, NTX increases the motility of the gastrointestinal tract and uterus, increases the secretion of the salivary and lachrymal glands, and causes a constriction of the pupil, and these effects are antagonized by atropine (Nitta, 1941). Therefore, these stimulating actions on mammalian tissues are cholinomimetic in nature exerted on the muscarinic receptors.

It then appears that NTX possesses both the cholinergic blocking action on the nicotinic receptors and the cholinomimetic action on the muscarinic receptors. It remains to be seen whether or not these two actions are exerted at different dose levels. Detailed dose-response relations for the two effects must be studied.

Since the NTX molecule contains one nitrogen and two sulfurs, it is very important that certain sulfhydryl compounds are known to antagonize the neuromuscular blocking action of NTX (Nagawa *et al.*, 1971). It was also found recently that several dithiol esters of NTX are converted into NTX in insects (Sakai and Sato, 1971). These compounds included 1,3-bis(carbamoylthio)-2-(N,N-dimethylamino)propane (cartap), 1,3-dithiocyanato-2-(N,N-dimethylamino)propane, 1,3-bis(methanesulfonylthio)-2-(N,N-dimethylamino)propane, and 1,3-bis(benzenesulfonylthio)-2-(N,N-dimethylamino)propane. Their insecticidal activity depends on the ability to form NTX. It appears that the disulfide bond of NTX plays some important role in binding to the receptor macromolecules in the end plate membrane. NTX and its derivatives will become useful tools for the study of the molecular mechanism of receptors.

It should be emphasized that cartap is one of the best examples of a marine toxin that has eventually been developed into a useful chemical with practical applications. Because of the strong cholinergic actions of NTX, potential usefulness of the toxin and its derivatives for clinical purposes should also be explored.

ACKNOWLEDGMENTS

This study was supported by grants from NIH (NS06855 and NS09272). The author is indebted to Professor Y. Hashimoto for his supply of nereistoxin samples. Thanks are also due to Mrs. Donna Crutchfield and Mrs. Delilah Munday for secretarial assistance.

REFERENCES

Albert, A. (1968). "Selective Toxicity." Methuen, London.

Callec, J., and Boistel, J. (1967). Les effets de l'acétylcholine aux niveaux synaptique et somatique dans le cas du dernier ganglion abdominal de la blatte *Periplaneta americana. C. R. Soc. Biol.* **161,** 442–446.

Chiba, S., and Nagawa, Y. (1971). Effects of nereistoxin and its derivatives on the spinal cord and motor nerve terminals. *Jap. J. Pharmacol.* **21,** 175–184.

Chiba, S., Saji, Y., Takeo, Y., Yui, T., and Aramaki, Y. (1967). Nereistoxin and its derivatives, their neuromuscular blocking and convulsive actions. *Jap. J. Pharmacol.* **17,** 491–492.

Cole, K. S. (1949). Dynamic electrical characteristics of the squid axon membrane. *Arch. Sci. Physiol.* **3,** 253–258.

Deguchi, T., and Narahashi, T. (1971). Effects of procaine on ionic conductances of end-plate membranes. *J. Pharmacol. Exp. Ther.* **176,** 423–433.

Deguchi, T., Narahashi, T., and Haas, H. G. (1971). Mode of action of nereistoxin on the neuromuscular transmission in the frog. *Pestic. Biochem. Physiol.* **1,** 196–204.

del Castillo, J., and Katz, B. (1954). Quantal components of the end-plate potential. *J. Physiol. (London)* **124,** 560–573.

del Castillo, J., and Katz, B. (1955). On the localization of acetylcholine receptors. *J. Physiol. (London)* **128,** 157–181.

Eisenberg, B., and Eisenberg, R. S. (1968). Selective disruption of the sarcotubular system in frog sartorius muscle. A quantitative study with exogenous peroxidase as a marker. *J. Cell Biol.* **39,** 451–467.

Eisenberg, R. S., and Gage, P. W. (1967). Frog skeletal muscle fibers: Changes in electrical properties after disruption of transverse tubular system. *Science* **158,** 1700–1701.

Eisenberg, R. S., Howell, J. N., and Vaughan, D. C. (1971). The maintenance of resting potentials in glycerol-treated muscle fibres. *J. Physiol. (London)* **215,** 95–102.

Fatt, P., and Katz, B. (1951). An analysis of the end-plate potential recorded with an intracellular electrode. *J. Physiol. (London)* **115,** 320–370.

Gage, P. W., and Armstrong, C. M. (1968). Miniature end-plate currents in voltage-clamped muscle fibres. *Nature (London)* **218,** 363–365.

Gage, P. W., and Eisenberg, R. S. (1967). Action potentials without contraction in frog skeletal muscle fibers with disrupted transverse tubules. *Science* **158,** 1702–1703.

Hagiwara, H., Numata, M., Konishi, K., and Oka, Y. (1965). Synthesis of nereistoxin and related compounds. I. *Chem. Pharm. Bull.* **13,** 253–260.

Hashimoto, Y., and Okaichi, T. (1960). Some chemical properties of nereistoxin. *Ann. N. Y. Acad. Sci.* **90,** 667–673.

Hirayama, K., Matsue, Y., and Komaki, Y. (1960). Toxicity of nereistoxin to aquatic animals. *Suisan-Zoshoku* **8,** 95–102.

Hodgkin, A. L., and Huxley, A. F. (1952a). Currents carried by sodium and potassium ions through the membrane of the giant axon of *Loligo. J. Physiol. (London)* **116,** 449–472.

Hodgkin, A. L., and Huxley, A. F. (1952b). The components of membrane conductance in the giant axon of *Loligo. J. Physiol. (London)* **116,** 473–496.

Hodgkin, A. L., and Huxley, A. F. (1952c). The dual effect of membrane potential on sodium conductance in the giant axon of *Loligo. J. Physiol. (London)* **116,** 497–506.

Hodgkin, A. L., and Huxley, A. F. (1952d). A quantitative description of membrane current and its application to conduction and excitation in nerve. *J. Physiol. (London)* **117,** 500–544.

Hodgkin, A. L., Huxley, A. F., and Katz, B. (1952). Measurements of current-voltage relations in the membrane of the giant axon of *Loligo. J. Physiol. (London)* **116,** 424–448.

Kerkut, G. A., Pitman, R. M., and Walker, R. J. (1969). Iontophoretic application of acetylcholine and GABA onto insect central neurones. *Comp. Biochem. Physiol.* **31,** 611–633.

Konishi, K. (1968a). New insecticidally active derivatives of nereistoxin. *Agr. Biol. Chem.* **32,** 678–679.

Konishi, K. (1968b). Studies on organic insecticides. Part X. Synthesis of nereistoxin and related compounds. III. *Agr. Biol. Chem.* **32,** 1199–1204.

Konishi, K. (1970a). Studies on organic insecticides. Part XI. Synthesis of nereistoxin and related compounds. IV. *Agr. Biol. Chem.* **34,** 926–934.

Konishi, K. (1970b). Studies on organic insecticides. Part XII. Synthesis of nereistoxin and related compounds. V. *Agr. Biol. Chem.* **34,** 935–940.

Marmont, G. (1949). Studies on the axon membrane. I. A new method. *J. Cell. Comp. Physiol.* **34,** 351–382.

Nagawa, Y., Saji, Y., Chiba, S., and Yui, T. (1971). Neuromuscular blocking actions of nereistoxin and its derivatives and antagonism by sulfhydryl compounds. *Jap. J. Pharmacol.* **21,** 185–197.

Nastuk, W. L. (1951). Membrane potential changes at a single muscle end-plate produced by acetylcholine. *Fed. Proc., Fed. Amer. Soc. Exp. Biol.* **10,** 96.

Nitta, S. (1934). Über Nereistoxin, einen giftigen Bestandteil von *Lumbriconereis heteropoda* Marenz (Eunicidae). *Yakugaku Zasshi* **54,** 648–652.

Nitta, S. (1941). Pharmakalogische Untersuchung des Nereistoxins, das vom Verf. im Körper des *Lumbriconereis heteropoda* (Isome) isoliert wurde. *Tokyo J. Med. Sci.* **55,** 285–301.

Numata, M., and Hagiwara, H. (1968). Synthesis of nereistoxin and related compounds. II. *Chem. Pharm. Bull.* **16,** 311–319.

O'Brien, R. D. (1967). "Insecticides: Action and Metabolism." Academic Press, New York.

Okaichi, T., and Hashimoto, Y. (1962a). The structure of nereistoxin. *Agr. Biol. Chem.* **26,** 224–227.

Okaichi, T., and Hashimoto, Y. (1962b). Physiological activities of nereistoxin. *Bull. Jap. Soc. Sci. Fish.* **28,** 930–935.

Sakai, M. (1964). Studies on the insecticidal action of nereistoxin, 4-N,N-dimethylamino-1,2-dithiolane. I. Insecticidal properties. *Jap. J. Appl. Entomal. Zool.* **8,** 324–333.

Sakai, M. (1966a). Studies on the insecticidal action of nereistoxin, 4-N,N-dimethylamino-1,2-dithiolane. II. Symptomatology. *Bochu-Kagaku* **31,** 53–61.

Sakai, M. (1966b). Studies on the insecticidal action of nereistoxin, 4-N,N-dimethylamino-1,2-dithiolane. III. Antagonism to acetylcholine in the contraction of rectus abdominis muscle of frog. *Bochu-Kagaku* **31,** 61–67.

Sakai, M. (1966c). Studies on the insecticidal action of nereistoxin, 4-N,N-dimethylamino-1,2-dithiolane. IV. Role of the anticholinesterase activity in the insecticidal action to house fly *Musca domestica* L. (Diptera: Muscidae). *Appl. Entomol. Zool.* **1,** 73–82.

Sakai, M. (1967). Studies on the insecticidal action of nereistoxin, 4-N,N-dimethylamino-1,2-dithiolane. V. Blocking action of the cockroach ganglion. *Bochu-Kagaku* **32,** 21–33.

Sakai, M. (1969). Nereistoxin and cartap: Their mode of action as insecticides. *Rev. Plant Protect. Res.* **2,** 17–28.

Sakai, M., and Sato, Y. (1971). Metabolic conversion of the nereistoxin-related compounds into nereistoxin as a factor of their insecticidal action. *Abstr., Int. Congr. Pesticide Chem., 2nd, 1971* p. 123.

Sakai, M., Sato, Y., and Kato, M. (1967). Insecticidal activity of 1,3-bis(carbamoylthio)-2-(N,N-dimethylamino)propane hydrochloride, cartap, with special references to the effectiveness for controlling the rice stem borer. *Jap. J. Appl. Entomol. Zool.* **11,** 125–134.

Takeuchi, A., and Takeuchi, N. (1959). Active phase of frog's end-plate potential. *J. Neurophysiol.* **22,** 395–411.

Takeuchi, A., and Takeuchi, N. (1960). On the permeability of end-plate membrane during the action of transmitter. *J. Physiol. (London)* **154,** 52–67.

Tasaki, I., Polley, E. H., and Orrego, F. (1954). Action potentials from individual elements in cat geniculate and striate cortex. *J. Neurophysiol.* **17,** 454–474.

Yamamoto, R. (1968). "Agricultural Chemistry." Nankodo, Tokyo.

Yamasaki, T., and Narahashi, T. (1960). Synaptic transmission in the last abdominal ganglion of the cockroach. *J. Insect Physiol.* **4,** 1–13.

CHAPTER V

Comparative Studies on Algal Toxins

JOHN J. SASNER, JR.

I. Introduction

Biological productivity is the direct result of the conversion of solar energy by biochemical transducing mechanisms contained in autotrophic organisms called "producers." In aquatic environments, the primary producers are the microscopic phytoplankton that bloom during periods when suitable nutrient and physical conditions exist. Photosynthetic producers constitute the basis of the food chain as well as the energy budget of fresh and salt water environments. The autotrophic microorganisms that play a vital role in productivity are also the source of many active chemical substances. Some of these are extracellular products called "external metabolites" or "ectocrines" (exocrines) (McLaughlin *et al.*, 1960; Lucas, 1955; Collier, 1958; Aaronson *et al.*, 1971). They may have antibacterial, antiviral, or growth-inhibiting activity (Nigrelli *et al.*, 1967; Baslow, 1969), and thus may affect other organisms at the same or higher trophic levels in the food chain. Extracellular products have been known for a long time, but only relatively recently has their potential importance to aquatic communities been discussed. Other active substances, called "endotoxins," are synthesized and retained within the microorganisms, and they exert their effects when consumed and passed through the food chain or when released into the water by cell breakage. These endotoxic substances are some of the most potent materials known.

Increasing interest in biochemical compounds from aquatic sources in general and from microorganisms specifically stems from two aspects of the recent "Products from the Sea" concept; first, the increased exploitation of the ocean and freshwater ponds as food sources via aquaculture and fish cultivation (including shellfish), and, second, the potential source of new materials for commercial or biomedical purposes. Extensive reviews by Halstead (1965), Russell (1965), der Marderosian (1969), Baslow (1969), and Schantz (1970) reveal the state of the art regarding the biological sources of toxins, their chemical and physiological properties, and their potentials as biochemical tools (see also Chapter I).

This chapter attempts to review and discuss some of the work completed and in progress concerning several aquatic biotoxins. O'Brien (1969) notes that toxic substances attract researchers because of their potency, specificity, and usefulness in determining natural functions. With this idea in mind, I have chosen to emphasize some of the biologically active compounds from unicellular organisms, primarily dinoflagellates and blue-green algae. However, other biotoxic products have been included where appropriate to the comparative approach. The toxins discussed have been selected to illustrate the methods employed in discovering their site and mode of action at the cellular level. Continued research should lead to a greater understanding of the normal functioning of cellular systems in much the same way that products from terrestrial plants (i.e., curare, eserine, atropine) have been used as investigative tools.

A. Red Tides

The source of biotoxins from microorganisms concerns, in some instances, unique ecological catastrophes. Intermittently, in marine waters, the delicate balance of nature is upset by phenomena commonly referred to as red tides or red water. These terms are used to indicate massive local growths or blooms of various algae or protozoa causing a discoloration of surface water which can spread over vast areas. The discoloration is not always red, as the term "red tide" would indicate, but can be brown, yellow, or green, depending on the pigmentation of the causative organism(s), their depth, and their concentrations in the plankton community. Massive blooms or red tide conditions have been observed, at irregular intervals, off the coasts of all continents, and are thus worldwide in distribution (Brongersma-Sanders, 1948; Hayes and Austen, 1951; Ballantine and Abbott, 1957; Halstead, 1965; Baslow, 1969). A great many of the protists causing such phenomena are dinoflagellates, which can usually be found in all oceans at all times of the year (Sverdrup *et al.*, 1942). The dinoflagellates and the diatoms comprise the bulk of the phytoplankton—the basis for all life in the sea (Ryther, 1955).

The biological community in which red tides occur is drastically affected by the catastrophic growth of these microorganisms. The most dramatic evidence of this is the massive mortalities of other organisms higher in the food chain (Davis, 1948; Ballantine and Abbott, 1957; Halstead, 1965). Fortunately, however, not all unicellular organisms in high concentrations, dinoflagellates included, produce such drastic effects (Collier, 1958; Ryther, 1955). The deleterious effects caused by massive microorganism blooms may be due to so-called secondary conditions resulting from the ecological imbalance of nutrients, oxygen deficiency, or hydrogen sulfide production from decomposing organic matter and increased bacterial concentration (Ballantine and Abbott, 1957; Connell and Cross, 1950). On the other hand, the liberation of toxic material(s) from unicellular organisms, particularly dinoflagellates, may produce a veritable "biological desert" from a previously abundant fauna. Estimates of 100 tons of dead fish per day were claimed for the west coast of Florida during the 1971 red tide caused by *Gymnodinium breve*.

Freshwater ponds, lakes, and rivers also undergo seasonal blooms of various algal species. The greatest toxic offenders are the blue-green algae. The stage in the eutrophication process can be directly associated with the frequency of freshwater algal blooms. Seasonal cycles or pulses occur in the plankton populations of freshwater environments, particularly in temperate lakes. Diatoms predominate in late winter and early spring; they are followed by pulses of green algae, and then blue-green algae reach peak concentrations during the warmest summer months (Palmer, 1962; Gruendling and Mathieson, 1969). Figure 1 represents the seasonal changes in the major algal components of the plankton in Winnisquam Lake, Laconia, New Hampshire (a eutrophic lake) during 1966 and 1967. Each point

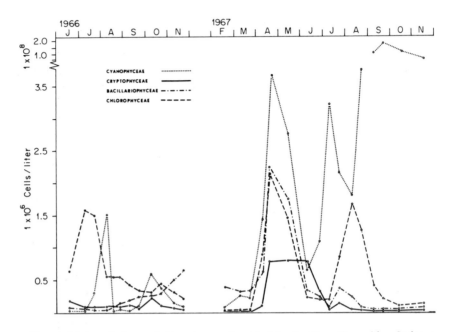

FIG. 1. Major algal populations in a eutrophic lake in New Hampshire during a phytoplankton bloom. (Adapted from Gruendling and Mathieson, 1969.)

represents the mean value of four depths within the top 10 m from three stations on the 1661-hectare lake. The blue-green alga, *Aphanizomenon flos aquae*, has been incriminated as a source of toxin in this and in other New Hampshire lakes (Sawyer *et al.*, 1968). The large pulse of cyanophyceans is due to species of *Aphanizomenon*, *Anacystis*, and *Anabaena*. During peak conditions, cell counts may be greater than 4.0×10^5/ml. Freshwater microorganism blooms are, in some ways, similar to those that occur in marine waters. They are dependent on chemical, physical, and biotic factors that may be more predictable in fresh than salt water. At least, the parameters that trigger and perpetuate the local massive growths of organisms can be more conveniently studied and perhaps controlled in the smaller freshwater situation.

The use of copper sulfate (0.5 ppm $CuSO_4 \cdot 5 H_2O$) as an algicide can be effective in temporarily reducing the population density of blooming algae in freshwater lakes. However, chemical control may not be useful in situations where toxic algae are present (Sawyer *et al.*, 1968). Rapid breakdown of great numbers of cells may release endotoxic substances and cause a fish kill.

Although processes of eutrophication cannot be reversed, they may be slowed by nutrient stripping of wastes before they enter the lake. Greeson (1969) summarized the methods used for retarding eutrophication. In addition, the treatment of phytoplankton blooms by physical mixing in the water column is currently being tested in small New Hampshire lakes. Large "circulators" (aerators) have been installed in the bottom of Kezar Lake (180 acres), North Sutton, N. H. for this purpose. The circulators are driven by compressed air and effectively intermix the top and bottom water in a manner similar to an aerator in an aquarium tank. The idea is to distribute nutrients and organisms throughout the water column and to prevent stratification (and algal concentration at the surface) during the summer months. Haynes (1971) has studied the effects of this macro-circulation on the chemical, physical, and biological characteristics of Kezar Lake.

The physical mixing process, as any chemical means of control, provides only temporary relief. However, such methods do allow extended recreational use of freshwater lakes that would be otherwise unattractive because of coloration and odor.

B. Trophic Level Relationships

Figure 2 is a diagrammatic scheme that shows some of the relationships between toxin-producing microorganisms and other organisms at different trophic levels. The basic principles are the same in both marine and freshwater environments. The primary producers (phytoplankton) elaborate a variety of extracellular substances, in addition to their own degradation products, which become part of the external pool of micronutrients, chelators, growth accelerators, inhibitors, and toxins. Bacterial action on the materials in the pool and suitable physical and chemical conditions may enhance the massive growth of one particular species and inhibit the growth of others. Ryther (1955) discusses the factors or conditions necessary to initiate marine blooms which are pertinent to freshwater forms as well. Common denominators in all blooms include (a) a seed population of organisms, (b) the proper chemical environment—organic and inorganic nutrients—and (c) suitable physical and hydrographic conditions for concentrating and maintaining nutrients and organisms. It cannot be assumed, however, that the conditions necessary to initiate or trigger phytoplankton blooms are the same as those required to perpetuate the extensive growth phenomena observed. It is suggested that some organisms and associated bacteria may, in high concentrations, condition the environment in such a way as to enhance their own growth (Starr *et al.*, 1957; Meyers *et al.*, 1959; Wilson and Collier, 1955).

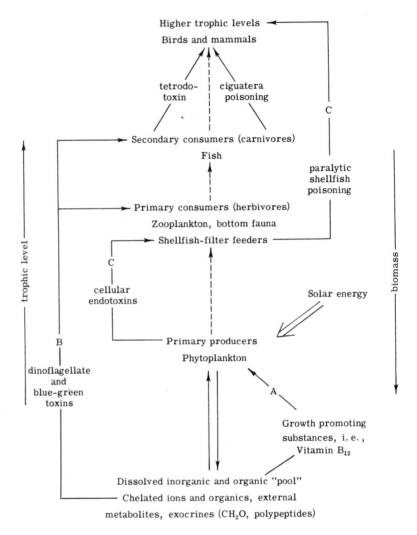

Fɪɢ. 2. Generalized scheme of trophic relationships in aquatic environments with special emphasis on the role of toxic microorganisms.

External metabolites have been considered as the source of potential nutrient pools, chelating agents for harmful trace metals, and cellular toxins (Lucas, 1947, 1949; McLaughlin *et al.*, 1960; Ryther, 1955). Organic compounds, synthesized in and liberated from photosynthetic protists, may be utilized by other organisms that feed back growth-promoting substances (Fig. 2 A). Collier (1958) suggests such a relationship between the Florida red tide dinoflagellate *Gymnodinium breve* and associated bacteria. Organic compounds produced by the dinoflagellate provide a substrate for bacterial metabolism which, in turn, produces vitamin B_{12}, a requirement for the growth of red tide organisms. Runoff from the land also adds growth-promoting factors to the nutrient supply, and has been implicated in the trigger stimulus for *G. breve* red tides (Slobodkin, 1953; Collier, 1958). On the other hand, external metabolites may be lethal to other organisms, and the subsequent decomposition of these affected forms feeds back nutrients that contribute to the extended growth of the toxin producers. Since such complex interrelationships exist between these organisms and their environment, it is important to determine the source of components contributed to the external metabolite pool. McLaughlin *et al.* (1960), Guillard and Wangersky (1958), Collier (1958), and Lewin (1956) have demonstrated the presence of numerous carbohydrate and polypeptide substances in cultures of unicellular organisms. In several cases of red tide conditions, microorganisms have been conclusively shown to be the source of toxic substances. Ray and Wilson (1957) have demonstrated this for *Gymnodinium breve*; Connell and Cross (1950) for *Gonyaulax monilata*; Burke *et al.* (1960) for *Gonyaulax catenella*; and Abbott and Ballantine (1957) for the British gymnodinoid *Gymnodinium veneficum*.

The evolutionary significance of red tide phenomena and associated conditions has not been discussed, but would be of definite academic interest. What advantage could be conferred upon a unicellular species by the ability to produce toxin? The effects of massive mortalities caused by red tides on the paleontological record is discussed by Gunter (1947). The fact that red tide conditions can have commercial significance in the fishing and tourist industry is evident from both scientific and popular literature (Lasker and Smith, 1954; St. Petersburg Times, July, 1971).

At least twenty-two dinoflagellate species have been implicated in poisonings during red tide blooms (Halstead, 1965). There are several ways that toxic dinoflagellates exert effects on animals higher in the food chain. Massive fish kills are caused by the release of poisons during the breakdown of cells after peak red ride conditions or via secretion of materials from living cells (external metabolites) into the water (Fig. 2 B). *Gymnodinium breve* and *Gonyaulax monilata*, both from the Gulf of Mexico, act in this way and also may affect many invertebrate species that occupy intermediate positions in the food chain (Sievers, 1969). Also, toxic dinoflagellates may exert their effect via intermediary consumers called "transvectors" which are apparently unaffected themselves. When these intermediary consumers (i.e., shellfish, bivalves) are ingested by animals higher in the food chain, shellfish poisoning may result (*Gonyaulax catenella, G. tamarensis*) (Fig. 2 C).

Beyond the descriptive phase, relatively little is known about (a) the conditions that trigger microorganism blooms, (b) the conditions that prolong these massive growths, (c) the materials (endo- or exo-) that are elaborated by phytoplankton during blooms, (d) the relationships of inter- and intraspecies effects (including bacterial) due to the production of external metabolites, (e) the pathways in the food chain that toxic materials may take, (f) the chemical identification and physiological activity associated with microorganism toxins.

C. Biotoxins—Source

The history and folklore of aquatic toxins has been extensively covered by Halstead (1965). Perhaps the best known marine biotoxins are ciguatera toxin, tetrodotoxin, and paralytic shellfish toxin. The first two are ichthyosarcotoxins, that is, they are related to the ingestion of fish flesh. The toxic material is apparently passed through the food chain beginning with toxic plant material and passing through several intermediary consumer stages (Randall, 1958). In the case of tetrodotoxin, the source has not been identified, but Halstead (1965 and earlier) reports an association with blue-green algae and food chain relationships similar to that of ciguatera toxin. Ciguatera poisoning has been linked to various intermediates in the food chain, principally species of blue-green algae. Ciguateralike toxins have also been reported from animals other than fish. Banner (1967) and McFarren et al. (1965) have implicated bivalve mollusks as possible sources of ciguatera. The term "cigua" toxin was first used to describe a malady associated with the ingestion of marine snails (Baslow, 1969). The fact that similar toxic effects have been produced from a variety of sources suggests that at least several ciguateralike toxins are present in the marine food chain. On the other hand, when chemical extraction procedures and bioassay techniques become standardized between research groups, it may be found that the same toxic materials are present at the various trophic levels. This might be particularly true if a common source of the toxin for for all implicated species is discovered.

Helfrich and Banner (1963) have already demonstrated that toxicity can be experimentally induced in nontoxic fish, and thereby passed through the food chain. In general, it appears that herbivorous animals ingest the toxic material, and are apparently unaffected by the presence of the toxin in their tissues. Predators then may pass the toxin through the food chain with little or no chemical change, and it can be stored by the transvectors for considerable periods of time.

According to McFarren *et al.* (1965), there are at least two toxic components that can be isolated from the red tide dinoflagellate *Gymnodinium breve*. The first is a ciguateralike component that is accumulated by filter-feeding shellfish. The bivalves act as "biological storage depots" before human consumption. The symptoms described by McFarren *et al.* (1965) are similar to those commonly associated with ciguatera poisoning from the ingestion of fish.They include loss of equilibrium, tingling sensations around the mouth, face, and extremities, paralysis, gastrointestinal distress, loss of sensory facilities, and, in mice, subsequent death after several hours. The other toxin is described as a fast-acting poison affecting neuromuscular systems with death associated with spastic twitching and subsequent respiratory failure. Several attempts to isolate and purify the active materials have been successful and will be discussed later. It appears that the toxin(s) from *G. breve* may manifest itself in massive fish mortalities or in shellfish toxicity (ciguateralike). It was thought that dinoflagellates causing one type of toxicity were different from those causing the other (Abbott and Ballantine, 1957). Members of the genus *Gonyaulax* appear to support this generality in that they have been implicated only in paralytic shellfish poisoning (although it is not ciguateralike). *Gymnodinium breve*, however, is an exception since toxic substances from this species have been associated with both massive fish kills and shellfish toxicity in the Gulf of Mexico (Ray and Wilson, 1957; McFarren *et al.*, 1965; Cummins *et al.*, 1971) (see also Chapter VI).

The mode of action of ciguatera toxin isolated from the red snapper, *Lutjanus bohar*, was claimed by Li (1965) to involve inhibition of cholinesterase in *in vitro* systems. Rayner *et al.* (1969 and earlier) refute this claim on the basis of pharmacological and chemical test results obtained with ciguatoxin. An interesting point in this regard is that the *Gymnodinium breve* fast-acting poison shows anticholinesterase-like activity when tested on various cholinergic systems (Sasner *et al.*, 1972). The relationship, if any, between the two is unclear, and should be investigated using common chemical and pharmacological systems.

Tetrodotoxin (TTX) and saxitoxin (clam poison) are perhaps the most studied poisons from the marine environment (Kao, 1966). In addition, ciguatoxin (reviewed by Baslow, 1969), the active materials from the dinoflagellate *Gymnodinium breve* (Martin and Chatterjee, 1970; Trieff *et al.*, 1971; Sasner *et al.*, 1972), and the complex of toxins from *Prymnesium parvum* (Shilo, 1967) have received considerable attention (see also Chapters VIII and IX). Only the latter species is not strictly marine, since it thrives in brackish and freshwater fish ponds in Europe and the Middle East. Biotoxins from the freshwater environment are becoming more noteworthy, particularly in some shallow ponds and lakes where processes of eutrophication are rapidly progressing. Gorham (1964), Prescott (1968), and Schantz (1970) summarize the toxicity of blue-green algae that have been linked to animal kills in the freshwater environment.

D. Biotoxins—Potential Utility

Animals are characterized by the possession of certain fundamental properties that set them apart from inanimate objects. The common denominators in the animal kingdom are metabolism, growth, reproduction, excitability, and motility. When the total life cycle of a particular organism or species is considered, the properties are essentially interdependent. From the point of view of the biochemist, immediate and continous energy requirements must be met in order to drive living systems, and, therefore, metabolism stands out as the property on which the others depend. However, animals act on their environment to gain energy sources (food) for metabolism, and, thus, the electrophysiologist or muscle biophysicist may consider sensory and motor properties (i.e., excitability) to be most important. This is not an attempt to designate one feature as being more significant than another, but to point up the dependency that exists between living characteristics. Metabolic poisons such as malonic acid, iodoacetic acid, or dinitrophenol, which block specific enzymes in small quantities, have been used to delineate biochemical pathways and energy flow in biological systems. We are discovering that biotoxins, such as tetrodotoxin, can also be used to analyze phenomena associated with excitable tissues. This area of research helps both the general and the comparative physiologist toward the goal of defining functional common denominators at the cell and membrane level.

In higher taxonomic groups of organisms, a division of labor exists whereby different tissues and cells become specialized for specific functions. Although fundamental properties are inherent in all cells to some degree, liver cells are specialized for metabolic processes, sex cells for growth and reproduction, muscle cells for excitability and contraction (motility), and nerve cells for excitability and conduction. It is therefore most rewarding to study excitable properties in nerve and muscle cells. Large organisms, e.g., vertebrates, use subsidiary systems (respiratory, circulatory, digestive, and excretory) to support physical processes associated with material exchange between cells, their bathing medium, and the external environment. Bernard, in 1859, first recognized these relationships, and Cannon, in 1929, discussed their role in the maintenance of homeostasis (Langley, 1965).

Biotoxins have been studied at the systems level by public health oriented researchers interested in the effects and possible antidotes for poisoning that usually occurs through the food chain. The best examples of this are ciguatera, puffer fish, and paralytic shellfish poisoning. For the general and comparative physiologist the primary interest concerns the mode of action and the specific site of action at the cell and membrane level. Since the main thrust of this treatise is directed toward cellular functions, emphasis will be placed on some of the techniques, general applications, and results at the tissue, cell, membrane level of biological organization. It is, perhaps, redundant to note that the fundamental properties that describe living animals also characterize cellular processes. Here we find additional common denominators among living cells such as bioelectrogenesis and chemical transmission processes which can be investigated by using toxins as tools, since it is at this level that toxins interfere with normal cellular processes. The goal is to understand cell and membrane properties in a wide variety of systems in order to establish new common features.

Nervous systems, in general, are characterized by the neuron doctrine (see Bullock and Horridge, 1965). They are composed of discrete cells that as all cells have different intra- and extracellular environments. This characteristic imparts to cells (nerve and muscle cells in particular) the property of excitability. The features that underlie excitable phenomena are integrally linked to membrane systems. Neuromuscular systems are particularly sensitive to the effects of many toxic substances. Their dependence on high metabolic activity and the chemical sensitivity of cellular membranes may be responsible for the deleterious and varied effects of biotoxins at this level.

II. Experimental Procedure and Discussion

A. Laboratory Culturing

Although it is important to verify the existence of a particular toxic substance in nature, laboratory cultures may provide much of the material for physiological testing. Many authors of scientific papers dealing with toxic algae describe their culturing techniques in a very few paragraphs. However, when one has experience in culturing, it is understood that a great deal of time and effort may be included in those few paragraphs. Extraction, purification, and chemical identification require such large amounts of material that mass cultivation is necessary.

Laboratory cultivation of microorganisms dates back to the nineteenth century. Early methods for isolating algae from associated bacteria by plating on gelatin and on agar are still useful especially for unicellular and filamentous forms. Many workers used an agar media that was inoculated while the agar was still liquid. The agar had to be broken to retrieve the individual cultures. By 1913, Pringsheim was growing blue-green algae in an axenic liquid media while studying their nutritive requirements. A great deal of early work was done, however, using solid media and bacteria-contaminated culture, and doubt may be cast on its validity. Studies on multicellular species often understimated the impact of bacteria in the culture media. However, several important contributions resulted from these early studies which are still useful today. Before the turn of the century, a technique of starting cultures by inoculation with single zoospores or flagellates using capillary pipettes was developed. Pringsheim (1921) suggested the method of washing which had been utilized previously for ciliated forms. This method consists of the serial transfer of isolated cells from one sterile solution to another (see Pringsheim, 1949; Droop, 1954; Boleyn, 1967). This effectively dilutes contaminants and will initiate axenic cultures in many cases. However, this method is not effective in purifying cells that may have bacteria attached to protective mucilagenous sheaths, such as in blue-green algae. Some recent work (Kraus, 1966) has demonstrated the potential of gamma radiation to initiate axenic cultures of blue-green algae. Utilization of antibiotics has also been effective in controlling bacteria (Droop, 1967). For a review of early work, see Pringsheim's (1949) introduction, and, for a discussion of algal isolation methods, see Lewin (1959).

The early workers discovered that several species of blue-green algae (*Nostoc, Anabaena, and Cylindrospermum*) grew successfully in phosphate-enriched water layered over soil. The utilization of soil and peat extracts to improve growth in laboratory cultures is important. Pringsheim (1949) suggested that the soil extracts were important in supplying soluble iron compounds and that peat extracts supplied hydrogen ions and various salts; both helped regulate pH of the media. Some culture media still utilize soil extracts, but many that have been recently developed are completely artificial.

The controlled mass cultivation of unicellular algae was attempted more than 20 years ago at Stanford Research Institute. Primary interest was generated by the green alga *Chlorella* as a potential source of food. Numerous investigations into the growth rates, nutrient requirements, physical parameters optimal for growth, and potential utility of the alga were initiated at this time (Burlew, 1953). The toxicology of compounds elaborated by aquatic microorganisms and their growth in the laboratory are relatively new and challenging areas of research, and require mass or bulk cultivation in the laboratory. Since blooms in nature are, at best, sporadic and since it is important to determine the causative organism, axenic cultivation is essential at some point in the study to determine the specific source of the active substances (biotoxins). Growth requirements and extrametabolite production can also be more accurately determined when axenic cultures are used.

The growth requirements of marine and freshwater microorganisms have been recently reviewed by Lewin (1962), Loeblich (1966), and Prescott (1968). Since the ultimate goal is to culture these organisms axenically, it has become necessary to investigate not only the inorganic, but the organic requirements as well. Artificial culture media may be divided into several major categories: (a) macronutrients, including a nitrogen source, (b) trace elements, (c) organic growth factors, and (d) a buffer system.

Macronutrients include C, H, O, N, Ca, Mg, S, K, Na, and P. These may be added to the media as various salts, or, if a natural media (e.g., seawater) is used, they may be already present (see Table I). The total salt concentration is dependent, of course, upon whether a freshwater or estuarine species is being cultured. One media called f/2-α, a modification of media f (Guillard and Ryther, 1962), is especially designed for testing salinity tolerance and growth under different salinity regimes (Droop, 1961). In cultures that include natural freshwater or distilled seawater, trace elements may still be added. Exact requirements for trace elements are generally not known. Since it is very difficult to completely remove any of these elements experimentally, it is correspondingly difficult to evaluate the actual requirements for them.

McLaughlin *et al.* (1960) reported that a wide variety of marine diatoms, cryptomonads, chrysomonads, euglenoids, and dinoflagellates in axenic culture require vitamin B_{12}, thiamine, and biotin. Freshwater organisms also require these same organic growth factors for prolific growth, although they may not be essential. The universal need for vitamin B_{12} in several photosynthetic groups has also been indicated by Provasoli (1958). It follows that ecological, *in vivo* considerations of the nutrition of these organisms must involve material interchange between species, i.e., external metabolites. The need of some for organic growth factors has been long recognized, though it seems essentially that the three mentioned are of particularly widespread importance (see Droop, 1962).

The pH of the media is often a crucial factor for several reasons. First, at higher pH nitrate uptake is favored, while at lower pH ammonia uptake increases. Second, higher values of pH tend to increase precipitation of calcium, magnesium, and iron phosphates. Third, and obviously important, is the pH that supports maximum growth. The components of the media must, when mixed, give a final pH that is conducive to growth and cell division.

Finally, the stability of the media over time is obviously crucial if a continuous growth-extraction schedule is desired. Three factors are important: (a) adequate supply of necessary chemicals to support increased biomass; (b) stability of pH; (c) buildup of growth-inhibiting or toxic substances (autotoxicity). The supply of chemicals necessary for growth in artificial media is naturally designed so as not to limit growth. The stability of pH has led to the addition of various buffers in the different media, but, for short-run experiments, a buffer may not be needed. For example, McLachlan (1964) showed that *Amphidinium carteri* grew as well in unbuffered media as in media buffered with glycylglycine. Natural seawater is buffered mainly by the bicarbonate ion. When it is autoclaved, the pH rises due to the release of CO_2, and precipitates may form that may deplete trace metal components. Therefore, organic buffers and synthetic seawater are now widely used. The third factor—buildup of growth-inhibiting substances—is an area that is only recently receiving attention.

Example of three popular marine media useful in the culture of various unicellular algae are given in Table I. The f media of Guillard and Ryther (1962), in particular, has been subsequently modified in different ways to serve different ends. McLaughlin *et al.* (1960) describe their MKD media as a maintenance media for extended logarithmic growth and give two other media: one (MMK) for maximum polysaccharide production and the other (MDV) designed specifically for testing for *N*-ethyl carbazole. The NH-15 medium (Gates and Wilson, 1960) was designed for *Gonyaulax monilata*, and is utilized in our laboratory and in others for culturing *Gymnodinium breve* and *Amphidinium carteri*. Media for the culture of freshwater forms, especially blue-green algae, appear in tabular form in Zehnder and Gorham (1960, Table 1, p. 648).

The measurement of growth in laboratory cultures can be accomplished by several methods. Culture density can be effectively estimated in test tube samples by optical density measurements matched against a predetermined standard curve (cell number versus OD). Direct count of samples from mass cultures can be made using a Sedgewick-Rafter counting cell. A 1.0-ml sample of culture is placed in the counting chamber and observed visually under the microscope. This method can be time consuming when the growth in many cultures is being monitored. The most accurate and effective way of determining growth in cell cultures is by means of the Coulter Counter (Coulter Electronics, Hialeah, Florida). This is an automatic, electric counting system that offers several advantages. It gives a rapid, precise count of the cells and, in addition, can discriminate particles (cells) of different sizes. The cell counts obtained by the various methods are conveniently expressed using growth curves.

TABLE I

MEDIA COMPOSITION FOR CULTIVATION OF MARINE ALGAE

Substance or property	f/2 (Guillard and Ryther, 1962)	MKD (McLaughlin et al., 1960)	NH-15 (modified after Gates and Wilson, 1960)
KNO$_3$	—	—	100 mg
NaNO$_3$	75 mg	50 mg	—
K$_2$HPO$_4$	—	10 mg	—
NaH$_2$PO$_4$·H$_2$O	5 mg	—	10 mg
Na$_2$SiO$_3$·9 H$_2$O	15–30 mg	10 mg	—
Na$_2$ EDTA	—	—	10 mg
Trace metals	f/2[a]	P-II[b] (3 ml)	NH-15[c] (5 ml)
NaCl	—	24 g	24 g
MgSO$_4$·7 H$_2$O	—	9 g	6 g
MgCl$_2$·6 H$_2$O	—	—	4.5 g
CaCl$_2$	—	300.0 mg	700.0 mg
KCl	—	700.0 mg	600.0 mg
Nitrilotriacetic acid	—	200.0 mg	—
Vitamin B$_{12}$	0.5 μg	10 μg	1.0 μg
Biotin	0.5 μg	10 μg	1.0 μg
Thiamine-HCl	0.1 mg	0.1 mg	10 mg
Supplement organic mix	—	MKD organics[d]	0.1 ml vit-8[e]
Tris	—	1 g	400 mg
pH	—	7.6–7.8	8.0
Sulfides soln.[f]	—	—	5 ml
Adenine-SO$_4$	—	—	1 mg
Fe sequestrene	5 mg	—	—
Water (to 1 liter)	NS[g]	GD[g]	GD[g]

[a] Composition: 10 μg CuSO$_4$·5 H$_2$O; 22 μg ZnSO$_4$·7 H$_2$O; 10 μg CoCl$_2$·6 H$_2$O; 180 μg MnCl$_2$·4 H$_2$O; 12.6 μg Na$_2$MoO$_4$·2 H$_2$O.

[b] Per ml—1.0 mg EDTA; 0.01 mg Fe; 0.2 mg B; 0.04 mg Mn; 5 μg Zn; 1 μg Co.

[c] In 100 ml—25 mg Fe tartrate; 30 mg H$_3$BO$_3$; 1 mg H$_2$SeO$_3$; 1.2 mg NH$_4$VO$_3$; 1.1 mg K$_2$CrO$_4$; 3.7 mg MnCl$_2$; 8.3 mg TiCl$_3$; 50 mg Na$_2$SiO$_3$; 4.0 mg ZrOCl$_2$; 1.5 mg BaCl$_2$.

[d] Composition: 20 μg pyridoxine-HCl; 20 μg folic acid; 1 mg urea; 50 mg DL-alanine; 50 mg Na$_2$ fumarate; 1 mg (NH$_4$)$_2$SO$_4$; 50 mg D-ribose.

[e] In 100 ml—20 mg thiamine; 50 μg biotin; 5 μg B$_{12}$; 250 μg folic acid; 1 mg PABA; 10 mg nicotinic acid; 80 mg thiamine; 50 mg choline; 100 mg inositol; 800 μg putrescine; 500 μg riboflavin; 4.0 mg pyridoxine; 2.0 mg pyridoxamine; 26.0 mg orotic acid.

[f] Use 5 ml per liter. Stock—200 mg NH$_4$Cl; 100 mg K$_2$HPO$_4$; 40 mg MgCl$_2$; 200 mg NaHCO$_3$; 150 mg Na$_2$S·9 H$_2$O raised to 1000 ml with distilled water.

[g] NS, natural seawater; GD, glass distilled. (Composite table reproduced with permission of the Natural Research Council of Canada from the *Canadian Journal of Microbiology*; The New York Academy of Sciences; and the authors.)

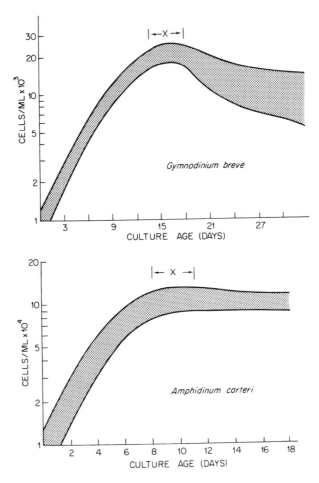

Fɪɢ. 3. Growth curves for two marine dinoflagellates, *Gymnodinium breve* and *Amphidinium carteri*. Both species were grown on the NH-15 medium (see Table I) of Gates and Wilson (1960). The curves represent the range of growth measured in 60 cultures. Toxin extractions were carried out when cultures reached the age indicated by X. (Reprinted with permission of Pergamon Press, 1972.)

Figure 3 demonstrates the growth curves for two dinoflagellate species (*Gymnodinium breve* and *Amphidinium carteri*) grown in our laboratory. Both species were cultured in the NH-15 medium described by Gates and Wilson (1960). The mass cultures were started with high density inocula (1000 ± 200 cells/ml) that provided a time advantage when large quantities of cellular material were required. This avoided an intial lag phase of slow growth which occurred when cultures were inoculated with fewer cells, and permitted harvesting of mature cultures sooner (approximately 14 days for *G. breve*). Paster and Abbott (1970) have shown that gibberellic acid stimulates growth in *G. breve* and also shortens or eliminates the initial lag phase of growth. Growth of marine blue-green algae is also potentiated by gibberellic acid (Ramamurthy, 1970).

The stage in the growth cycle at which the cells are harvested can be critical in cultures of toxic microorganisms. Gentile and Maloney (1969) showed that toxicity increased in cultures of *Aphanizomenon flos aquae* at high cell densities. The authors observed that increased potency of toxic extracts was related to decreased light intensity during growth. Using *Gymnodinium breve* cultures, we have found that extracts harvested soon after peak cell density is reached show consistent potency, but become irregular shortly thereafter. Ether extracts of *G. breve* cultures during the period indicated by X in Fig. 3 yielded 5.4 ± 0.4 mg of material per 10^6 cells, and had a potency of approximately 1.5 mouse units/mg. When cultures were allowed to exceed this time period (X), the potency of extracts was erratic (Thurberg, 1972).

When conditions permit, it may be possible to obtain toxic materials from natural blooms. This can be accomplished by using chemical extraction methods or continuous flow centrifugation of natural waters. Ether extracts of *G. breve* were obtained from seawater samples collected during the red tide in the Tampa–St. Petersburg, Florida area during the summer of 1971. Likewise, we have harvested *Aphanizomenon flos aquae* from several New Hamsphire lakes during blooms when high concentrations of organisms (4.0×10^8 cells/liter) caused water coloration and musty odor. In this case, DeLaval Separators were taken to the site of the bloom and used to spin the cells from hundreds of liters of water per day. Harvesting from *in vivo* situations can be important in comparative chemical analysis of toxic materials, and must be done to prove the identity of biotoxins in nature.

B. Bioassay

Biological methods are used to determine, and sometimes standardize, the potency of toxins or toxic preparations that are unavailable in chemically pure form. The time of onset of a response after toxic stress is related to the dose level used. There are many methods described in the literature that have utilized whole organisms, tissues, and cell preparations to determine the activity and potency of active materials in nature. Shilo and Aschner (1953) used tadpoles (*Rana* and *Bufo*) and minnows (*Gambusia*) to test materials from the phytoflagellate *Prymnesium parvum*. Shilo and

Rosenberger (1960) tested the toxin from the same source on erythrocytes, Ehrlich ascites cells, HeLa cells, human amnion cells, and the Chang strain of liver cells (see Shilo, 1967). Cornman (1947) tested dinoflagellate extracts on cleavage in sea urchin eggs (*Arbacia*), and found that cell division was retarded. Abbott and Ballantine (1957) tested alcohol extracts from cultures of *Gymnodinium veneficum* on representatives of all the major invertebrate phyla plus *Amphioxus*, fish, frogs, and mice. These authors chose a fish (*Gobius virescens*) for comparing the toxicity of whole cultures and extracts because of the apparent sensitivity of the goby to *G. veneficum* toxin. Several authors (Sawyer *et al.*, 1968; Sasner *et al.*, 1972; Spikes, 1971; Thurberg, 1972; Abbott and Ballantine, 1957) have made use of isolated nerve–muscle, heart, and intestinal smooth muscle preparations to test the activity and potency of various microorganism toxins. Protozoan cultures have been useful in the bioassay of several vitamins and growth factors (Ford, 1953; Baker *et al.*, 1962; Hall, 1965). In addition, protozoans have been utilized for the bioassay of toxins (Hutner *et al.*, 1961; Hutner, 1964).

The time required to kill mice, fish, and various other organisms is the most widely used criterion for measuring the potency of microorganism toxins. The use of death time (or survival time) reduces variables that may exist when behavioral or physiological anomalies are employed, particularly when testing whole organisms. These variables usually concern individual differences between test organisms, in the experimenter's methods, and in the interpretation of the observed changes. In addition, when large numbers of tests are necessary to satisfy statistical requirements, it can be difficult and time consuming to monitor behavioral or physiological responses. Thus, the criterion most widely used, particularly for comparative work, is the time from treatment to death (see Chapter VI).

While the end point (death) may be clear cut, the dose levels, testing procedures, and interpretation of potency or lethality of active samples has not been. This can be crucial when attempting to compare information obtained from several laboratories working on the same toxins. Russell (1966) cited twenty-four different treatments of bioassay data used in about 200 scientific publications dealing with the potency of animal venoms. There has also been some lack of unity in the presentation of assay information on the active materials from unicellular sources. However, two means of expressing and comparing potency have been widely used. These are the LD_{50} and the mouse unit (MU) (see Chapter VI).

The LD_{50} is the dose level that will cause 50% mortality of the test animals. The administration of the toxic material may be via ingestion, intravenous, or intraperitoneal injection in mammals or other vertebrates.

When fish are used, they can be either injected with (IP) or immersed in the toxic solution. Russell (1966) and, earlier, Trevan (1927) pointed out that the effective use of the LD_{50} requires that at least thirty animals be tested in order to satisfy 95% confidence limits. Thus, preliminary testing to find the effective dose range and the use of large numbers of test animals may require that significant amounts of precious toxin be used up in this procedure. However, accurate estimation of the LD_{50} value has been accomplished with Weil's Tables (Weil, 1952) used by McFarren *et al.* (1965) and the probit transformation method of Miller and Tainter (1944) used by Trieff *et al.* (1971) in studies on the active substances from the dinoflagellate, *Gymnodinium breve.*

At least two different interpretations of the mouse unit have been used to determine the potency or toxicity of bivalve tissues during periods when they may be filter-feeding toxic dinoflagellates. McFarren *et al.* (1965), when testing the ciguateralike poison from *Gymnodinium breve*, defined the mouse unit as the LD_{50} effective in 20-g mice in $15\frac{1}{2}$ hours. Although only a limited number of cases has been studied, the authors report that 40–50 mouse units may produce illness in persons eating toxic oysters.

One of the most widely used units for potency is the mouse unit described by Sommer and Meyer (1937) to evaluate the amount of paralytic shellfish poison (PSP) in Alaskan butter clams. One mouse unit was defined, in this case, as the amount of poison that will kill a 20-g mouse in 10–20 minutes. The type of PSP associated with the dinoflagellates *Gonyaulax catenella* and *G. tamarensis* and the butter clam (saxitoxin) has been routinely assayed in natural populations of mollusks because of the potential hazard to human health. [See Halstead (1965) and Chapter VI for the assay procedure and its historical development.] State and federal agencies use this effective monitoring method to protect potential consumers on both coasts of North America. The method is based on a reference standard of purified poison obtained from the United States Public Health Service, against which partially extracted field samples of bivalves are compared (Halstead, 1965; Schantz, 1970, and earlier).

C. Physiological Methods

1. BIOELECTROGENESIS

The cell is the source of bioelectric potentials, and depends upon an intact active membrane system for ionic or chemical gradients. Although the osmotic concentration of materials in the intra- and extracellular environment may be nearly equal, the excitatory properties observed in cells are dependent on the unequal distribution of these materials. According to the ionic theory of bioelectrogenesis (reviewed by Grundfest, 1967; J. W. Woodbury, 1966), changes in the permeability properties of the membrane provide the basis for excitatory and inhibitory phenomena. In addition, at rest, the selective permeability of the membrane and associated active transport (energy requiring, metabolically driven) accounts for a resting membrane potential that may be 50–100 mV depending on the type of cell. The inside is negative relative to the outside.

Figure 4 illustrates the general electric and ionic conditions that determine the resting state in nerve and muscle cells. During resting conditions, the membrane is moderately permeable to K^+ ions and relatively impermeable to Na^+ ions. This results in a large gradient for Na^+ ions that tend

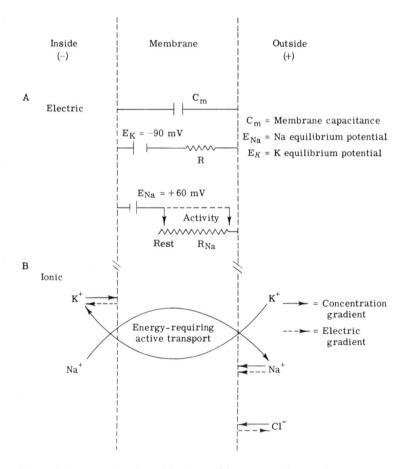

Fig. 4. Scheme of electric and ionic conditions across the membrane at rest.

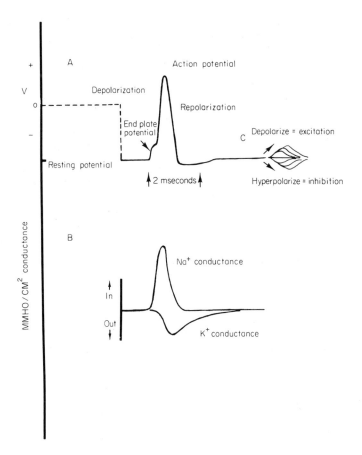

FIG. 5. Scheme of electric and ionic conditions across the membrane during activity. See text for explanation.

to flow down the concentration and electric gradients that have been established. Because of the membrane's impermeability, this movement is retarded, and only a small Na+ current is observed, this small current being counteracted by the Na+ pump system. The membrane permeability allows K+ to diffuse out of the cell, but this flow is retarded by the electric gradient.

During activity, the physiochemical properties of the membrane are briefly altered. While the permeability to K+ ions remains essentially similar to the resting membrane state, the permeability to Na+ ions greatly increases. Since the membrane is the major retarding force to this ion, the brief increase in permeability allows Na+ to rush down its concentration and electric gradients. The electric difference of 90 mV across the membrane is destroyed (depolarization, Fig. 5 A) and reversed by 20–30 mV in the opposite direction (Nastuk and Hodgkin, 1950). At the peak of this depolarization phase, the membrane resumes the permeability properties of the resting condition. Figure 5 B illustrates the conductance of ions during depolarization and repolarization (Hodgkin, 1958).

The sequence of ionic events includes (a) depolarization caused by Na^+ ions diffusing into the cell down both concentration and electric gradients and (b) repolarization: relative impermeability of the membrane to Na^+ is restored, and K^+ ions diffuse down both concentration and transient electric gradients established by the movement of the Na^+ ions. This activity, called an action potential, is an all or none phenomenon, nondecrimentally propagated along the cell membrane to the synaptic or end plate region. Action potentials (more precisely, volleys of action potentials) represent the signals that may be integrated at either higher CNS levels or peripheral sensory and motor systems. These signals may excite or inhibit activity in contiguous cells. (For a review, see Katz, 1966.)

2. COMMUNICATION BETWEEN CELLS

The messages carried by action potentials are not conducted by ionic current flow between cells. With the exception of tight junctions and functional syncytia, most neuromuscular systems employ some type of gap or synaptic junction. Transmitter substances are released from presynaptic terminals of one cell (nerve) and diffuse across the synaptic junction (end plate) to active sites on the adjacent postsynaptic membrane (muscle). In the resting state, a low level of activity results from the continuous release of transmitter by the presynaptic terminals. This low level activity results in local miniature end plate potentials (mepp's) that are characteristic of subthreshold changes in ion conductance at postsynaptic sites. Increases in both Na^+ and K^+ conductances usually result in excitation via depolarization. An increase in the conductance of K^+ and/or Cl^- ions (but not Na^+) results in hyperpolarization of the postsynaptic terminals and, hence, inhibition (Fig. 5 C). (See also Chapters III and IV.)

Electrophysiological measurements on nerve and muscle cells are a valuable means of determining the site and mode of action of aquatic microorganism poisons. Studies using toxins from a variety of biological sources indicate the sensitivity of excitable membranes (Abbott and Ballantine, 1957; Parnas and Abbott, 1965; Kao, 1966; Sasner, 1965; Evans, 1971) to these active materials. The general effects of biotoxins on neuromuscular preparations concern several factors. First, the destruction of excitability by prolonged membrane depolarization may indirectly involve the alteration or destruction of active transport systems responsible for the maintenance of ionic gradients or, on the other hand, alteration of the membrane properties may result in a general change in ion conductance pathways. Second, the blockage of excitability with no depolarization may be related to the blockage of specific ionic pathways. Third, the alteration of the complex transmitter system in the nerve–muscle end plate offers a wide range of possibilities. Such effects could involve transmitter synthesis, transmitter release, enzyme control, or competition for active sites. In addition, direct effects of the toxin on postjunctional membranes (excitatory or inhibitory) might be involved.

3. Measurement of Excitable Phenomena

In several instances, standard bioassay techniques using injection of whole animals (mice, fish, amphibians) indicates involvement of the skeletal neuromuscular system. Uncontrolled twitching, loss of coordination, and respiratory irregularity are commonly observed upon injection of mice with some of the dinoflagellate and blue-green algal toxins investigated thus far. To study the effects of biotoxins at the cellular level, it is important to measure resting and action potentials from nerve and muscle preparations.

Figure 6 represents the recording system used for measuring intracellular (transmembrane) potentials. Using a micropipette puller (Model MI, Industrial Science Ass., Inc., Ridgewood, N. J.), it is possible to draw out very fine-tipped glass microelectrodes (0.5-μm diameter or less). When prop-

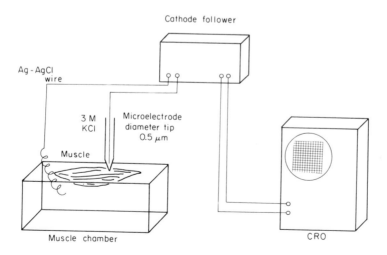

Fig. 6. Apparatus for measuring resting potentials in single muscle fibers.

erly prepared and mounted in a micromanipulator, these are suitable for penetrating single cells (Ling and Gerard, 1949). Electric continuity is achieved by filling the microelectrodes with 3 M KCl and by inserting a fine wire (Ag–AgCl or tungsten) into the wide end. Since it is impossible to observe and therefore to measure the microelectrode tip under a compound microscope, it is necessary to use electric methods to determine its characteristics. The resistance at the tip is directly related to its diameter. A useful microelectrode will have a high tip resistance (10–20 megohms). It is, therefore, necessary to record through a cathode-follower circuit or an electrometer having a very high input resistance (10^{10} ohms or greater). [For a review of glass microelectrodes and their utility in physiological monitoring, see LaVallee *et al.* (1969), Frank and Becker (1964), and Agin and Holtzman (1966).] Glass microcapillary electrodes can also be used to measure transient electric events at the motor end plate region. Spontaneous electric activity called miniature end plate potentials (mepp's) can be recorded from resting nerve–muscle preparations. These low amplitude (< 1 mV) signals occur, on the average, at a frequency of one per second, and are due to the release of acetylcholine (transmitter) at irregular intervals by presynaptic nerve endings. Activity potentials called end plate potentials (epp's) can also be recorded from motor end plates. Each action potential reaching the end plate via the nerve causes a localized postsynaptic depolarization that is ten to twenty times the amplitude of the mepp's described above. The amplitude of end plate potentials can be decreased with the application of curare, which blocks the postsynaptic electric activity leading to muscle contraction. Thus, the electric events in the nerve and end plate can be separated from the mechanical events in the muscle using curare on a motor nerve–muscle preparation. (See also Chapters III and IV.)

Action potentials can also be monitored effectively using the system shown in Fig. 6, provided the source of stimulation is some distance from the microelectrode. In some instances, it is desirable to stimulate the cell internally. This can be accomplished using a second glass microcapillary with a larger tip diameter (resistance ~ 5 megohms) as the stimulating electrode. Electric activity can generally be illustrated more easily from nerve and muscle preparations with external recording electrodes. These are usually sensing (receiving) from a bundle of cells in contact with the electrodes, and record compound action potentials.

Muscles and nerves have membranes that are specialized for the rapid and repeated conduction of electrical activity. In addition, muscles are biological machines that convert the chemical energy derived from metabolic processes into force or tension development. By allowing the muscle to work against a transducer system, the tension developed and work performed under the influence of foreign chemicals can easily be measured. All three muscle types (skeletal, smooth, and cardiac) have been useful in determining the mode of action of biotoxins. The comparative approach has been particularly useful in systems where transmitter substances differ—such as in the different parts of the autonomic nervous system in vertebrates.

It is appropriate that I choose amphibian skeletal muscle to illustrate some of the methodology. There is probably more known about amphibian skeletal muscle than any other type in the animal kingdom. This amphibian preparation provides a reproducible system still widely used in muscle physiology. The sartorius muscle, for example, is composed of long parallel fibers, is thin enough (~ 1 mm) to allow gas exchange when excised, and performs well at low temperatures where transient physicochemical phenomena are slowed (see Fig. 8 A). The frog sartorius muscle has been used extensively as a research tool, particularly by Professor A. V. Hill, his students, and associates. (For a review, see Hill, 1965; Mommaerts et al., 1961; Wilkie, 1968.) Work in our laboratory has demonstrated the potential use of this nerve–muscle system as a research tool, particularly because of its sensitivity to dinoflagellate and blue-green algal poisons.

For definitive experiments it is desirable to maintain a constant temperature, to stimulate all muscle fibers simultaneously, and to use both experimental and control muscles from the same animal at the same time. Figure 7 illustrates a multielectrode system that meets all of the above requirements. An outer Lucite chamber, not shown in the diagram, serves as a temperature control jacket for the electrode assembly. With a refrigeration unit, the temperature can be maintained at $0° \pm 0.1°C$. The inner bathing chamber is divided longitudinally to keep the experimental (toxic) and control solutions separate. It can be raised or lowered quickly by a rack and pinion positioning device. This permits continuous bathing of the muscles between successive stimuli in air. Solution changes and aeration are accomplished from the top of the assembly through fine tubing. Stimulation occurs via multielectrodes of 0.008-inch silver wire, stretched across the Lucite block, 3 mm apart. Other materials, for example, stainless steel, may be used for the electrodes. Alternate wires are connected in parallel to common terminals. This permits simultaneous excitation of the two muscles along their entire length. In addition, it allows the use of both indirect and direct stimulation of the paired sartorius muscles. This is accomplished because of the different excitation characteristics of amphibian nerve and muscle. Indirect stimulation of the nerve endings within the excised muscle is accomplished by a very short pulse width of approxi-

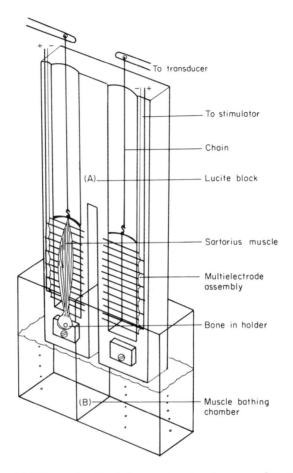

To transducer

To stimulator

Chain

(A)   Lucite block

Sartorius muscle

Multielectrode assembly

Bone in holder

(B)   Muscle bathing chamber

FIG. 7. Multielectrode stimulating system for frog sartorius muscles.

mately 10-μseconds duration. Direct stimulation (via muscle) is accomplished with a 1-msecond pulse width. The muscle cells require a longer pulse width before responding, and thus show different excitation properties when compared with nerve cells. When current pulses of short duration are used, the quantity of current (K) to just excite is constant (current $\times$ time $= K$) for a given preparation. Sartorius muscle fibers require a larger quantity of current than the nerve cells that innervate them. These relationships are expressed in strength–duration curves that are useful in describing excitability characteristics of different tissues (Davson, 1964). The pulse width required to stimulate the nerve endings and not muscle cells can be determined or proved with the use of curare. Figure 10 illustrates the separation of the response to indirect and direct stimulation in the frog sartorius preparation. The nerves conduct action potentials to the end plate; however, the transmitter's (acetylcholine) depolarizing effect via postsynaptic end plate potentials is blocked. Excitation does not reach the muscle via the nerve, although direct stimulation is still effective. In order to measure nerve action potentials, it is necessary to dissect out the nerve attached to the muscle.

There are several transducers available for accurately measuring the tension developed by the muscles. We use Grass FT03C Force-Displacement Transducers and RCA 5734 Mechano-electrical Transducers with the output signals displayed on a cathode ray oscilloscope (CRO) or write out recorder. The rack and pinion system of old microscopes provides an inexpensive means of positioning the transducer above the muscles and allows the adjustment of the muscle length necessary to record maximum tension development.

The recording systems described above permit the determination of the general site of action of toxic materials on peripheral motor systems. With some general modifications, they can be used for measuring activity (electric and mechanical) in hearts and smooth muscles of the intestinal tract.

Studies on the effects of microorganism toxins will serve to illustrate the utility of the methods just described. The cellular or membrane effects of these toxins are not uniformly understood, but the comparative biochemical and physiological approach has demonstrated important similarities and differences in their actions.

4. ELECTROMECHANICAL STUDIES

As mentioned above, it is imperative that definitive studies on the effects of active materials be done with pure samples. This may be difficult to do initially, and several investigators have used crude or partially purified samples for preliminary physiological testing. Dinoflagellate toxins from two gymnodinoid species serve as a good example. T. J. Starr (1958), Sasner (1965), and Sievers (1969) demonstrated the toxicity of unextracted cultures of *Gymnodinium breve* to a wide variety of invertebrate species and fish. Physical destruction of the cells increased the potency of the solutions, as death times in fish were two to four times faster when compared to toxicity in solutions containing whole cells (Sasner, 1965). Injection of sublethal doses from toxic extracts into the dorsal lymph sac of frogs produced a period of hyperexcitability followed by a progressive loss of response to tactile stimulation. Muscle fibrillations were particularly evident in the posterior appendages. Respiration rates increased, slowed, and be-

came very irregular for a period of 30-50 minutes, after which overt signs
of stress gradually disappeared. Frogs given lethal doses were used for
preliminary neuromuscular studies. Within 10 minutes after active respiration ceased, sartorius muscles were tested and found to respond to
direct stimulation only. Sciatic nerve action potentials were of low amplitude and gradually decreased to zero and could not be "driven" to respond
with greater stimulus strength or increased duration. The sartorius muscle still responded to direct stimulation. The sciatic nerves were affected
similarly, whether desheathed or with the protective myelin sheath layers
intact.

Nerve–muscle preparations from untreated amphibians were used to
probe further into the possible mode of action of *G. breve* unpurified (crude)
toxic samples. Figure 8 A shows the range of variability in the isotonic
twitch response of the control sartorius muscles at a low temperature. The
degree of tension development and time course of the contraction and relaxation phases showed little change over a 3-hour control test period.
Figure 8 B illustrates the effect of *G. breve* toxin on the twitch response
evoked by indirect stimulation. There was a rapid and irreversible loss
of mechanical activity after nerve stimulation. Direct stimulation produced
responses long after indirect stimuli became ineffective. The particular
records shown in Fig. 8 were chosen to show differences in the time course
of the mechanical response of sartorius muscles at two temperatures. At
0°C the response takes more than twice as long ($\sim$250 mseconds at 0°C
versus $\sim$600 mseconds at 20°C).

At least three possibilities are suggested by this apparent differential
effect: (a) that the toxin is more specific or harmful to nerve than to muscle tissue; (b) that there are tissue barriers limiting diffusion of the
toxin into the muscle cells; or (c) that the toxin acts at the nerve–muscle
junction. It is interesting to point out, in this regard, that a toxic extract
that was potent enough to abolish the action potential in a bullfrog sciatic nerve (sheathed, $\sim$1 mm in diameter) within 5 minutes took more
than 30 minutes to completely abolish a muscle twitch elicited by direct
stimulation in a sartorius muscle ($\sim$1 mm thick).

The reversibility of the toxic effect was tested on several sartorius muscle preparations. No recovery of the response to indirect stimulation was
ever observed at temperatures of 20°C. However, a significant recovery
of the muscle response to direct stimulation was recorded. In addition,
the response to indirect stimuli always decreased three to four times faster
than to direct stimulation. The directly stimulated muscle decreased its
twitch amplitude in 1 hour to approximately 30% of its control or normal
twitch amplitude, and then was soaked in regular frog Ringer for a period

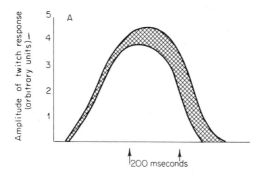

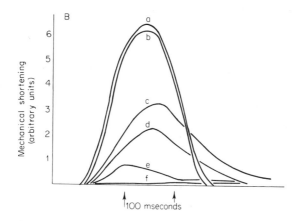

Fig. 8. (A) Response variation in control sartorius muscles. Mechanical records were made over a 3-hour period at 15 minute intervals. Temperature 0°–1°C. (B) Response of sartorius muscles exposed to *Gymnodinium breve* toxin. a, Control response; b, c, d, e, f, after 2, 4, 6, 10, 15 minutes in toxin. Temperature 20°C.

of 4 hours. After this soak-out period, the muscle responded at approximately 75% of its original twitch amplitude.

The conventional way to elucidate synaptic events normally uses electrophysiological measurement of end plate and miniature end plate potentials in skeletal muscle fibers. However, the action of the crude *G. breve* toxin on the end plate, even when completely curarized, caused violent muscle fibrillations making intracellular and/or external end plate recording difficult without mechanical interference. Spontaneous end plate activity increased in frequency from 1–2/second to 9–11/second and in amplitude from 3–6 mV to 4–12 mV within 30 seconds after toxin applicacation. After 2–4 minutes, end plate activity was completely abolished. At this time, the muscle was no longer responsive to indirect stimulation, although contractions via direct stimulation and nerve action potentials appeared unaltered.

Muscle resting potential values decreased from 75 mV to within a few millivolts of zero during a 15- to 40-minute exposure to crude *G. breve* toxin. The transmembrane potential drop coincided with the loss of mechanical activity in sartorius muscles.

Preliminary experiments with crude *G. breve* toxin provided the following information: (a) the primary site of action involves the nervous and muscular systems; (b) the toxin acts on membranes by blocking action potentials; (c) amphibian nerves appear to be more sensitive to the toxin than the muscle cells which they innervate; (d) the mode of action on the membrane is via depolarization.

Our results were compared with those of Abbott and Ballantine (1957) using crude extracts from unialgal cultures of *Gymnodinium veneficum*, a toxic form from the British coast. They reported the harmful effects of *G. veneficum* toxin on more than thirty-five species of invertebrate and vertebrate animals. The gross effects observed in whole organisms implicated the neuromuscular system.

Tests on frog sartorius muscles showed that the mechanical response to both indirect and direct stimulation was rapidly abolished in the presence of *G. veneficum* toxin. The rate of rise (tension development) and the fall in tension (relaxation) became slower and were dependent on the duration of exposure to toxin. Unlike our results with *G. breve*, they found that end plate potentials were evident for a short time after indirect stimuli were no longer effective, but they (epp's) also decreased. When epp's were blocked, the muscle was not reponsive to direct stimulation either; however, the nerves were still capable of conducting action potentials. These effects were apparently reversible. Sciatic nerves gave good action potentials in the presence of toxin for a long period of time. However, crab leg nerves, which are nonmyelinated, were blocked. When the myelin sheath was removed from the frog sciatic nerve, it too was rapidly blocked. Intracellular measurements showed that the toxin caused a fairly rapid loss of the transmembrane potential in the presence of *G. veneficum* toxin. The inability of the toxin to block sheathed nerves was probably because of the large size of the active molecule that could not penetrate the myelin sheath to affect the nerve membrane. The toxin from *G. veneficum* is a general depolarizing agent that perhaps acts on the Na^+ exchange mechanism by allowing equilibration of this ion down concentration and electric gradients.

Thus, the toxins from *G. breve* and *G. veneficum* cause membrane depolarization and thereby block excitability. However, there is good evidence that the active materials from each species are different. *Gymnodinium veneficum* toxin blocked the mechanical response of the sartorius muscle before affecting end plate potentials and nerve action potentials. Only after the myelin sheath was removed did the toxin affect the nerve fibers. The toxin from *G. breve*, on the other hand, was more effective on the nerve and end plate, rather than on the muscle fibers.

McFarren *et al.* (1965) found the presence of two toxins in field and laboratory extracts from *G. breve*. Martin and Chatterjee (1969) also found two active fractions (see also Chapter VI). Apparently one is a slow-acting, ciguateralike substance, while another separate material is a fast-acting neurotoxin. Recently, we have isolated and purified a fast-acting neurotoxin from *G. breve* cultures and a red tide bloom in the Gulf of Mexico (Sasner *et al.*, 1972; Alam, 1972). This toxic component is represented in the flow diagram in Fig. 9 as Fraction IVa.

Electrophysiological studies like those described above show that Fraction IVa from *G. breve* cultures and natural blooms renders nerves and muscles inexcitable to a wide variety of electrical stimuli. The toxin's effect on these tissues was observed to be a function of exposure time, temperature, and toxin concentration (0.5 μg to 0.1 mg IVa per milliliter of frog Ringer). Figure 10 A demonstrates the effect of Fraction IVa on the isometric contraction of frog sartorius nerve–muscle preparations. Immediate fibrillations and spontaneous tension development occurred upon bathing the preparation in toxin–Ringer (10 μg/ml). Both indirect and direct stimulation caused an initial increase in the amplitude of isometric twitches. This enhancement of mechanical activity is characteristic of materials that depolarize either at the synapse (i.e., decamethonium or succinylcholine-like activity) or the muscle cell membrane. Alternate stimulation through the nerve and then the muscle showed a differential effect of the toxin which closely parallels the effects described for the crude toxin. The mechanical response of the muscle to nerve stimulation was rapidly abolished (20 minutes in 10 μg/ml). Direct stimulation, on the other hand, resulted in a more gradual decline in tension development (at least 50% of control amplitude after 30 minutes in 10 μg/ml toxin). Toxin concentrations below 1 μg/ml did not significantly affect the amplitude of sartorius muscle twitches using direct stimulation, although indirect responses were blocked. These results indicate that the sartorius

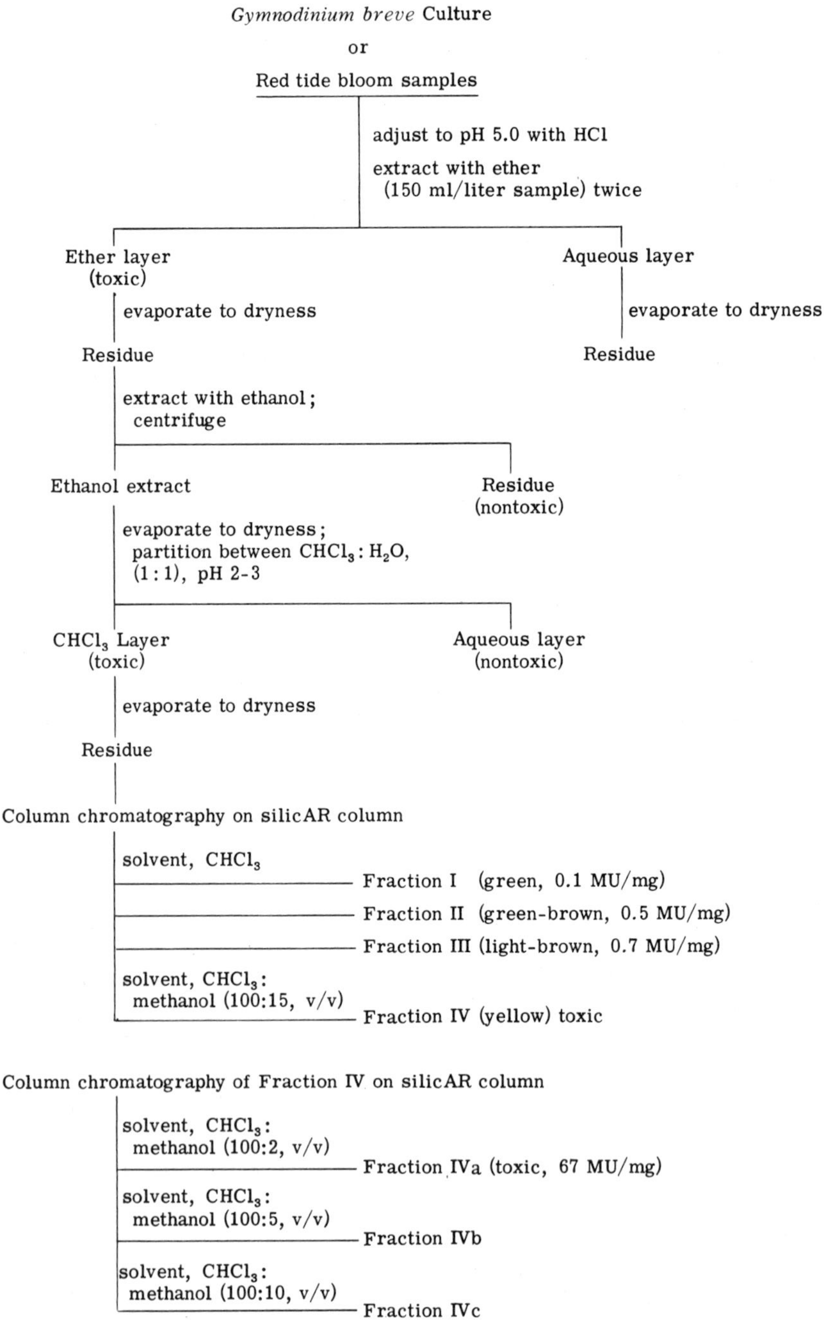

Gymnodinium breve Culture
or
Red tide bloom samples

— adjust to pH 5.0 with HCl
  extract with ether
  (150 ml/liter sample) twice

Ether layer   Aqueous layer
(toxic)

— evaporate to dryness   — evaporate to dryness

Residue   Residue

— extract with ethanol;
  centrifuge

Ethanol extract   Residue
                                                   (nontoxic)

— evaporate to dryness;
  partition between $CHCl_3 : H_2O$,
  (1:1), pH 2-3

$CHCl_3$ Layer   Aqueous layer
(toxic)   (nontoxic)

— evaporate to dryness

Residue

Column chromatography on silicAR column

— solvent, $CHCl_3$

———————————————— Fraction I   (green, 0.1 MU/mg)
———————————————— Fraction II (green-brown, 0.5 MU/mg)
———————————————— Fraction III (light-brown, 0.7 MU/mg)

— solvent, $CHCl_3$:
  methanol (100:15, v/v)
———————————————— Fraction IV (yellow) toxic

Column chromatography of Fraction IV on silicAR column

— solvent, $CHCl_3$:
  methanol (100:2, v/v)
———————————————— Fraction IVa (toxic, 67 MU/mg)

— solvent, $CHCl_3$:
  methanol (100:5, v/v)
———————————————— Fraction IVb

— solvent, $CHCl_3$:
  methanol (100:10, v/v)
———————————————— Fraction IVc

Fig. 9

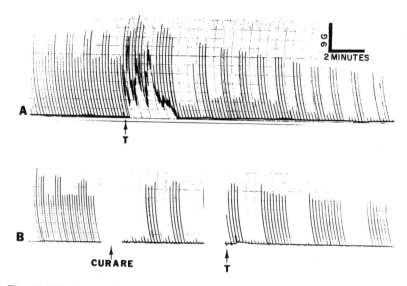

FIG. 10. Effect of *Gymnodinium breve* toxin on isometric twitches of frog nerve–muscle preparation. Stimulation with alternate indirect (0.05-msecond pulse width) and direct (5.0 msecond) single pulses. (A) Muscle treated with toxin (T) only. (B) Muscle pretreated with *d*-tubocurarine chloride (2 μg/ml) before toxin. T, Fraction IVa, 10 μg/ml. Temperature 20°C. (Reprinted with permission of Pergamon Press, 1972.)

nerve and/or the end plate is the primary site of action of Fraction IVa from *G. breve*.

Nerve–muscle preparations that were bathed in curare (2–10 μg *d*-tubocurarine chloride per milliliter of Ringer) before the addition of toxin showed two major differences when compared with uncurarized muscles (Fig. 10 B). Fibrillations were either greatly reduced or completely abolished in muscles pretreated with curare. Electric stimulation (either direct or indirect) did not produce enhanced twitch responses that were characteristic of uncurarized muscles. These experiments suggested that the toxin acted on the end plate, and its effect was blocked by curare. They further suggest that the primary site of action may be at the postsynaptic terminal, and its mode of action may be as a depolarizing agent. However, in choliner-

FIG. 9. Flow diagram for the fractionation of *Gymnodinium breve* toxin. Fraction IVa is a potent neuromuscular toxin. (Adapted from Alam, 1972.)

gic systems, at least four possibilities are compatible with these results:

1. A toxin that acts directly on the presynapse by enhancing the release of additional transmitter (i.e., acetylcholine)
2. A toxin that acts directly on the postsynapse thus potentiating the effect of acetylcholine
3. A toxin that inhibits the normal breakdown of the transmitter (i.e., anticholinesterase) thus causing a temporal potentiation (depolarization) at the postsynapse
4. A toxin that causes a general depolarization of nerve and muscle membranes

One, two, and three above would be inhibited by curare, while four should be unaffected by this synaptic receptor blocking agent.

Transmembrane resting potential values were recorded from frog sartorius muscles after their contraction amplitude was reduced at least 50% by the application of Fraction IVa. Resting potential values did not change significantly upon exposure to toxin (10 μg/ml) for at least 1 hour. A minimum of twenty individual fibers were penetrated and measured from each muscle. Control muscles had a transmembrane resting potential of 81 $\pm$ 8 mV, while toxin-treated muscles measured 77 $\pm$ 8 mV. These results negate the possibility of a general membrane-depolarizing agent and support a more specific, localized site of action of the toxin.

While the response of sartorius muscles to direct stimulation could be reversed by removal of the toxin and bathing in frog Ringer, the response to indirect stimulation was never reversible at the concentrations used in our experiments. In addition, frog sciatic nerves (either sheathed or desheathed) were completely and irreversibly blocked when bathed for 15–20 minutes in *G. breve* Fraction IVa (5 μg/ml).

A comparison of the effects obtained with crude *G. breve* toxin and the purified Fraction IVa indicate many similarities between the two samples. However, the fact that one depolarizes membranes and the other does not may indicate the presence of at least two active substances with different modes of action. Unfortunately, the measurement of mepp's and epp's has not as yet been completed in the presence of Fraction IVa. The results using amphibian skeletal muscle have revealed the potential presence of a multiple toxin system in *G. breve* which is apparently different from the toxin described for *G. veneficum* by Abbott and Ballantine (1957).

The neurotoxin from the phytoflagellate *Prymnesium parvum* is also a potent material. The physiological effects on neuromuscular preparations have been studied by Parnas and Abbott (1965). Injection of the toxin into amphibians and small mammals produced sensory block and motor paralysis. Skeletal muscles, however, were responsive to direct stimulation after intoxication. Using the frog sciatic nerve–sartorius muscle preparation described above, the investigators showed that *P. parvum* toxin blocked muscle tension development from indirect stimulation, while responses to direct stimulation were unaltered. These results suggested that the nerve and/or the motor end plate was the primary site of action of the toxin. Action potential measurements from sciatic nerves were essentially unaffected by the toxin, thereby localizing the end plate as the sensitive part of the system. End plate potentials recorded from curarized muscles were completely blocked. The toxin was synergistic with curare, i.e., it did not cause postsynaptic depolarization. The specific site of action was determined by measuring the sensitivity of the motor end plate to acetylcholine applied iontophoretically by means of a micropipette (Del Castillo and Katz, 1955a). The toxin did not possess any cholinesterase activity that would destroy the acetylcholine before it could exert its depolarizing effect on the motor end plate. Induced epp's (via acetylcholine) were abolished in the presence of *P. parvum* toxin, suggesting that transmitter receptor sites of the postsynapse are blocked, perhaps, by means of a curare-like mechanism in vertebrate motor systems. This nondepolarizing blocking action is also effective on crustacean neuromuscular preparations that are not cholinergic. The toxin from *P. parvum* may be a potential tool for comparative studies on neuromuscular transmission. (See also Chapters VIII and IX for further discussion.)

The active materials derived from axenic cultures of *Gonyaulax catenella*, the hepatopancreas of the mussel *Mytilus californianus* (mussel poison), and the siphon of the Alaskan butter clam *Saxidomus giganteus* (saxitoxin) have received considerable attention. The main focus has been to determine the site and mode of action of the toxin(s) and to establish the relationship, if any, between the active substances from the microorganisms in culture and the tissues of the two bivalve species. The systemic effects of mussel poison and saxitoxin have been known for some time (Murtha, 1960). (For a review, see Kao, 1966; Baslow, 1969.) Cellular and membrane effects have been proved only recently.

The experimental design of Kao and Nishiyama (1965) provides another good model to show how biotoxins are studied at the cellular membrane level. Using mammalian preparations, they found rapid neuromuscular paralysis after injection of mussel or clam toxins. Tetanic nerve stimulation and acetylcholine injections into the artery supplying the test muscle caused a short-lived transient response that might suggest that the end plate was the site of action and that the mode of action was curarelike. This conclusion had been reached by earlier investigators (Fingerman *et al.*, 1953).

End plate potentials recorded with intracellular microelectrodes were briefly reduced and then completely blocked under the influence of clam and mussel poison (see Bolton *et al.*, 1959). In order to record epp's intracellularly, one will remember that pretreatment of the nerve muscle preparation with curare is necessary. Curare reduces the amplitude of the epp to a level where recording is possible without exciting the muscle to contract, thereby breaking the fine glass microelectrode. Since no depolarization of the membrane was observed, the results obtained suggest that the toxins may act synergistically with curare to block end plate activity. The synaptic block was readily reversible. During recovery, nervous stimulation produced irregular responses—some stimuli being effective in causing reduced epp's, other stimuli producing no response. This irregular activity at the end plate suggested possible failure of the presynapse where acetylcholine is released and not of the postsynapse where the transmitter exerts its effect. When the epp's were abolished by the toxin and acetylcholine was applied to the end plate iontophoretically (see Del Castillo and Katz, 1955a,b), depolarization resulted. The fact that the end plate could be activated by adding transmitter from an external source indicated that the release of acetylcholine was involved in the specific site of action of the toxin. Presynaptic activity was checked by monitoring the miniature end plate potentials. These were recorded from uncurarized and resting (nonstimulated) muscle preparations. This spontaneous electrical activity is the result of regular transmitter release from the presynaptic nerve terminal. End plate activity increased and then decreased after the addition of toxin. When epp's and mepp's were recorded from the same end plates, however, the former were blocked, but the latter were still evident. This difference indicated that the axon was the site of action of clam and mussel poison. It also supports the view that epp's are directly linked to electric and ionic changes in the presynaptic nerve cell, although mepp's may not be linked directly to nerve membrane activity.

The action potentials of frog sciatic nerves were blocked by the toxin without alteration of the resting potential. Also, action potential conduction was blocked in sartorius muscles. Current–voltage records obtained with intracellular electrodes showed that depolarizing current would not initiate spikes, and the membranes under the influence of toxin could pass a large outward (sixfold increase) current without causing activity. In simple terms, the membrane, when depolarized, responded in the same way as cells with no external Na^+ in the bathing medium. Since the inrush of Na^+ is responsible for spike initiation (see Fig. 5 B), it appeared that the Na^+ conductance was blocked by the toxin. The K^+ and Cl^- conductances were not affected. Thus, the primary site of action was on the excitable membrane and not on the end plate (synapse), as was previously suggested.

The reversible effects of pure samples of saxitoxin, mussel poison, and *Gonyaulax catenella* toxin on nerve action potentials were reviewed by Evans (1971). Schantz *et al.* (1966) had concluded that the toxins from the three sources are biochemically identical. The physiological studies of Evans (1971) support this conclusion.

D. Pharmacology

Another approach to the study of active chemicals and their effects on living systems falls into the realm of neuropharmacology. This constitutes a broad field of investigation. It includes the synaptic control of all muscle types and the direct effects of chemicals (drugs) on nerve and muscle cells. (For a general review, see Florey, 1966.) The toxicities of naturally occurring substances are useful indicators of biological activity. In addition, their specificity and potency may mimic or selectively block the transmitters that control the normal functioning of effectors. Although many of the toxins are as yet unknown to the synthetic chemist, they provide new opportunities to explore biological function using pharmacological methods.

The action of neurotransmitters is affected by several potent poisons from terrestrial plants. Table II lists some of the most commonly exploited poisons that have been useful in pharmacology. Their specific effects involve changes in transmitter synthesis and release at presynaptic terminals (hemicholine, botulinum) and enzyme inhibition or competition for active sites on postsynaptic membranes (curare, eserine, atropine). Most of the pharmacological information accumulated to date concerns cholinergic systems. These are widespread throughout the vertebrate and invertebrate animal groups (Crescitelli and Geissman, 1962; Florey, 1967).

Cholinergic systems, as indicated above, are sensitive to several toxins from marine and freshwater microorganisms. Mammalian gut preparations have been widely used for bioassay of active chemicals. In addition, the myogenic hearts of amphibians and mollusks and the neurogenic hearts of crustaceans offer sensitive tools for testing. However, the information obtained by the general application of a biotoxin on a transmitter system must be considered nonspecific. The action of normal transmitter substances (for example, acetylcholine in molluscan hearts) has been known for some time. However, as Florey (1967) notes, the effects of such transmitters are described using the mechanical characteristics and rate changes which they provoke in the effector organ. One must use such characteristics with caution when interpreting the specific site of action of

TABLE II

SUMMARY OF POISONS FROM TERRESTRIAL PLANTS

Compound	Plant source	Chemical formula	MW	Physiological action
Curare (*d*-tubo-curarine Cl)	*Chondodendron tomentosum*	$C_{38}H_{44}O_6N_2 \cdot Cl_2$	695.7	Postsynaptic blocking agent in skeletal neuro-muscular systems
Eserine (physotigmine)	African calabar bean *Physostigma venenosum*	$C_{15}H_{21}N_3O_2$	275.3	Anticholinesterase, potentiates ACh activity
Atropine	*Atropa belladonna*	$C_{17}H_{23}NO_3$	289.4	Blocks ACh effects in parasympathetic systems
Muscarine	Mushrooms, *Amanita muscarina*	$C_8H_{19}NO_3$	177.2	ACh mimic in visceral smooth and cardiac muscle, blocked by atropine
Nicotine	Tobacco leaves, *Nicotiana tabacum*	$C_{10}H_{14}N_2$	162.2	ACh-like activity in skeletal muscle, blocked by curare
Caffeine	Tea, coffee, nate leaves, cola nuts	$C_8H_{10}O_2$	194.2	Produces muscle contraction via Ca^{2+} release without membrane depolarization
Picrotoxin (cocculin)	East Indian shrub, *Anamirta coculus*	$C_{30}H_{34}O_{13}$	602.5	Convulsant, resembles strychnine; blocks inhibitory transmitter (GABA) in crustacean nerve-muscle systems
Ouabain	Seeds of South American trees, *Acanthera ouabaio* and *Strophanthus gratus*	$C_{29}H_{44}O_{12}$	584.6	Glycoside, metabolic inhibitor; blocks ion trans-port systems

a particular substance at the level of the cell and membrane, where, of course, the effects take place. This is not to discredit the pharmacological approach; it is only to suggest caution in the interpretation of membrane effects from mechanical data. In fact, the pharmacological approach can be very informative. The activity of a substance from the marine dinoflagellate, *Amphidinium carteri*, serves as a good example. One of the students in my laboratory tested extracts from *A. carteri* cultures on the heart of *Mercenaria mercenaria* (formerly called *Venus*). This is a particularly sensitive preparation for acetylcholine and other choline compounds (Prosser, 1940; Pilgrim, 1954). It responds with a negative inotropic action, and *A. carteri* extracts caused such an effect (Fig. 11 C). Since the sensitivity

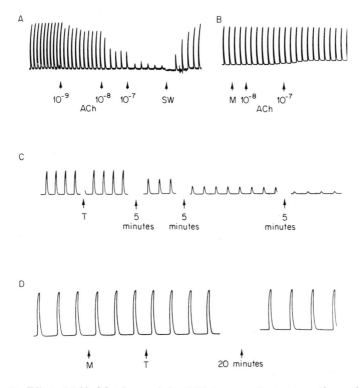

Fig. 11. Effect of ACh, Mytolon, and *Amphidinium carteri* extracts on the mechanical activity of bivalve hearts. (A) Mechanical activity of isolated *Mercenaria mercenaria* heart. SW, Seawater wash. Temperature 20°C. (B) Same as (A): M, Mytolon chloride (0.1 mg/ml). (C) Same as (A): T, *A. carteri* extract (100 mg/ml). (D) Same as (A): heart pretreated with mytolon followed by *A. carteri* extract as in (C). (Adapted from Thurberg, 1972.)

of the *Mercenaria* heart to choline compounds is, in part, determined by temperature and other factors, it was necessary to check the response of the bivalve hearts to acetylcholine. Figure 11 A shows the effect of increasing concentrations of acetylcholine on the hearts used in our laboratory (see Thurberg, 1972). This inhibitory reaction is not blocked by atropine as in vertebrate hearts; instead, Mytolon (benzoquinonium chloride) is the effective blocking agent for choline inhibition in molluscan hearts (Fig. 11 B). Heart preparations pretreated with Mytolon were protected from the inhibitory effects of *A. carteri* cell extracts (Fig. 11 D). The extraction and purification of a choline compound from this dinoflagellate is included in Chapter VII of this treatise.

We have recently suggested an anticholinesterase-like activity for one

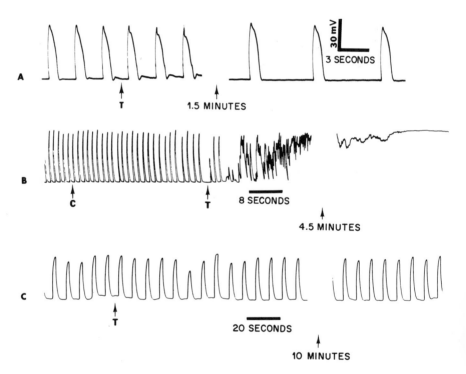

Fig. 12. Effect of *Gymnodinium breve* toxin on amphibian, crustacean, and bivalve heart activity. (A) Frog ventricular action potentials. Fraction IVa (T) added (0.5 µg/g body weight) via ventral abdominal vein. Temperature 20°C. (B) Mechanical activity of *Cancer* heart *in vivo*, Fraction IVa (5 µg/0.1 ml). Temperature 14°C. (C) Mechanical activity of *M. mercenaria* heart *in vivo*. Fraction IVa (100 µg/0.1 ml) injected into ventricle (T). Temperature 14°C. (Adapted from Thurberg, 1972.)

of the active substances (Fraction IVa, above) from the dinoflagellate, *Gymnodinium breve* (Sasner *et al.*, 1972). Figure 12 A demonstrates the effect of the toxin ὁn the action potential of the frog heart. With a "hanging microelectrode" (N. W. Woodbury and Brady, 1956), it is possible to monitor heart rate as well as changes in the characteristic vertebrate cardiac action potential (J. W. Woodbury *et al.*, 1966) under the influence of test substances. This is possible because the heart muscle acts as a functional syncytium. It contains tight electric junctions with no synaptic gaps or chemical transmitter mechanisms between contiguous cardiac muscle cells. Injection of toxin (0.5 μg/g body weight) via the ventral abdominal vein slowed the heart rate, although no significant alteration of the characteristic action potential plateau was observed. After injection of the toxin, the body musculature underwent violent fibrillations. Higher doses (2.5–5 μg/g body weight) caused a cessation of mechanical activity in diastole, with some apparent membrane depolarization. When similar amounts of *G. breve* toxin were injected into frog hearts previously atropinized (1 μg atropine sulfate per gram body weight), no effect was observed on either the action potential or frequency of heartbeat. Thus, Fraction IVa from *G. breve* appears to act in a synergistic manner with curare in peripheral motor systems (described previously), and is antagonized by atropine in vertebrate cardiac systems.

Mechanical recordings from crustacean and molluscan hearts treated with Fraction IVa indicate a differential effect on these two tissues. Toxin (5 μg in 0.1 ml seawater) topically applied to neurogenic crab hearts (*Cancer irroratus, Carcinus maenus*) *in vivo* caused an increase in frequency and prolonged irregular tension development (Fig. 12 B). Myogenic molluscan hearts (*Mercenaria mercenaria*) showed no alteration of mechanical activity even when increased dosages (twentyfold increase) were injected directly into the ventricle (Fig. 12 C). The toxin when applied to the crab heart caused an immediate increase in frequency of beat and irregular tension development before systolic arrest. It is difficult to explain this effect on the basis of an anticholinesterase-like activity for the toxin. Although the crustacean heart is extremely sensitive to acetylcholine, this substance is not considered to be the natural transmitter (Florey, 1967 and earlier). In addition, the increased activity (rate and tension development) is blocked by pyridine-2-aldoxime methiodide, i.e., 2-PAM (Thurberg, 1972). Many organophosphate insecticides and nerve gases also possess anticholinesterase activity, and their effects are similarly reversed in the presence of 2-PAM (Holmstedt, 1959). The restoration of cholinesterase activity is possible only when a potentially reversible complex between enzyme and inhibitor exists. Pre- and posttreatment of amphibian skeletal muscle preparations with 2-PAM did not alter the effect of *G. breve* toxin. The differential effects of dinoflagellate toxins is by no means clear, particularly with respect to neurogenic hearts. The active substances, however, show specificity and are effective in small quantities. When more comparative work is done, they may prove to be useful tools in elucidating natural transmitter systems and membrane effects in a wide variety of effector systems.

Tetrodotoxin and saxitoxin slow the crab heart before diastolic arrest, but have no effect on the bivalve heart in similar concentrations (4 μg/ml). The specific effects associated with these biotoxins are due to blockage of the conductance pathway for Na^+ ions. Similarly, bivalve hearts are unaffected by the toxin from *G. breve*, although we do not know if similar mechanisms are involved. The apparent immunity of bivalve hearts to these active materials has not been explained. However, it may be associated with the ability of clams to act as biological storage depots for toxin(s) accumulation related to paralytic shellfish poisoning in humans. Kao (1966) suggests that different ionic mechanisms may be responsible for the excitable properties in unaffected mollusks. Thurberg (1972) has reported that *Mercenaria* hearts did not beat normally when Na^+ was replaced in the bathing medium. This apparent immunity of bivalve tissues to paralytic shellfish poison and *G. breve* toxin should be investigated further.

While there have been relatively few definitive studies on dinoflagellate toxins, there is even less known about the active materials from the blue-green algae. The toxins from *Anacytis cyanea* (formerly *Microcystis aeruginosa*) and *Aphanizomenon flos aquae* are both potent materials that alter the excitable properties of nerve–muscle systems. *Aphanizomenon flos aquae* toxin blocks tension development in amphibian skeletal muscle, stimulated either directly or indirectly. The blockage of action potentials occurs without alteration of the transmembrane potential (Sawyer *et al.*, 1968). Jackim and Gentile (1968) reported chemical similarities between paralytic shellfish poison and *A. flos aquae* toxin. Preliminary studies in our laboratory suggest mechanisms of action similar to that of saxitoxin and tetrodotoxin. However, voltage clamp studies must be accomplished to determine if the blockage of Na^+ ion channels is the specific mode of action of this blue-green algal toxin.

Table III summarizes the general types of response produced by a variety of active materials from aquatic microorganisms: (1) the destruction of excitability by membrane depolarization—this is characteristic of the impure culture extracts from *Gymnodinium veneficum* and *G. breve*; (2) the destruction of excitability with no depolarization—this is characteristic

TABLE III

SUMMARY OF TOXIC MICROORGANISM SPECIES

Genus and species	Location	Chemical characteristics	Biological characteristics	Reference
Gymnodinium veneficum	British waters	H_2O and alcohol soluble; ether and $CHCl_3$ insoluble; nondialyzable; high mw	Depolarizes membranes, permeability alteration to Na^+ ions	Abbott and Ballantine (1957)
Gymnodinium breve	Gulf of Mexico	Several toxic fractions; ether and $CHCl_3$ soluble; low MW's 279–694	Depolarizes membranes; RBC hemolysis; anti-AChE-like; ciguatera-like; neurotoxin	Spikes (1971); Sasner et al. (1972); McFarren et al. (1965)
Gonyaulax catenella	Central–north Pacific coasts, US and Canada	H_2O soluble; MW 372; tetrahydropurine	PSP; blocks membrane Na^+ conductance	Kao (1966)
Amphidinium carteri	Atlantic temperate waters	Choline-containing compounds	ACh-like activity	Ikawa and Taylor (Chap. VII)
Prymnesium parvum	Europe and Middle East freshwater, Mediterranean Sea	Several toxic fractions	Neurotoxin; blocks end plate transmission; hemolytic agent	Parnas and Abbott (1965); Shilo (1967)
Aphanizomenon flos aquae	Temperate lakes of US and Canada	Similar but not identical to saxitoxin; H_2O soluble	Neurotoxin; blocks action potentials; no depolarization	Sawyer et al. (1968); Jackim and Gentile (1968)
Anacystis cyanea	Lakes of north US and Canada	Cyclic polypeptide; 10 amino acids; MW 1200; H_2O soluble.	Neurotoxin; fast death factor	Prescott (1968); Palmer (1962)

of *Gonyaulax catenella*, *Gymnodinium breve* (Fraction IVa), *Aphanizomenon flos aquae*, and *Anacystis cyanea* and may involve blockage of specific ion conductance pathways (this type of mechanism has been proved for saxitoxin and tetrodotoxin); (3) the alteration of transmission properties between excitable cells—active substances from *Amphidinium carteri*, *G. breve* (Fraction IVa), and *Prymnesium parvum* affect postsynaptic end plate phenomena in cholinergic systems.

III. Concluding Remarks

In any field of investigation, the tools and techniques available determine the extent to which pertinent questions may be asked as well as the level at which they may be answered. The measurement of electric and ionic characteristics of excitable membrane systems is a relatively new tool to physiologists. Revolutionary changes in the theories concerning the ionic basis of electrogenesis in cells and junctional (synaptic) transmission between cells were made during the last 20 years. Katz (1966) presents an excellent review of this productive era in neuromuscular physiology. As demonstrated above, toxicologists have made use of this information to study the specific sites and modes of action of several aquatic poisons. The specificity of active materials and the sensitivity of excitable membranes to them must be established before toxins can be useful as physiological tools. Tetrodotoxin and perhaps saxitoxin are among the few marine poisons that have been studied to this extent. Only a limited number of definitive studies have been accomplished to date because they require purification and chemical identification of the toxic material. Since toxic blooms or red tides have occurred only sporadically in nature, are short lived, and may contain substances from a variety of sources, laboratory cultivation is usually necessary. Thus, the investigator's interests must include either microorganism cultivation or collaboration with other workers to obtain toxic material, as well as interests in membrane physiology—an apparently rare combination.

From the approach of the comparative physiologist, biotoxins may prove useful in the determination of similarities and differences in electrogenic and transmitter mechanisms in a wide variety of organism systems. Tetrodotoxin, for example, has already been widely used in blocking Na^+ conductance across nerve and muscle membranes. The effect of this toxin is more specific than procaine and other anesthetics which, in addition to Na^+, also affect K^+ conductance. It will be interesting to see if the dinoflagellate toxins that cause general membrane depolarization (e. g., *Gymnodinium*) produce their effects by altering membrane permeability and/or by inactivating the ionic pump active transport mechanism. If the latter is the case, the depolarizing toxins may act as metabolic poisons. However, if the former can be proved, the depolarizing effects may be antagonized by tetrodotoxin, saxitoxin, or their analogs which block ionic channels.

There are also many questions to be asked and answered regarding Ca^{2+} dependent membrane systems in invertebrate organisms, in cardiac tissues, in end plate phenomena, and in skeletal and smooth muscle. Of equal interest is the apparent immunity of some living systems to potent biotoxins that are extremely damaging to others. Tetrodotoxin in the puffer fish, ciguateralike toxins in fish and mollusks, saxitoxin and other dinoflagellate poisons which do not apparently affect their primary consumers are harmful to organisms higher in the food chain. The chemical and physiological relationships of tetrodotoxin, tarichatoxin, saxitoxin, and active materials from blue-green algae should be clarified. All of these are apparently chemically different, but they produce similar effects by blocking ion conductance in membranes.

Although the potency of low molecular weight poisons from terrestrial plants has been realized for centuries, only their general mode of action was understood until recently when a physicochemical basis for excitability was established. Now we are adding a variety of new low molecular weight materials to the chemical cabinet which appear to be both potent and specific for inhibiting or exciting natural systems. It is clear that flagellate and blue-green algal toxins affect ionic mechanisms of electrogenesis associated with the membrane and the transmitter system exerting chemical control between contiguous cells. Although compounds from marine sources still have to prove their biomedical value, they offer interesting molecules for the chemist and pharmacologist as well as the membrane physiologist.

ACKNOWLEDGMENTS

Part of the work on which this article is based was supported by Research Grant FD-00138 from the United States Public Health Service, also by a grant from the Office of Water Resources Research, United States Department of the Interior as authorized under the Water Resources Research Act of 1964, Public Law 88-379. I gratefully acknowledge the assistance of Mrs. Sheri Clark in the preparation of this manuscript.

REFERENCES

Aaronson, S., DeAngelis, B., Frank, O., and Baker, H. (1971). Secretion of vitamins and amino acids into the environment by *Ochromonas danica. J. Phycol.* **7,** 215–218.

Abbott, B. C., and Ballantine, D. (1957). The toxin from *Gymnodinium veneficum* Ballantine. *J. Mar. Biol. Ass. U.K.* **36**, 169–189.

Agin, D., and Holtzman, D. (1966). Glass microelectrodes: The origin and elimination of tip potentials. *Nature (London)* **211**, 1194–1195.

Alam, M. (1972). "Algal Toxins." Ph.D. Thesis, University of New Hampshire, Durham.

Baker, H., Frank, O., Matovitch, V. B., Pasher, I., Aaronson, S., Hutner, S. H., and Lobotka, H. (1962). A new assay method for biotin in blood, serum, urine, and tissues. *Anal. Biochem.* **3**, 31–39.

Ballantine, D., and Abbott, B. C. (1957). Toxic marine flagellates: their occurrence and physiological effects on animals. *J. Gen. Microbiol.* **16**, 274–281.

Banner, A. H. (1967). Marine toxins from the Pacific. I. Advances in the investigations of fish toxins. *In* "Animal Toxins" (F. E. Russell and P. R. Saunders, eds.), pp. 157–165. Pergamon, Oxford.

Baslow, M. H. (1969). "Marine Pharmacology." Williams & Wilkins, Baltimore, Maryland.

Boleyn, J. (1967). A simple pipette control for isolating planktonic algae. *Can. J. Microbiol.* **13**, 1129–1130.

Bolton, B. L., Bergner, A. D., O'Neill, J. J., and Wagley, D. F. (1959). Effect of shellfish poison on end-plate potentials. *Bull. Johns Hopkins Hosp.* **105**, 233–238.

Brongersma-Sanders, M. (1948). The importance of upwelling water to vertebrate paleontology and oil geology. *Verh. Kon. Ned. Akad. Wetensch., Afd. Natuurk., Sect. 2* **45**, No. 4.

Bullock, T. H., and Horridge, G. A. (1965). "Structure and Function in the Nervous Systems of Invertebrates." Vol. I. Freeman, San Francisco, California.

Burke, J. M., Marchisotto, J., McLaughlin, J. J. A., and Provasoli, L. (1960). Analysis of the toxin produced by *Gonyaulax catenella* in axenic culture. *Ann. N.Y. Acad. Sci.* **90**, 837–842.

Burlew, J. S., ed. (1953). "Algal Culture from Laboratory to Pilot Plant," Publ. No. 600. Carnegie Institution of Washington, Washington, D.C.

Collier, A. (1958). Some biochemical aspects of red tides and related oceanographic problems. *Limnol. Oceanogr.* **3**, 33–39.

Connell, C. H., and Cross, J. B. (1950). Mass mortality of fish associated with the protozoan *Gonyaulax* in the Gulf of Mexico. *Science* **112**, 359–363.

Cornman, I. (1947). Retardation of *Arbacia* egg cleavage by dinoflagellate-contaminated seawater (red tide). *Biol. Bull.* **93**, 205.

Crescitelli, F., and Geissman, T. A. (1962). Invertebrate pharmacology: Selected topics. *Annu. Rev. Pharmacol.* **2**, 143–192.

Cummins, J. M., Jones, A. C., and Stevens, A. C. (1971). Occurrence of toxic bivalve molluscs during a *Gymnodinium breve* "red tide." *Trans. Amer. Fish. Soc.* **100**, 112–116.

Davis, C. C. (1948). *Gymnodinium brevis* sp. nov., a cause of discolored water and animal mortality in the Gulf of Mexico. *Bot. Gaz.* **109**, 358–360.

Davson, H. (1964). "A Textbook of General Physiology." Little, Brown, Boston, Massachusetts.

Del Castillo, J., and Katz, B. (1955a). On the localization of acetylcholine receptors. *J. Physiol. (London)* **128**, 157–181.

Del Castillo, J., and Katz, B. (1955b). Local activity at a depolarized nerve–muscle junction. *J. Physiol. (London)* **128**, 396–411.

der Marderosian, A. (1969). Marine pharmaceuticals. *J. Pharm. Sci.* **58**, 1–33.

Droop, M. R. (1954). A note on the isolation of small marine algae and flagellates for pure cultures. *J. Mar. Biol. Ass. U.K.* **33**, 511–514.

Droop, M. R. (1961). Some chemical considerations in the design of synthetic culture media for marine algae. *Bot. Mar.* **2**, 231–246.

Droop, M. R. (1962). Organic micronutrients. *In* "Physiology and Biochemistry of Algae" (R. A. Lewin, ed.), pp. 141–159. Academic Press, New York.

Droop, M. R. (1967). A procedure for routine purification of algal cultures with antibiotics. *Brit. Phycol. Bull.* **3**, 295–297.

Evans, M. H. (1971). A comparison of the biological effects of paralytic shellfish poisons from clam, mussel and dinoflagellate. *Toxicon* **9**, 139–144.

Fingerman, M., Forester, R. H., and Stover, R. H. (1953). Action of shellfish poison on peripheral nerve and muscle. *Proc. Soc. Exp. Biol. Med.* **84**, 643–646.

Florey, E. (1966). "An Introduction to General and Comparative Animal Physiology." Saunders, Philadelphia, Pennsylvania.

Florey, E. (1967). Neurotransmitters and modulators in the animal kingdom. *Fed. Proc. Fed. Amer. Soc. Exp. Biol.* **26**, 1164–1178.

Ford, J. E. (1953). The microbiological assay of vitamin B_{12}. The specificity of the requirement of *Ochromonas malhamensis* for cyanocobalamin. *Brit. J. Nutr.* **7**, 299–306.

Frank, K., and Becker, M. C. (1964). Microelectrodes for recording and stimulation. *Phys. Tech. Biol. Res.* **5**, 22–87.

Gates, J. A., and Wilson, W. B. (1960). The toxicity of *Gonyaulax monilata* Howell to *Mugil cephalus*. *Limnol. Oceanogr.* **5**, 171–174.

Gentile, J. H., and Maloney, T. E. (1969). Toxicity and environmental requirements of a strain of *Aphanizomenon flos-aquae* (L.) Ralfs. *Can. J. Microbiol.* **15**, 165–173.

Gorham, P. R. (1964). Toxic algae. *In* "Algae and Man" (D. F. Jackson, ed.), pp. 307–336. Plenum, New York.

Greeson, P. E. (1969). Lake eutrophication—a natural process. *Water Resour. Res.* **5**, 16–30.

Gruendling, G. K., and Mathieson, A. C. (1969). Phytoplankton populations in relation to trophic levels of lakes in New Hampshire. *U.S. Water Resour. Res. Cent., Res. Rep.* No. 1.

Grundfest, H. (1967). Some comparative biological aspects of membrane permeability control. *Fed. Proc. Fed. Amer. Soc. Exp. Biol.* **26**, 1613–1626.

Guillard, R. R. L., and Wangersky, P. J. (1958). The production of extracellular carbohydrate by some marine flagellates. *Limnol. Oceanogr.* **3**, 449–454.

Guillard, R. R. L., and Ryther, J. H. (1962). Studies on marine planktonic diatoms. I. *Cyclotella nana* Hustedt and *Detonula confervacea* (Cleve) Gran. *Can. J. Microbiol.* **8**, 229–239.

Gunter, G. (1947). Catastrophism in the sea and its paleontological significance with special reference to the Gulf of Mexico. *Amer. J. Sci.* **239**, 825–835.

Hall, R. P. (1965). "Protozoan Nutrition." Blaisdell, New York.

Halstead, B. W. (1965). "Poisonous and Venomous Marine Animals of the World," 3 vols. US Govt. Printing Office, Washington, D.C.

Hayes, H. L., and Austen, T. S. (1951). The distribution of discolored sea water. *Tex. J. Sci.* **3**, 530–541.

Haynes, R. (1971). "Some Ecological Effects of Artificial Circulation on a Small. Eutrophic New Hampshire Lake." Ph.D. Thesis, University of New Hampshire, Durham.

Helfrich, P., and Banner, A. H. (1963). Experimental induction of ciguatera toxicity in fish through diet. *Nature (London)* **197**, 1025–1026.

Hill, A. V. (1965). "Trails and Trials in Physiology." Arnold, London.

Hodgkin, A. L. (1958). Ionic movements and electrical activity in giant nerve fibers. *Proc. Roy. Soc., Ser. B* **148**, 1–37.

Holmstedt, B. (1959). Pharmacology of organo-phosphorous cholinesterase inhibitors. *Pharmacol. Rev.* **11**, 567–688.

Hutner, S. H. (1964). Protozoa as toxicological tools. *J. Protozool.* **11**, 1–6.

Hutner, S. H., Provasoli, L., and Baker, H. (1961). Development of microbiological assays for biochemical, oceanographic, and clinical use. *Microchem. J., Symp. Ser.* **1**, 95–113.

Jackim, E., and Gentile, J. (1968). Toxins of a blue-green alga: Similarity to saxitoxin. *Science* **162**, 915–916.

Kao, C. Y. (1966). Tetrodotoxin, saxitoxin and their significance in the study of excitation phenomena. *Pharmacol. Rev.* **18**, 997–1049.

Kao, C. Y., and Nishiyama, A. (1965). Actions of saxitoxin on peripheral neuromuscular systems. *J. Physiol. (London)* **180**, 50–66.

Katz, B. (1966). "Nerve, Muscle and Synapse." McGraw-Hill, New York.

Kraus, M. D. (1966). Preparation of pure blue-green algae. *Nature (London)* **211**, 310.

Langley, L. L. (1965). "Homeostasis." Van Nostrand-Reinhold, Princeton, New Jersey.

Lasker, R., and Smith, G. W. (1954). Red tide. *U.S. Fish Wildl. Serv., Fish. Bull.* **55**, 173–176.

LaVallee, M., Schanne, O. F., and Hebert, N. C., eds. (1969). "Glass Microelectrodes." Wiley, New York.

Lewin, R. A. (1956). Extracellular polysaccharides of green algae. *Can. J. Microbiol.* **2**, 665–672.

Lewin, R. A. (1959). The isolation of algae. *Rev. Algol.* **3**, 181–197.

Lewin, R. A., ed. (1962). "Physiology and Biochemistry of Algae." Academic Press, New York.

Li, K. M. (1965). Ciguatera fish poison: A cholinesterase inhibitor. *Science* **147**, 1580–1581.

Ling, G., and Gerard, R. W. (1949). The normal membrane potential of frog sartorius fibers. *J. Cell. Comp. Physiol.* **34**, 383–396.

Loeblich, A. R., III. (1966). Aspects of the physiology and biochemistry of the Pyrrhophyta. *Phykos* **5**, 216–255.

Lucas, C. E. (1947). The ecological effects of external metabolites. *Biol. Rev.* **22**, 270.

Lucas, C. E. (1949). External metabolites and ecological adaptation. *Symp. Soc. Exp. Biol.* **111**, 336–356.

Lucas, C. E. (1955). External metabolites in the sea. *Pap. Mar. Biol. Oceanogr.* (Deep-Sea Res.), **3** (Suppl.), 139–148.

McFarren, E. F., Tanabe, H., Silva, F. J., Wilson, W. B., Campbell, J. E., and Lewis, K. H. (1965). The occurrence of a ciguatera-like poison in oysters, clams and *Gymnodinium breve* cultures. *Toxicon* **3**, 111–123.

McLachlan, J. (1964). Some considerations of the growth of marine algae in artificial media. *Can. J. Microbiol.* **10**, 769–782.

McLaughlin, J. J. A., Zahl, P. A., Nowak, A., Marchisotto, J., and Prager, J. (1960) Mass cultivation of some phytoplanktons. *Ann. N.Y. Acad. Sci.* **90**, 856–865.

Martin, D. F., and Chatterjee, A. B. (1969). Isolation and characterization of a toxin from the Florida red tide organism. *Nature (London)* **221**, 59.

Martin, D. F., and Chatterjee, A. B. (1970). Some chemical and physical properties of two toxins from the red tide organism, *Gymnodinium breve*. *U.S. Fish Wildl. Serv., Fish. Bull.* **68**, 433–443.

Meyers, S. P., Baslow, M. H., Bein, S. J., and Marks, C. E. (1959). Studies on *Flavobacterium piscicida* Bein. I. Growth, toxicity and ecological considerations. *J. Bacteriol.* **78**, 225–230.

Miller, L. C., and Tainter, M. L. (1944). Estimation of the ED_{50} and its error by means of logarithmic-probit graph paper. *Proc. Soc. Exp. Biol. Med.* **57**, 261–264.

Mommaerts, W. F. H. M., Brady, A. J., and Abbott, B. C. (1961). Major problems in muscle physiology. *Annu. Rev. Physiol.* **23**, 529–576.

Murtha, E. F. (1960). Pharmacological studies of poisons from shellfish and puffer fish. *Ann. N.Y. Acad. Sci.* **90**, 820–836.

Nastuk, W. L., and Hodgkin, A. L. (1950). The electrical activity of single muscle fibers. *J. Cell. Comp. Physiol.* **35**, 39–73.

Nigrelli, R. F., Stempien, M. F., Jr., Ruggieri, G. D., Liguori, V. R., and Cecil, J. T. (1967). Substances of potential biomedical importance from marine organisms. *Fed. Proc. Fed. Amer. Soc. Exp. Biol.* **26**, 1197–1204.

O'Brien, R. D. (1969). Poisons as tools in studying the nervous system. *Essays Toxicol.* **1**, 1–59.

Palmer, C. M., (1962). Algae in water supplies. *U.S., Publ. Health Serv., Publ.* **657**.

Parnas, I., and Abbott, B. C. (1965). Physiological activity of the ichthyotoxin from *Prymnesium parvum*. *Toxicon* **3**, 133–145.

Paster, Z., and Abbott, B. C. (1970). Gibberellic acid: A growth factor in the unicellular alga *Gymnodinium breve*. *Science* **169**, 600–601.

Pilgrim, R. L. C. (1954). The action of acetylcholine on the heart of lamellibranch molluscs. *J. Physiol. (London)* **125**, 208–214.

Prescott, G. W. (1968). "The Algae: A Review." Houghton, Boston, Massachusetts.

Pringsheim, E. G. (1921). Algenkultur. *In* "Handbuch der biologischen Arbeit methoden" (E. Abderhalden, ed.), Sect. XI, Part 2, p. 377. Urban & Schwarzenberg, Berlin.

Pringsheim, E. G. (1949). "Pure Cultures of Algae." Cambridge Univ. Press, London and New York.

Prosser, C. L. (1940). Acetylcholine and nervous inhibition in the heart of *Venus mercenaria*. *Biol. Bull.* **78**, 92–102.

Provasoli, L. (1958). Growth factors in unicellular marine algae. *In* "Perspectives in Marine Biology" (A. A. Buzzati-Traverso, ed.), pp. 385–403. Univ. of California Press, Berkeley.

Ramamurthy, V. D. (1970). Experimental study relating to red tide. *Mar. Biol.* **5**, 203–204.

Randall, J. E. (1958). A review of ciguatera tropical fish poisoning with a tentative explanation of its cause. *Bull. Mar. Sci. Gulf Carib.* **8**, 236–267.

Ray, S. M., and Wilson, W. B. (1957). The effects of unialgal and bacteria-free cultures of *G. brevis* on fish and notes on related studies with bacteria. *U.S., Fish Wildl. Serv., Spec. Sci. Rep.—Fish.* **211**.

Rayner, M. D., Baslow, M. H., and Kasaki, T. I. (1969). Marine toxins from the Pacific. VI. Ciguatoxin: Not an *in vivo* anticholinesterase. *J. Fish. Res. Bd. Can.* **26**, 2208–2210.

Russell, F. E. (1965). Marine toxins and venomous and poisonous marine animals. *Advan. Mar. Biol.* **3**, 255–384.

Russell, F. E. (1966). To be, or not to be . . . the LD_{50}. *Toxicon* **4**, 81–83.

Ryther, J. H. (1955). Ecology of autotrophic marine dinoflagellates with reference to red water conditions. *In* "Luminescence of Biological Systems," (F. H. Johnson, ed.), pp. 387–414. Amer. Ass. Advance. Sci., Washington, D.C.

Sasner, J. J., Jr. (1965). "A Study of the Effects of a Toxin Produced by the Florida Red Tide Dinoflagellate, *Gymnodinium breve* Davis." Ph.D. Thesis, University of California, Los Angeles.

Sasner, J. J., Jr., Ikawa, M., Thurberg, F., and Alam, M. (1972). Physiological and chemical studies on *Gymnodinium breve* Davis toxin. *Toxicon* 4, 163–172.

Sawyer, P. J., Gentile, J. H., and Sasner, J. J., Jr. (1968). Demonstration of a toxin from *Aphanizomenon flos-aquae.* (L.) Ralfs. *Can. J. Microbiol.* 14, 1199–1204.

Schantz, E. J. (1970). Algal toxins. *In* "Properties and Products of Algae" (J. E. Zajic, ed.), pp. 83–96. Plenum, New York.

Schantz, E. J., Lynch, J. M., Vayvada, G., Matsumoto, K., and Rapoport, H. (1966). The purification and characterization of the poison produced by *Gonyaulax catenella* in axenic culture. *Biochemistry* 5, 1191–1195.

Shilo, M. (1967). Formation and mode of action of algal toxins. *Bacteriol. Rev.* 31, 180–193.

Shilo, M., and Aschner, M. (1953). Factors governing the toxicity of cultures containing the phytoflagellate *Prymnesium parvum* Carter. *J. Gen. Microbiol.* 8, 333–343.

Shilo, M., and Rosenberger, R. F. (1960). Studies on the toxic principles formed by the chrysomonad *Prymnesium parvum* Carter. *Ann. N.Y. Acad. Sci.* 90, 866–876.

Sievers, A. M. (1969). Comparative toxicity of *Gonyaulax monilata* and *Gymnodinium breve* to annelids, crustaceans, molluscs and a fish. *J. Protozool.* 16, 401–404.

Slobodkin, L. B. (1953). A possible initial condition for red tides on the coast of Florida. *J. Mar. Res.* 12, 148–155.

Sommer, H., and Meyer, K. F. (1937). Paralytic shellfish poisoning. *Arch. Pathol.* 24, 560–598.

Spikes, J. J. (1971). "The Extraction, Concentration and Biologic Effects of a Toxic Material from *Gymnodinium breve.*" Ph.D. Thesis, University of Texas, Galveston.

Starr, T., Jones, M. E., and Martinez, D. (1957). The production of vitamin B_{12}-active substances by marine bacteria. *Limnol. Oceanogr.* 2, 114–119.

Starr, T. J. (1958). Notes on a toxin from *Gymnodinium breve. Tex. Rep. Biol. Med.* 16, 500–507.

Sverdrup, H. V., Johnson, M. W., and Fleming, R. H. (1942). "The Oceans." Prentice-Hall, Englewood Cliffs, New Jersey.

Thurberg, F. P. (1972). "The Comparative Effects of Aquatic Biotoxins on Cardiac Systems." Ph.D. Thesis, University of New Hampshire, Durham.

Trevan, J. W. (1927). The error of determination in toxicity. *Proc. Roy. Soc., Ser. B* 101, 483–514.

Trieff, N. M., Spikes, J. J., Ray, S. M., and Nash, J. B. (1971). Isolation and purification of *Gymnodinium breve* toxin. *In* "Toxins of Plant and Animal Origin" (A. de Vries and E. Kochva, eds.). Gordon and Breach, London.

Weil, C. S. (1952). Tables for convenient calculation of median effective dose (LD_{50} or ED_{50}) and instructions in their use. *Biometrics* 8, 249–263.

Wilkie, D. R. (1968). "Muscle." Studies in Biology. No. 11, St. Martins Press, New York.

Wilson, W. B., and Collier, A. (1955). Preliminary notes on the culturing of *Gymnodinium brevis* Davis. *Science* 21, 394–395.

Woodbury, N. W., and Brady, A. J. (1956). Intracellular recording from moving tissues with flexibly mounted ultramicroelectrode. *Science* 123, 100–101.

Woodbury, J. W. (1966). 1. The cell membrane: Ionic and potential gradients and active transport. 2. Action potential: Properties of excitable membranes. *In* "Physiology and Biophysics" (T. C. Ruch and H. D. Patton, eds.), pp. 1–58. Saunders, Philadelphia, Pennsylvania.

Woodbury, J. W., Gordon, A. M., and Conrad, J. T. (1966). Muscle. *In* "Physiology and Biophysics" (T. C. Ruch and H. D. Patton, eds.), pp. 113–152. Saunders, Philadelphia, Pennsylvania.

Zehnder, A. and Gorham, P. R. (1960). Factors influencing the growth of *Microcystis aeruginosa* Kutz. Emend. Elenkin. *Can. J. Microbiol.* **6,** 645–660.

CHAPTER VI

The Effects of Gymnodinium breve Toxin on Estuarine Animals

K. A. STEIDINGER, M. A. BURKLEW, AND R. M. INGLE

I. Introduction

A. Ecological Background Data

Gymnodinium breve, Florida's red tide organism, was described in 1948 by C. C. Davis. Subsequent outbreaks could then be attributed to this unarmored dinoflagellate, yet outbreaks as far back as 1844 are suspect.

The 1916 red tide* along Florida's west coast was described by Taylor (1917) who included mention of an irritant "gas." Woodcock (1948) and Ingle (1954) demonstrated that seawater containing dense populations of *G. breve* when physically disrupted (e.g., heated) caused irritation to eyes and throat, producing tearing and coughing. Irritation was not due to a gas, but rather to toxic particles of lysed *G. breve* cells airborne in sea spray. Therefore, it can be assumed, but not verified, that the 1916 and earlier marine mortalities were caused by *G. breve* blooms in coastal waters.

Since 1844, discolored seawater and marine mortalities (mainly fish) have been reported twenty-four times from 1854 to 1971. The areas affected, as well as the severity, vary, but the general area of potential outbreaks extends from Apalachee Bay to the Florida Keys. Gulf of Mexico waters off of southern Texas and northern Mexico have also experienced red tides (Wilson and Ray, 1956). However, major outbreak areas center around Tampa Bay and Charlotte Harbor, large drowned-river valley estuaries. The most severe red tide outbreaks occurred in 1947–1948 and in 1953, after or during heavy rainfall and land runoff, and did not penetrate upper estuarine waters.

A causal relationship of rainfall and land runoff to red tides was made 20 years ago (Slobodkin, 1953; University of Miami Marine Laboratory, 1954), but recent research has helped clarify the relationship. Laboratory studies by Wilson (1966) showed that in defined media additives—particularly chelated iron—stimulated *G. breve* growth. With this new evidence, researchers turned to field data records, and, knowing that land runoff is rich in humic substances that chelate iron and other trace elements naturally, they were able to propose a method of prediction. The predictability of Florida red tides off the Charlotte Harbor area is based on iron content in the Peace River. If and when it reaches 235,000 pounds over a 3-month period (Ingle and Martin, 1971), a red tide in the coastal waters is forecast. This does not exclude the possibility of red tides occurring during low runoff periods, nor does it imply that iron is a "triggering" factor (Martin *et al.*, 1971).

Growth-promoting substances are obviously involved in stimulating red tide outbreaks; however, other factors such as temperature, salinity, basic nutrient requirements (e.g., nitrogen, phosphorus, vitamins, sulfides), water stability, clarity, and movement, and atmospheric conditions must be within their respective optima. All these factors are particularly significant to the topic under discussion—the effect of *G. breve* toxin on es-

---

* In the context of this paper, red tide refers to streaks of discolored water and associated marine mortality.

tuarine animals. In essence, many estuarine animals, whether they are endemic populations or transitory, are never subjected to *G. breve* (GB) toxin because of a salinity "barrier" (Ray and Aldrich, 1965; Morton and Burklew, 1969). *Gymnodinium breve* blooms are usually limited to waters of 31–37‰ (parts per thousand) salinity (Rounsefell and Nelson, 1964), even though the organism does well under culture conditions between 27 and 37‰ (Aldrich and Wilson, 1960). Salinities below 24‰ were inhibitory. Most Florida west coast estuaries do not have salinities favorable to *G. breve* blooms, and the organism rarely penetrates farther than outer reaches of bays. However, after long periods of drought, red tides have penetrated upper reaches of estuaries (e.g., Old Tampa Bay, summer, 1971). The dinoflagellates thrived under higher than normal salinities, favorable nutrient, water, and weather conditions (e.g., high concentrations of NH_4^+, organic N, and phosphates; tidal action and gentle winds moving and concentrating parcels of *G. breve*; poor flushing rates). Under such conditions, one would expect sessile populations or infauna to be the most susceptible to toxicity. Yet observations showed that motile populations (primarily vertebrates) suffer the worst casualties—particularly sluggish bottom dwellers. If there is a gradual buildup of red tide, the first visible signs are dead catfish, mullet, eels, and horseshoe crabs. Five possible interrelated explanations can be offered as to why these bottom animals are affected first: (1) *G. breve* blooms start on the bottom (possibly from a resident cyst population) in coastal waters and move into bays with tides and winds; (2) *G. breve* populations are more concentrated on the bottom, particularly during the night in shallow waters; (3) the toxin may be associated with lysed *G. breve* cells and particles and is therefore more concentrated in sediments and interfacial water; (4) different species have degrees of susceptibility to varying levels of GB toxin; (5) large active swimmers may be able to detect and successfully avoid heavy *G. breve* concentrations.

Research on site and mode of action confirmed that GB toxin affected the neuromotor systems in a complex manner. Therefore, susceptible animals subjected to lethal concentrations of toxin were initially paralyzed and eventually succumbed from respiratory failure. However, casual observations, as well as laboratory studies (Sievers, 1969), indicated that the nervous systems of many invertebrates (e.g., lamellibranchs, crustaceans, certain annelids) are apparently not affected even when cell densities were 10^6–10^7/liter, yet death was noted. These observations do not contradict one another if death can be attributed to oxygen depletion or physical asphyxiation rather than to toxicity at a neuromuscular locus. Blooms of any nature can deplete oxygen in seawater by the increased respiratory

TABLE I

Species List of Dead Animals Found During Red Tide Outbreaks[a,b]

Vertebrates

Scientific name	Common name
Achirus lineatus (6)	Lined sole
Aluterus schoepfi (5, 6)	Orange filefish
Anchoa mitchelli (5, 6)	Bay anchovy
Archosargus probatocephalus (3, 6)	Sheepshead
Arius felis (3, 4, 5, 6)	Sea catfish
Astroscopus y-graecum (5, 6)	Southern stargazer
Bagre marinus (3, 4, 5, 6)	Gafftopsail catfish
Bairdiella chrysura (5)	Silver perch
Balistes capriscus (4, 5)	Gray triggerfish
Balistes vetula (3, 4)	Queen triggerfish
Bascanichthys teres (6)	Sooty eel
Brevoortia patronus (3, 6)	Gulf menhaden
Calamus sp. (4)	Porgy family
Caranx crysos (3, 4)	Blue runner
Caranx hippos (3, 5, 6)	Crevalle jack
Centropomus undecimalis (3)	Snook
Chaetodipterus faber (3, 5, 6)	Atlantic spadefish
Chilomycterus schoepfi (3, 5)	Striped burrfish
Chlorscombrus chrysurus (3)	Atlantic bumper
Cynoscion arenarius (5, 6)	Sand seatrout
Cynoscion nebulosus (3, 5, 6)	Spotted seatrout
Decapterus punctatus (3, 5)	Round scad
Diodon holocanthus (6)	Balloonfish
Diplectrum formosum (5)	Sand perch
Echeneis naucrates (6)	Sharksucker
Elops saurus (3, 5, 6)	Ladyfish
Epinephelus morio (5)	Red grouper
Epinephelus nigritus (3)	Warsaw grouper
Eucinostomus gula (3)	Silver jenny
Floridichthys carpio (5)	Goldspotted killifish
Fundulus similis (5, 6)	Longnose killifish
?Gymnothorax moringa (3)	Spotted moray
?Gymnothorax vicinus (3)	Purplemouth moray
Haemulon aurolineatum (5)	Tomtate
Haemulon parrai (3)	Sailors choice
Haemulon plumieri (4, 5)	White grunt
Haemulon sciurus (3)	Bluestriped grunt
Harengula pensacolae (3, 4, 5)	Scaled sardine
Hemiramphus sp. (6)	Halfbeak family
Hyporhamphus unifasciatus (3)	Halfbeak
Istiophorus platypterus (5)	Sailfish
Lactophrys trigonus (6)	Trunkfish

TABLE I (Cont.)

Vertebrates

Scientific name	Common name
Lactophrys quadricornis (3, 5)	Scrawled cowfish
Lagodon rhomboides (3, 4, 5, 6)	Pinfish
Leiostomus xanthurus (3, 5)	Spot
Lepisosteus sp. (1)	Gar family
Lutjanus griseus (4)	Gray snapper
Megalops atlantica (3)	Tarpon
Menidia beryllina (5)	Tidewater silverside
Menticirrhus americanus (3, 5)	Southern kingfish
Menticirrhus littoralis (3)	Gulf kingfish
Monocanthus hispidus (3)	Planehead filefish
Mugil cephalus (3, 5, 6)	Striped mullet
Mycteroperca bonaci (3, 6)	Black grouper
Myrophis punctatus (3, 6)	Speckled worm eel
Mystriophis intertinctus (3, 5, 6)	Spotted spoon-nose eel
Ogcocephalus vespertilio (3, 4, 5, 6)	Longnose batfish
Oligoplites saurus (3, 5, 6)	Leatherjacket
Ophichthus gomesi (5, 6)	Shrimp eel
Ophichthus ocellatus (6)	Palespotted eel
Ophidion holbrooki (5, 6)	Bank cusk-eel
Opisthonema oglinum (5)	Atlantic thread herring
Opsanus tau (3, 5)	Oyster toadfish
Orthopristis chrysoptera (4, 5, 6)	Pigfish
Paralichthys albigutta (4, 5)	Gulf flounder
Peprilus alepidotus (4, 6)	Harvestfish
Peprilus burti (3)	Gulf butterfish
Peprilus triacanthus (3, 6)	Butterfish
Pogonias cromis (3, 5)	Black drum
Pomacanthus arcuatus (3)	Gray angelfish
Porichthys porosissimus (6)	Atlantic midshipman
Prionotus scitulus (3, 5)	Leopard searobin
Pristigenys alta (5)	Short bigeye
Sciaenops ocellata (3)	Red drum
Scomberomorus maculatus (3, 4, 6)	Spanish mackerel
Scorpaena sp. (4)	Scorpiofish family
Sphoeroides maculatus (3, 4)	Northern puffer
Sphoeroides nephelus (5, 6)	Southern puffer
Sphoeroides testudineus (3)	Checkered puffer
Sphyraena barracuda (3)	Great barracuda
Strongylura marina (3)	Atlantic needlefish
Strongylura notata (5)	Redfin needlefish
Symphurus plagiusa (3)	Blackcheek tonguefish
Synodus foetens (5, 6)	Inshore lizardfish
Trachinotus carolinus (5, 6)	Florida pompano
————	Porpoise (3)
————	Turtles (3)

TABLE I (Cont.)

SPECIES LIST OF DEAD ANIMALS FOUND DURING RED TIDE OUTBREAKS[a,b]

Aves	
Scientific name	Common name
———	Cormorant[c] (1)
———	Ducks[c] (1)
———	Frigate bird[c] (1)
———	Gulls[c] (1)
———	Terns[c] (1)
———	Vultures[c] (1)

Invertebrates	
Scientific name	Common name
Arbacia sp.[d] (2)	Sea urchin
Balanus sp.[d] (3)	Barnacle
Callinectes sapidus[d] (3)	Blue crab
Crassostrea virginica[d] (3)	American oyster
Donax variables[d] (3)	Coquina
Ircinia sp.[d] (2)	Sponge
Limulus polyphemus (2, 3, 4)	Horseshoe crab
Penaeus sp.[d] (3)	Shrimp

[a] Fish names (both scientific and common) were verified in Bailey (1970).

[b] Numbers in parentheses indicated references: (1) Walker (1884); (2) Taylor (1917); (3) Gunter *et al.* (1948); (4) Springer and Woodburn (1960); (5) Finucane *et al.* (1964); (6) Moe (1964).

[c] Certain animals may be affected via the food chain or by taking in water containing *G. breve*, e.g., birds with salt glands.

[d] Species may suffer mortality not attributable directly to GB toxin, but rather to associated adverse conditions, e.g., oxygen depletion.

activity of the bloom organism itself or by high bacterial activity associated with decomposition of the affected organisms. It is quite conceivable that barnacles, mollusks, polychaetes, corals, sponges, isopods, etc. situated in shallow waters would necessarily die from the resultant anaerobic conditions. Table I lists organisms killed directly or indirectly during red tide outbreaks, and includes both neritic and estuarine animals.

An aspect of research that deserves further attention pertains to ecological effects of red tide outbreaks on migratory species. Many marine animals seek out the protection and productivity of estuaries to breed or develop through their juvenile stages. However, analyses of commercial landings after red tides indicated that commercial fisheries were not affected (Torpey and Ingle, 1966).

In addition to the specificity of GB toxin to certain invertebrates and vertebrates, it appears that different species have different levels of susceptibility. Kills of larger fish and mammals have been reported only during moderate to severe outbreaks (or under pen or aquaria confinement). It is not known whether these animals were more susceptible because of disease, weakened condition, territoriality, confinement, or because of food preference. Certain fish and birds feed selectively on filter-feeding mollusks, polychaetes, or even directly on phytoplankton blooms, and therefore can be affected through the food chain. Birds killed during red tides may have succumbed because they consumed contaminated food or because they were able to drink salt water. Although such birds are capable of excreting salts through glands, during red tides consumption of water containing *G. breve* could prove fatal. Ray and Aldrich (1965) demonstrated that oysters exposed to high *G. breve* concentrations when force-fed to chicks produced toxic symptoms and even death.

Man himself is endangered by red tides indirectly through the food chain—specifically through shellfish. Oysters, clams, coquina, and other filter-feeding bivalves in Florida estuarine waters exposed to *G. breve* blooms or to the toxin threaten man's equilibrium and digestive tranquility if consumed. Fortunately, the effects on humans appear to be mild and temporary. No human deaths have been reported from eating Florida shellfish exposed to red tide blooms.

In contrast, there have been over 220 human fatalities attributed to paralytic shellfish poisoning throughout the world (Halstead, 1965). This particular poisoning is caused by the ingestion of toxic filter-feeding shellfish, e.g., mussels and clams. Occurrences of paralytic shellfish poisoning are directly associated with blooms of various toxic dinoflagellates, particularly *Gonyaulax* species (i.e., *G. catenella, G. acatenella,* and *G. tamarensis*). The chemical and physical properties of paralytic shellfish poison, PSP, the toxin isolated from shellfish tissue, and a toxin isolated from *G. catenella* (saxitoxin) are almost identical. The poisonous condition in shellfish is usually temporary; however, the Alaska butter clam apparently accumulates and stores the toxin over periods of years, and rates of detoxification are slow (Ray, 1971). Unlike GB toxin, PSP or saxitoxin is water soluble, and, when shellfish are cooked or steamed and the liquor discarded, the chances of fatality are reduced.

The exposure to toxic *Gonyaulax*, or the accumulation thereof, is usually not fatal to Pacific mussels, scallops, and queens; however conchs, clams (e.g., *Venus*), and the sea star *Asterias* have suffered mortalities (Ray, 1971).

B. Characterization of Gymnodinium breve Toxin

The breakthrough in studying GB toxin came when Wilson and Collier (1955) developed media suitable for growing *G. breve*. Since then, various media (both defined and enriched seawater) have been developed and used for mass culture. The advantages of one over another concern differences in duration of the lag phase and total population density desired. Ray and Wilson (1957) and Starr (1958), working with different density cultures or cell-free supernates, were the first to publish on effects of GB toxin. They showed that several fish had different susceptibilities and that lysis of *G. breve* cells caused by temperature extremes, pH and salinity changes, filtration, addition of heavy metals, or age of cultures increased toxicity of the media. The greater the cell density or toxic units, the lower was the average death time of the test animal (Starr, 1958); also, the larger a particular test animal, the greater was its resistance. Mouse bioassay experiments using extracted toxins (shellfish or culture) support these general observations (Figs. 1 and 2).

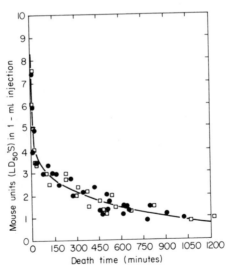

Fig. 1. Relation of dose to death time (IP injection) of mice. ●, Mean of ten mice; □, median of ten mice. (After McFarren *et al.*, 1965.)

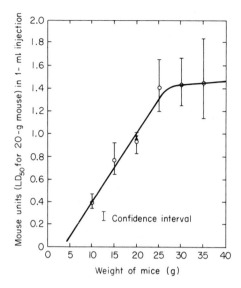

FIG. 2. Relation of mouse weight to LD_{50} dose. O, Males; X, females. (After McFarren *et al.*, 1965.)

Martin and Chatterjee (1969) were the first to publish findings on the chemical characterization and physical properties of the toxin. Later, Martin and Chatterjee (1970) and Cummins and Stevens (1970) published the bulk of their results which is summarized in Table II. Both papers present the isolation of two toxic fractions, and, according to Cummins and Stevens, their "slow acting" fraction corresponds to Martin and Chatterjee's substance II. Unfortunately, these data conflict. The opposing results probably represent differences in extraction procedures and the degree of purification or stability of the preparations. It is also conceivable that pH differences during extraction or the extractants used could have yielded artifacts.

Recently, Spikes (1971), using thin-layer chromatography, and Trieff *et al.* (1971), using dry column chromatography (DCC), were able to isolate one GB toxin. Trieff and co-workers found that the toxic fraction between R_f 0.105 and 0.40 (3.3 LD_{50} mg/kg), when further separated by thin-layer chromatography (TLC), yielded a toxic fraction at R_f 0.50 (7.8 LD_{50}), indicating that the additional purification (TLC) lowered toxicity. They speculated that the TLC solvent system, including 0.5% 6 N NH₄OH, altered potency. Trieff *et al.* (1971) also pointed out that their results for the DCC + TLC isolation agreed well with Martin and Chatterjee's substance II, i.e., similar elemental analyses (C, H, O, and P) and

TABLE II

COMPARATIVE RESULTS OF CHEMICAL AND PHYSICAL CHARACTERIZATION OF *Gymnodinium breve* AND *Gonyaulax catenella* TOXINS

Character	Martin and Chatterjee (1970)		Cummins and Stevens (1970)		Shantz et al. (1966)
	Toxic substance II (major fraction)	Toxic substance I	"Slow-acting" toxic substance (major fraction)	"Fast-acting" toxic substance	*Gonyaulax catenella* toxin
Empirical formula	$C_{90}H_{162}O_{57}P$	—	$C_{102}H_{157}NO_7$	—	$C_{10}H_{17}N_7O_4 \cdot 2\ HCl$
Molecular weight	650 (chloroform solvent)	—	1050 (benzene solvent)	—	372
Solubility	CCl_4–chloroform (pH 4)	Ether–ethanol	CCl_4; ether (pH 3); chloroform (pH 3)	Ether (pH 3); chloroform (pH 3)	Water; lower alcohols
Lability	—	Heat labile; volatile at reduced pressures	—	—	Heat labile; pH labile; alkali labile
Absorption spectra	265–270 mμ (CCl_4 solvent)	—	210–250 mμ (ethanol solvent)	—	None in UV or visible above 220 mμ
State	Solid	Oily solid	Oil (crude); powder (purified)	—	Solid

Melting point	Low melting		140°–155°C		
Color	Light yellow	Light yellow	Yellow (crude); gray (purified)		White
Endotoxin	Yes	Yes			
Optical activity	[α] at 25°C + 546 mμ, 68.2 (varied depending on treatment)	—	—	—	—
Optical rotation	+68 at 546 mμ		—		+128 at 589 mμ
R_f	0.83–0.90 (depending on eluent)	0.63–0.72 (depending on eluent)	0.78–0.83 (depending on eluent)	—	0.26–0.30 (Jaffe reagent)
Characteristic groups	No carbonyl groups; suggested major fragment: OP(OCH=CH₂) (OCH₂=CH₂)	Carbonyl groups	Hydroxyl radical (3430 cm); carbonyl group (1730 cm)	Carboxyl group	Alkyl guanidine group; no carbonyl group
Culture versus field samples	Similar results	Similar results	Similar results	Similar results	—

molecular weight (694 versus 650). However, it still remains to be shown which researchers are working with which toxin and just how many toxins are involved, particularly since Sasner *et al.* (1972) describe a single anticholinesterase-like GB toxin not containing phosphorus and having a low molecular weight of 279.

Ironically, GB toxin (from shellfish and culture) was first equated to ciguatoxin because of its effects on bioassay animals (McFarren *et al.*, 1965). Ciguatoxin, which is prevalent in certain tropical and semitropical fish, depending on geographic distribution and feeding habits, was initially reported to contain phosphorus, but later testing revealed nitrogen (Scheuer *et al.*, 1967). These authors suggested that ciguatoxin was "apparently a lipid containing quaternary nitrogen, hydroxyl and carbonyl functions," and raised the question as to whether it was readily decomposed or actually represented more than one toxic fraction. The latter speculation appears reasonable in the light of recent work showing that the toxin exhibits more than just anticholinesterase activity (Rayner *et al.*, 1968).

In essence, then, the structural configuration of GB toxin(s) is not known, and the empirical formula(s) needs further verification. On the other hand, the toxin of *Gonyaulax catenella* is better characterized, and the complete structure has recently been proposed (Wong *et al.*, 1971). Saxitoxin differs from *Gymnodinium breve* toxins not only physically and chemically, but pharmacologically as well.

C. Toxic Signs

GB toxin, whether injected intraperitoneally, fed, or merely encountered in seawater, produces remarkably similar toxic signs and, as mentioned above, has effects on various systems which are somewhat like those of ciguatoxin. The stepwise visual signs of poisoning can be expressed for mullet, mice, kittens, and humans.

Mullet: (1) violent twisting and corkscrew swimming, (2) further contractions and tail curvature, (3) loss of equilibrium, (4) quiescence, (5) sudden convulsions leading to death (Starr, 1958).

Mice: (1) irritability, (2) inactivity, (3) instability, (4) hindquarter paralysis, (5) labored breathing (dyspnea), (6) general paralysis, (7) prostration which can lead to hyperactivity and death or to recovery (Cummins and Stevens, 1970).

Kittens: (1) unusual playfulness, (2) instability, (3) hindquarter paralysis and head shaking, (4) general paralysis, (5) loss of equilibrium and then recovery within 2 days (McFarren *et al.*, 1965).

Humans: (1) tingling sensations in mouth and digits, (2) ataxia, (3) hot–

cold reversal, (4) slowed pulse, (5) pupil dilation (mydriasis), (6) mild diarrhea followed by recovery within 2 days (McFarren *et al.*, 1965).

The degree of reaction depends, of course, on the quantity of toxin administered, but the actual signs appear to follow the same progression. The lower the dose, the more likely will be the recovery. Although test animals referred to are vertebrates, a few invertebrates have been studied. Sievers (1969) reported the following sequence for *Neanthes succinea*, a marine annelid: decreased movement followed by ragged parapodia, eversion of the proboscis, and finally death. Another polychaete studied by Sievers (*Polydora websteri*) showed no reaction to GB toxin.

D. Mode and Site of Action

As discussed in greater detail in Chapters III and IV, there are four ways in which synaptic junctions can be blocked: (1) competitive inhibition, e.g., curare; (2) nerve conduction block; (3) transmitter release block; (4) uptake block or blockage of another step in resynthesis of transmitter leading to transmitter depletion. In this context, toxins (or chemicals) act as depolarizing desensitizing agents or competitive inhibitors, such as curarelike agents. Depolarizing agents are capable of destroying or lowering membrane potentials and blocking nerve impulse transmission. Depolarizing agents affect the ability of the nerve terminals and/or muscle membranes to generate action potentials. Curarelike agents compete for the same sites that acetylcholine molecules occupy on the muscle side of motor end plates prior to generation of an end plate potential leading to impulse propagation. In the latter instance, inactivation of the enzyme acetylcholinesterase, which hydrolyzes acetylcholine into acetic acid and choline, allows the buildup of acetylcholine until it reaches a level capable of depolarizing the motor end plate. Therefore, anticholinesterase drugs can, at least in theory, be used as antidotes. However, there are no known antidotes for the other type of blockage—synaptic or general depolarizing agents. Washing, breakdown, or excretion are the only means of detoxification, and in many cases irreversible damage has already occurred. *Gymnodinium breve* toxin(s) are thought to belong to the first group, depolarizing agents, and in this sense are similar to *G. veneficum* (Ballantine and Abbott, 1957). Dinoflagellate toxins affect ionic transport and membrane potentials, but saxitoxin (*Gonyaulax* toxin) differs from the *Gymnodinium* toxins by not causing any depolarization in all types of excitable cells so far studied (Kao, 1966). (See also Chapter V.)

GB toxin decreased or eliminated the resting and/or action potential of nerves, muscles, and skin tissue (Figs. 3 and 4), and because of its small molecular size was able to penetrate sheathed nerves as rapidly as un-

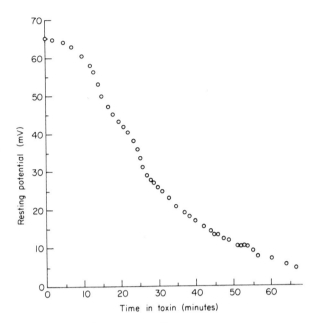

Fig. 3. The effect of *Gymnodinium breve* toxin on the resting potential across frog skin. (After Sasner, 1965.)

sheathed nerves (Sasner, 1965). In addition, GB toxin, even though involved in the alteration of Na^+–K^+ flux, did not inhibit ATPase activity. Perhaps, as in *Gonyaulax* toxin, the effect was on membrane permeability and not on the Na^+–K^+ pump. Sasner's early work on frog tissue pointed out that the site of action was not at synapses exclusively; he demonstrated this by showing the loss in action potentials in sciatic nerve preparations where no synapses occur. The effect of general depolarization was found in all tissues tested: frog skin, frog striated muscle, invertebrate and vertebrate nerves, and *Mytilus* smooth muscle. However, Sasner *et al.* (1972) recently demonstrated that one isolated GB fraction was not a generalized depolarizing agent, but rather synaptic (probably at the end plate). Various tests indicated anticholinesterase activity (see Sasner, Chapter V). Sasner's recent work (e.g., anticholinesterase activity, low molecular weight, no phosphorus) may appear contrary to other research (Cummins and Stevens, 1970; Martin and Chatterjee, 1970; Spikes, 1971; Trieff *et al.*, 1971), but, again, data could indicate that (1) several toxins were involved, (2) extraction, isolation, and purification were critical, or (3) researchers were working with different physiological strains of *Gym-*

nodinium breve. It may even be that endosymbionts, such as bacteria, were responsible for the variety of results found in the literature.

Ciguatoxin also depolarizes muscle membranes, but perhaps to a lesser extent than does GB toxin. It first produces contractions and then inhibits an action potential that should be elicited by artificial stimulation (Cheng *et al.*, 1969). Ciguatoxin does show anticholinesterase activity, but it also produces additional toxic signs, even when the anticholinesterase activity is inhibited. One wonders if there are two or more fractions in ciguatoxin, as is the case with GB toxin. (See also Chapter VII for further discussion.)

When one considers the different animals killed by GB toxin, it becomes apparent that vertebrates are the most affected and invertebrates the least affected. Here lies a key to the possible site of activity and future research.

The statement that invertebrates are the least affected not only needs verification but also clarification. Sasner (1965), the first to report on GB toxin activity, showed that the Pacific mussel, *Mytilus californianus*, was killed by high concentrations of *Gymnodinium breve* (1.5–2 × 10⁶ cells/ liter) and that the site of action was the pedal ganglia. Even though *G. breve* and *Mytilus* would never come in contact in nature (*G. breve* is endemic to the Gulf of Mexico and Caribbean), the observation was significant because it implied that bivalves are adversely affected. Siever's (1969)

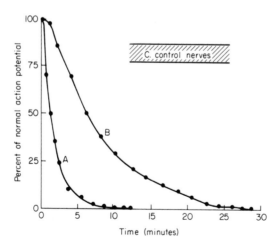

Fig. 4. Effect of toxin on frog sciatic nerve action potentials. (A) Time course of action potential decay in strong toxic solution. (B) Same as (A), but with toxic solution diluted 50% with frog Ringer. (C) Range of variation recorded in control nerves, which were bathed in Ringer containing uninoculated media. (After Sasner, 1965.)

work indicated the opposite—bivalves can accumulate GB toxin, but suffer no mortality. Her studies utilized *Crassostrea virginica*, an oyster common to east coast and Gulf estuarine waters and a major fishery species for Gulf coast states. The question arises, why are two pelecypods affected differently? The answer may reflect different anatomical sites of toxin action, the involvement of ionic mechanisms, or perhaps the existence of alternate metabolic pathways in the detoxication process.

Morphologically and physiologically, nerve fibers and nervous systems of divergent animal groups differ dramatically. The most outstanding differences between invertebrates and vertebrates involve the degree of nervous system centralization. One wonders if this modifies the effect of the toxin. Humans who consume shellfish exposed to GB toxin suffer hot and cold reversals, vertigo, and a slowed pulse—symptoms of CNS poisoning. However, they also experience ataxia, dilated pupils, mild diarrhea, and tingling sensations—symptoms of a peripheral toxicity, i.e., neuromuscular, autonomic, and gastrointestinal distress.

According to Spikes (1971), GB toxin acted on somatic motor nerves or the spinal cord areas. The effects were what could be expected of a depolarizing blocking agent: asynchronous action potentials and muscle fasciculations (contractions) and then blockage to volleys or bursts. Additional toxic signs (cardiovascular) in dogs were increased heartbeat, increased autonomic and ventricular fibrillation, and triphasic blood pressure changes $(\downarrow, \uparrow, \downarrow)$.

Spikes' results indicated that GB toxin affected the myocardium in rats, while Sasner (1965) showed that even after respiratory failure (frogs) the heart was still beating. In conclusion, Spikes thought that death (mice, rats, and frogs) was due to respiratory failure by the following sequence: (1) evoking of action potentials, (2) inhibition of potentials by depolarization of somatic motor nerves, (3) generalized skeletal muscle fasciculation and, finally, respiratory failure.

II. Experimental Procedure

A. Suggested Research

One of the first problems that comes to mind in toxicity studies is methodology. Most researchers work with partially purified, toxic substances that may yield only partial results. Abbott and Ballantine (1957) showed that pH of extraction (*Gymnodinium veneficum*) affected interpretation of mode of action. In addition, only "selected" tissue types have been used, e.g., frogs, lobsters, clams, mice, rats, dogs. Although useful for illustrating basic physiological phenomena, only a few of the animals used would ever come in contact with GB toxin in nature. Because certain animals, particularly fish and several invertebrates (e.g., *Limulus polyphemus*) are apparently more susceptible, it is suggested that researchers turn to test animals such as black drum, catfish, mullet, and particularly the common horseshoe crab. Literature on *Limulus* is extensive, and the experimental suitability of such tissue types no doubt equals squid axons and frog skin. Therefore, it is heartily recommended that the horseshoe crab, because of its apparent susceptibility to GB toxin and because of the ease in handling, be used for future toxicity research.

Unfortunately, there is little information on the effects of GB toxin(s) specifically on estuarine animals. The only deserving species presently receiving attention is the oyster, *Crassostrea virginica*. The Marine Research Laboratory, Florida Department of Natural Resources, has studied *C. virginica* for the last 20 years, primarily as a commercial bivalve, but more recently as a biological indicator organism. Past red tide studies involved monitoring shellfish toxicity and *G. breve* abundance to recommend closing and opening of commercial shellfish beds. Eldred *et al.* (1964) were the first to qualitatively correlate the presence and abundance of *G. breve* with the presence and levels of shellfish toxicity *in situ*.

Our recent work indicates that oysters cleanse themselves fairly rapidly (R. P. Saunders and M. A. Burklew, unpublished) and that commercial beds can be opened 1–2 months after the disappearance of red tide (Morton and Burklew, 1969; Steidinger and Ingle, 1972). Subsequently, a laboratory-oriented program was designed to answer the following questions. (1) How long does it take an oyster to detoxify in a *G. breve*-free environment? (2) Are the concentration of *G. breve* and the length of time that oysters are exposed to this concentration directly related to shellfish toxicity levels? (3) Is the oyster in any way adversely affected by the toxin, e.g., growth, reproduction, mortality? (4) What organ(s) store the toxin? (5) What are the different potential toxicity levels between various bivalve species? With these questions in mind, it is obvious that high quality shellfish, not contaminated by pesticides, heavy metals, or other undesirables, should be used.

To run such experiments it is necessary to culture *G. breve* in mass quantities. Sasner (see Chapter V) gave an introduction to culture principles, techniques, and media which will not be repeated here. However, various recent references give culturing accounts for *G. breve* that can be used to supplement Sasner's presentation (Wilson, 1966; Cummins and Stevens, 1970; Brydon *et al.*, 1971). Once *G. breve* is available, preconditioned healthy oysters can be exposed to a continual supply of GB toxin (i.e., *G. breve* cells in culture media) for various experimental periods. Occasionally, fouling will occur, and experiments must be repeated. In addition it is difficult to design controls for such experiments involving rates of detoxification. Cummins and Stevens (1970) used toxic oysters exposed to saltwater spray as their control, and results indicated this to be an excellent approach.

Toxicity of oyster meat is evaluated using the mouse bioassay technique of McFarren et al. (1965). Sasner (Chapter V) discusses the use and application of LD_{50} and mouse units. The mouse bioassay has been used to quantify and differentiate various marine toxins, but it is important that techniques be standardized so results are comparable and meaningful.

Another facet of GB toxicity that needs clarification is site of absorption or penetration. Do fish take up GB toxin through the gut or through respiratory tissues? Abbott and Ballantine (1957) suggested that *G. veneficum* toxin is taken up through gill surfaces. In addition, organic chemists could determine whether GB toxin(s) is the same, chemically and physically, as the toxic substance extracted from shellfish.

B. Mouse Unit Bioassay Method

1. Clean, shuck, and drain twelve to fifteen oysters to obtain 100–150 g of meat.

2. Homogenize oyster meat in electric blender at high speed for 5 minutes.

3. Transfer 100 g of homogenate to a 400-ml beaker; then add 5 g of NaCl and 1 ml of 6 N HCl (acid coagulates protein to make extraction easier). Stir to mix.

4. Heat mixture to boiling, stirring frequently for 5 minutes.

5. Cool homogenate, and transfer to a 250-ml centrifuge bottle. *All subsequent steps should be done in an explosion-proof hood with good ventilation.*

6. Add 100 ml of diethyl ether to the bottle containing homogenate, and shake vigorously. Use a rubber stopper covered with aluminum foil.

7. Centrifuge at 2000 rpm for 10–12 minutes in an explosion-proof centrifuge.

8. Transfer upper clear liquid portion to a 1000-ml separatory funnel, keeping solids in the centrifuge bottle. Shake the funnel, and drain the emulsion phase back into bottle. Transfer the ether phase to a 400-ml beaker.

9. Add 100 ml of ether to the bottle, centrifuge, and separate again until the process has been repeated a total of four times.

10. Pour the combined ether extracts into a tared 400-ml beaker.

11. Evaporate in a steam bath (or under continuously running hot

water) until all traces (smell) of ether are removed. An oily residue will remain.

12. Dilute the oily residue up to 9.17 g with Wesson oil (1 ml = 0.917 g) for a 1:10 dilution. Mix well.

13. Inject 1 ml of preparation IP into each of three mice (male, Swiss-Webster strain, available from Camm Research, Wayne, N. J.). Mice should weigh 20 ± 1 g; however, mice between 10 and 25 g can be used.

14. If mice die within 110–360 minutes, use Table III to determine mouse units (MU). If mice die prior to 110 minutes, make further dilu-

TABLE III

Initial Mouse Units Corresponding to Death Time and Correction Factors for Different Weight Mice[a]

Death time for 20-g mice (minutes)	Mouse units per ml	Mouse weight correction	
		Weight of mice (g)	Correction factor
8	10.0	10	0.39
10	9.0	11	0.45
12	8.0	12	0.51
14	7.0	13	0.57
16	6.0	14	0.63
18	5.0	15	0.69
20	4.5	16	0.75
30	4.0	17	0.81
38	3.8	18	0.87
45	3.6	19	0.94
60	3.4	20	1.00
83	3.2	21	1.06
105	3.0	22	1.12
140	2.8	23	1.18
180	2.6	24	1.24
234	2.4	25	1.30
300	2.2	26	1.36
360	2.0	27	1.39
435	1.8	28	1.41
540	1.6	29	1.42
645	1.4	30	1.43
780	1.2	—	—
930	1.0	—	—

[a] Values taken directly from McFarren *et al.* (1965).

tions of the remaining extract (e.g., 5:1 or 3:1) until a dilution kills mice between 110 and 360 minutes, then inject three mice IP (1 ml), and consult Table III.

15. Continuous observation for $15\frac{1}{2}$ hours (930 minutes) will give the highest sensitivity possible with this test (10 MU/100 g tissue), while the procedure used here (360 minutes) and recommended by Cummins and Hill (1969) is sensitive only to 20 MU/100 g of tissue, but it is more practical. Mice should be observed (not necessarily continuously) for a 24-hour period.

C. Calculations

To calculate the corrected MU values, consult Table III to determine (1) initial MU for specific death time and (2) a correction factor for actual weight used, since original calculations are based on 20-g mice. Multiply MU (initial) by weight correction factor by 10 (original dilution) by other dilution factors (if attempted). The final corrected MU can be used to find the mean MU (three mice were used). If dealing with greater-than or less-than values, e.g., 930 minutes (death may have occurred while the subject was not under observation), the median rather than the mean MU is reported. All results infer per 100 g. This bioassay procedure, first developed by McFarren *et al.* (1965) and later standardized by Cummins and Hill (1969), is an accepted procedure, and is used by various public health laboratories and research institutions involved in Florida shellfish toxicity.

III. Discussion

The mode of GB toxin activity has been partially established; it depolarizes excitable membranes. But exactly how does it interfere with ionic transport and $Na^+–K^+$ flow? Is it ion specific or membrane specific? Does it interfere with conversion of ADP to ATP? Research in this direction would not only yield valuable information on GB toxicity, but could conceivably reveal new aspects or concepts on membrane phenomena. In addition, Paster and Abbott (1969) and Padilla and Martin (Chapter IX) have isolated a hemolytic substance from GB toxin. This hemolytic fraction may also be useful in studying membrane phenomena and other cellular functions. Another possible avenue for research is comparison of GB toxin(s) to ciguatoxin(s). Present data indicate that the two may have some substances or activity in common. Ciguatoxin(s) possibly has its origin in toxic blue-green algae, e.g., *Schizothrix calcicola* (Banner, 1967). However, one obvious difference between blue-green algae toxin and GB toxin is the effect on fish: GB toxin kills fish, while the other is taken up and accumulated with no ill effects. Perhaps the toxin of the blue-green algae is metabolically altered into another toxic substance(s), becoming ciguatoxin. It is not far afield to correlate blue-green toxins and dinoflagellate toxins, for Jackim and Gentile (1968) recently showed that the toxin of *Aphanizomenon flos aquae*, a freshwater blue-green alga, was similar to PSP (saxitoxin) produced by *Gonyaulax catenella* (see also Chapter VII).

For thousands of years, useful and harmful natural poisons have been used to relieve pain, induce sleep, and even kill wild prey or human beings. Considering the alkaloid derivatives of terrestrial plants, there is much promise for marine toxins. Today, marine biotoxins, once they are chemically and physically characterized, can be synthesized and used as selective therapeutic drugs. GB toxin certainly must have its applications; however, because it affects a variety of systems, it may have limited use. In dilute concentrations, GB toxin might be useful as a pain depressant (analgesic), skeletal muscle relaxant, or as a treatment for certain diseases.

One wonders about the adaptive significance or evolutionary development of toxins. For example, tetrodotoxin does not affect the animal (puffer) from which it is isolated, yet PSP does affect puffer nerves. Does GB toxin serve any function for its producer? *Gymnodinium breve* is a single-celled protist, and it is difficult to rationalize that the toxin is a defensive mechanism. However, *G. breve*, like some other phytoplankton species, could benefit from the poison by inhibiting competitors or by conditioning its environment for more prosperous growth. The question then remains unanswered, but it is a more difficult and rhetorical question than those being asked about site activity and possible pharmacological use.

ACKNOWLEDGMENTS

This is Florida Department of Natural Resources Marine Research Laboratory Contribution No. 180.

REFERENCES

Abbott, B. C., and Ballantine, D. (1957). The toxin from *Gymnodinium veneficum* Ballantine. *J. Mar. Biol. Ass. U.K.* **36**, 169–189.
Aldrich, D. V., and Wilson, W. B. (1960). The effect of salinity on growth of *Gymnodinium breve* Davis. *Biol. Bull.* **119**, 57–64.
Bailey, R. M., ed. (1970). "A List of Common and Scientific Names of Fishes from The United States and Canada," 3rd ed., Spec. Publ. No. 6. Amer. Fish. Soc., Washington, D. C.

Ballantine, D., and Abbott, B. C. (1957). Toxic marine flagellates; their occurrence and physiological effects on animals. *J. Gen. Microbiol.* **16**, 274–281.

Banner, A. H. (1967). Marine toxins from the Pacific. I. Advances in the investigation of fish toxins. *In* "Animal Toxins" (F. E. Russell and P. R. Saunders, eds.), pp. 157–165. Pergamon, Oxford.

Brydon, G. A., Martin, D. F., and Olander, W. K. (1971). Laboratory culturing of the Florida red tide organism, *Gymnodinium breve*. *Environ. Lett.* **1**, 235–244.

Cheng, K. K., Li, K. M., Quinctillis, Y. H., and Ma, C. (1969). The mechanism of respiratory failure in ciguatera poisoning. *J. Pathol.* **97**, 89.

Cummins, J. M., and Hill, W. F., Jr. (1969). Method for the bioassay of *Gymnodinium breve* toxin(s) in shellfish. (After McFarren *et al.*, 1965.) *Gulf Coast Mar. Health Sci. Lab., Spec. Rep.* **69-3**, 1–6.

Cummins, J. M., and Stevens, A. A. (1970). "Investigations on *Gymnodinium breve* Toxins in Shellfish," Pub. Health Serv. Bull. U.S. Dept. of Health, Education and Welfare, Washington, D. C.

Eldred, B., Steidinger, K., and Williams, J. (1964). Preliminary studies of the relation of *Gymnodinium breve* counts to shellfish toxicity. *In* "A Collection of Data in Reference to Red Tide Outbreaks During 1963," pp. 23–52. Fla. Bd. Conserv. Mar. Lab., St. Petersburg, Fla.

Finucane, J. H., Rinckey, G. R., and Saloman, C. H. (1964). Mass mortality of marine animals during the April 1963 red tide outbreak in Tampa Bay, Florida. *In* "A Collection of Data in Reference to Red Tide Outbreaks During 1963," pp. 97–107. Fla. Bd. Conserv. Mar. Lab., St. Petersburg, Fla.

Gunter, G., Williams, R. H., Davis, C. C., and Smith, F. G. (1948). Catastrophic mass mortalities of marine animals and coincident phytoplankton bloom on the west coast of Florida, November 1946 to August 1947. *Ecol. Monogr.* **18**, 309–324.

Halstead, B. (1965). "Poisonous and Venomous Marine Animals of the World," Vol. 1. US Govt. Printing Office, Washington, D. C.

Ingle, R. M. (1954). Irritant gases associated with red tide. *Univ. Miami Mar. Lab., Spec. Serv. Bull.* **9**, 1–4.

Ingle, R. M., and Martin, D. F. (1971). Prediction of the Florida red tide by means of the iron index. *Environ. Lett.* **1**, 69–74.

Jackim, E., and Gentile, J. (1968). Toxins of a blue-green alga: Similarity to saxitoxin. *Science* **162**, 915.

Kao, C. Y. (1966). Tetrodotoxin, saxitoxin and their significance in the study of excitation phenomena. *Pharmacol. Rev.* **18**, 997–1049.

McFarren, E. F., Tanabe, H., Silva, F. J., Wilson, W. B., Campbell, J. E., and Lewis, K. H. (1965). The occurrence of a ciguatera-like poison in oysters, clams and *Gymnodinium breve* cultures. *Toxicon* **3**, 111–123.

Martin, D. F., and Chatterjee, A. B. (1969). Isolation and characterization of a toxin from the Florida red tide organism. *Nature (London)* **221**, 59.

Martin, D. F., and Chatterjee, A. B. (1970). Some chemical and physical properties of two toxins from the red tide organism, *Gymnodinium breve*. *U.S., Fish Wildl. Serv., Fish. Bull.* **68**, 433–443.

Martin, D. F., Doig, M., III, and Pierce, R., Jr. (1971). Distribution of naturally occurring chelators (humic acids) and selected trace metals in some west Florida streams, 1968–1969. *Fla. Dep. Natur. Resour. Mar. Res. Lab., Prof. Pap. Ser.* **12**, 1–52.

Moe, M. A., Jr. (1964). A note on a red tide fish kill in Tampa Bay, Florida during April 1963. *In* "A Collection of Data in Reference to Red Tide Outbreaks During 1963," pp. 122–125. Fla. Bd. Conserv. Mar. Lab., St. Petersburg, Fla.

Morton, R. A., and Burklew, M. A. (1969). Florida shellfish toxicity following blooms of the dinoflagellate *Gymnodinium breve*. *Fla. Dep. Natur. Resour. Mar. Res. Lab.*, *Tech. Ser.* **60**, 1–26.

Paster, Z., and Abbott, B. C. (1969). Hemolysis of rabbit erythrocytes by *Gymnodinium breve* toxin. *Toxicon* **7**, 245.

Ray, S. M., and Aldrich, D. V. (1965). *Gymnodinium breve*: Induction of shellfish poisoning in chicks. *Science* **148**, 1748–1749.

Ray, S. M., and Wilson, W. B. (1957). Effects of unialgal and bacteria-free cultures of *Gymnodinium brevis* on fish. *U.S., Fish Wildl. Serv., Fish. Bull.* **123**, 469–496.

Ray, S. M. (1971). Paralytic shellfish poisoning: A status report. *In* "Current Topics in Comparative Pathobiology" (T. C. Cheng, ed.), Vol. 1, pp. 171–200. Academic Press, New York.

Rayner, M. D., Kosaki, T. I., and Fellmeth, E. L. (1968). Ciguatoxin: More than an anticholinesterase. *Science* **150**, 70–71.

Rounsefell, G., and Nelson, W. (1964). Status of red tide research in 1964. *U.S., Fish Wildl. Serv., Tech. Rep.* **64-1**, 1–192.

Sasner, J. J., Jr. (1965). "A Study of the Effects of a Toxin Produced by the Florida Red Tide Dinoflagellate, *Gymnodinium breve* Davis." Ph.D. Thesis, University of California, Los Angeles.

Sasner, J. J., Jr., Ikawa, M., Thurberg, F., and Alam, M. (1972). Physiological and chemical studies on *Gymnodinium breve* Davis toxin. *Toxicon* **10**, 163–172.

Schantz, E. J., Lynch, J. M., Vayvada, G., Matsumoto, K., and Rapoport, H. (1966). The purification and characterization of the poison produced by *Gonyaulax catenella* in axenic culture. *Biochemistry* **5**, 1191–1195.

Scheuer, P. J., Takahashi, W., Tsutsumi, J., and Yoshida, T. (1967). Ciguatoxin: Isolation and chemical nature. *Science* **155**, 1267–1268.

Sievers, A. (1969). Comparative toxicity of *Gonyaulax monilata* and *Gymnodinium breve* to annelids, crustaceans, molluscs and a fish. *J. Protozool.* **16**, 401–404.

Slobodkin, L. B. (1953). A possible initial condition for red tides on the west coast of Florida. *J. Mar. Res.* **12**, 148–155.

Spikes, J. J. (1971). "The Extraction, Concentration and Biologic Effects of a Toxic Material from *Gymnodinium breve*." Ph.D. Thesis, University of Texas, Galveston.

Springer, V. G., and Woodburn, K. D. (1960). An ecological study of the fishes of the Tampa Bay area. *Fla. Bd. Conserv. Mar. Lab., Prof. Pap. Ser.* **1**, 1–104.

Starr, T. J. (1958). Notes on a toxin from *Gymnodinium breve*. *Tex. Rep. Bio. Med.* **16**, 500–507.

Steidinger, K. A., and Ingle, R. M. (1972). Observations on the 1971 summer red tide in Tampa Bay, Florida. *Environ. Lett.* **3**, 271–278.

Taylor, H. F. (1917). Mortality of fishes on the west coast of Florida. *Rep. U.S. Commer. Fish. Doc.* **848**, 1–24.

Torpey, J., and Ingle, R. M. (1966). The red tide. *Fla. Bd. Conserv. Mar. Lab., Educ. Ser.* **1**, 1–25.

Trieff, N. M., Verkatasubramanian, M. M., and Ray, S. M. (1971). Purification of *Gymnodium breve* toxin–dry column chromatographic technique (in press).

University of Miami Marine Laboratory. (1954). "Red Tide Studies, January to June 1954," No. 54–19 to the Florida State Board of Conservation. University of Miami, Coral Gables, Fla.

Walker, S. T. (1884). Fish mortality in the Gulf of Mexico. *Proc. U.S. Nat. Mus.* **6,** 105–109.

Wilson, W. B. (1966). The suitability of seawater for the survival and growth of *Gymnodinium breve* Davis, and some effects of phosphorus and nitrogen on its growth. *Fla. Bd. Conserv. Mar. Lab., Prof. Pap. Ser.* **7,** 1–42.

Wilson, W. B., and Collier, A. (1955). Preliminary notes on the culturing of *Gymnodinium breve* Davis. *Science* **121,** 394–395.

Wilson, W. B., and Ray, S. M. (1956). The occurrence of *Gymnodinium brevis* in the western Gulf of Mexico. *Ecology* **36,** 388.

Woodcock, A. H. (1948). Note concerning human respiratory irritation associated with high concentrations of plankton and mass mortality of marine organisms. *J. Mar. Res.* **7,** 56–62.

Wong, J. L., Oesterlin, R., Rapoport, H. (1971). The structure of saxitoxin. *J. Amer. Chem. Soc.* **93,** 7344–7345.

CHAPTER VII

Choline and Related Substances in Algae

MIYOSHI IKAWA AND RICHARD F. TAYLOR

I. Introduction

A. Role of Choline in General Cellular Processes

Choline in one form or another occurs widely in fungal, algal (other than blue-green), higher plant, and animal cells. This substance appears to be absent in the blue-green algae (Ikawa *et al.*, 1968), and its occurrence in bacteria seems to be the exception rather than the rule (Ikawa, 1967). Choline is found predominantly in living cells as a constituent of phospholipids and sphingolipids. These lipids include phosphatidylcholine (lecithin) [I], which is one of the most abundant phospholipids in plant and animal cells and is a major component of biological membranes; phosphatidalcholine [II], a plasmalogen that is abundant in the membranes of animal muscle and nerve cells, and sphingomyelin [III], which occurs in especially large amounts in the membranes of animal nerve and brain tissue. Phospholipase A_1, which is present in a number of animal venoms,

$$
\begin{array}{c}
\text{CH}_2\text{OOCR} \\
|\\
\text{R'COOCH} \\
|\quad\quad\text{O} \\
\text{CH}_2\text{OPOCH}_2\text{CH}_2\overset{+}{\text{N}}(\text{CH}_3)_3 \\
|\\
\text{O}^-
\end{array}
\qquad
\begin{array}{c}
\text{CH}_2\text{OCH=CHR} \\
|\\
\text{R'COOCH} \\
|\quad\quad\text{O} \\
\text{CH}_2\text{OPOCH}_2\text{CH}_2\overset{+}{\text{N}}(\text{CH}_3)_3 \\
|\\
\text{O}^-
\end{array}
$$

[I]   [II]

$$
\begin{array}{c}
\text{CH=CH(CH}_2)_{12}\text{CH}_3 \\
|\\
\text{HOCH} \\
|\\
\text{RCONHCH} \\
|\quad\quad\text{O} \\
\text{CH}_2\text{OPOCH}_2\text{CH}_2\overset{+}{\text{N}}(\text{CH}_3)_3 \\
|\\
\text{O}^-
\end{array}
\qquad
\begin{array}{c}
\text{CH}_2\text{OOCR} \\
|\\
\text{HOCH} \\
|\quad\quad\text{O} \\
\text{CH}_2\text{OPOCH}_2\text{CH}_2\overset{+}{\text{N}}(\text{CH}_3)_3 \\
|\\
\text{O}^-
\end{array}
$$

[III]   [IV]

such as snake venom, will cause the partial hydrolysis of phosphatidylcholine [I] to lysophosphatidylcholine (lysolecithin) [IV]. The latter compound is a powerful surface-active agent and causes the hemolysis of red blood cells.

It has been long known that on a low protein diet choline deficiency can cause fatty livers and hemorrhagic kidneys in experimental animals. The reason that choline is essential as a dietary factor became apparent when it was established that choline serves as a source of methyl groups for methionine synthesis and of one carbon (C_1) fragments through the tetrahydrofolic acid (THFA) coenzyme system (see Scheme 1). Methionine is required for the syntheses of S-adenosylmethionine, which is the essential component in a number of biological methylation reactions including

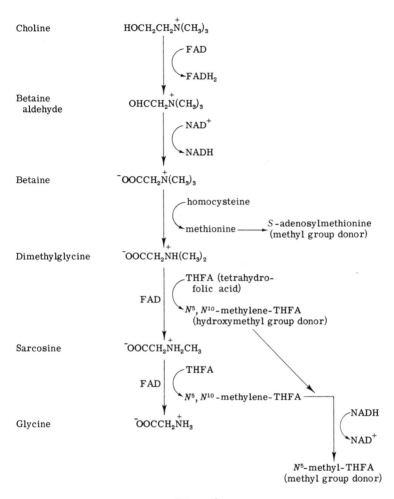

Scheme 1

the synthesis of phosphatidylcholine [I] from phosphatidylethanolamine [V].

Choline O-sulfate (sulfurylcholine, choline sulfate) [VI] occurs widely, having been found in fungi, algae, lichens, and higher plants. Active uptake mechanisms for this compound have been demonstrated in fungi (Bellenger *et al.*, 1968) and in higher plants (Nissen and Benson, 1961, 1964). Choline O-sulfate can also serve as the sole sulfur source for a number of microorganisms. Therefore, the function of this compound in a transport role is suggested.

$$
\begin{array}{ccc}
\begin{array}{l}
\text{CH}_2\text{OOCR} \\
\;\;\;| \\
\text{R}'\text{COOCH} \\
\;\;\;| \quad\;\; \text{O} \\
\;\;\;| \quad\;\; \| \\
\text{CH}_2\text{OPOCH}_2\text{CH}_2\text{NH}_2 \\
\qquad\;\;\; | \\
\qquad\;\;\; \text{O}^-
\end{array}
&
\xrightarrow[\text{methionine}]{3\;\;S\text{-adenosyl-}}
&
\begin{array}{l}
\text{CH}_2\text{OOCR} \\
\;\;\;| \\
\text{R}'\text{COOCH} \\
\;\;\;| \quad\;\; \text{O} \quad\;\;\; + \\
\;\;\;| \quad\;\; \| \\
\text{CH}_2\text{OPOCH}_2\text{CH}_2\overset{+}{\text{N}}(\text{CH}_3)_3 \\
\qquad\;\;\; | \\
\qquad\;\;\; \text{O}^-
\end{array}
\\
[\text{V}] & & [\text{I}]
\end{array}
$$

Although choline O-phosphate (phosphorylcholine) [VII] is a component of phospholipids and sphingolipids, it has also been shown to occur in non-lipoidal form in living organisms. Maizel et al. (1956) found the major phosphate ester in plant saps to be choline O-phosphate, and suggested that the compound may act as a phosphate carrier because of its solubility in organic solvents and its ability to penetrate plant membranes. The choline that has recently been found in the cell wall of a choline-requiring strain of Pneumococcus (Tomasz, 1967) was shown to occur in the pneumococcal C-substance, which was demonstrated to be a choline O-phosphate-containing ribitol teichoic acid (Brundish and Baddiley, 1968).

$$
\begin{array}{ccc}
\begin{array}{l}
\;\;\;\;\text{O} \\
\;\;\;\;\| \\
^-\text{OSOCH}_2\text{CH}_2\overset{+}{\text{N}}(\text{CH}_3)_3 \\
\;\;\;\;\| \\
\;\;\;\;\text{O}
\end{array}
& \qquad &
\begin{array}{l}
\;\;\;\;\text{O} \\
\;\;\;\;\| \\
^-\text{OPOCH}_2\text{CH}_2\overset{+}{\text{N}}(\text{CH}_3)_3 \\
\;\;\;\;| \\
\;\;\;\;\text{O}^-
\end{array}
\\
[\text{VI}] & & [\text{VII}]
\end{array}
$$

B. Special Cellular Roles of Choline and Related Substances

It is in special intercellular and transmembrane processes, which are the basis of neurophysiological phenomena, that choline derivatives and other nitrogenous bases assume an essential role or have very profound effects. Table I lists some of the compounds that affect these processes. It is evident that substances derived from strongly basic compounds such as choline, other quaternary nitrogen compounds, and guanidine are indeed of great importance. Of special interest here are choline esters which show two distinct types of activity at parasympathetic and somatic neuromuscular junctions. These are the normal depolarizing cholinergic activities caused by such compounds as acetylcholine, propionylcholine, butyrylcholine, succinyldicholine, urocanylcholine, senecioylcholine, and acetyl-β-methylcholine (Welsh and Taub, 1948; Bowman et al., 1967; Ariens and Simonis, 1967) and the anticholinergic activity of choline esters with

TABLE I

SITE OR MODE OF ACTION OF TRANSMITTER SUBSTANCES AND OF SOME INHIBITORS
OF THE NERVOUS SYSTEM[a,b]

Site or mode of action	Compound	Chemical nature of compound
Transmitters and mimics		
At neuromuscular junctions of the sympathetic nervous system	Noradrenaline	Primary amine
At neuromuscular junctions of the parasympathetic nervous system	ACh	Choline ester
	Muscarine	Quaternary N base
At neuromuscular junctions of the somatic nervous system	ACh	Choline ester
	Nicotine	Tertiary amine
At ganglionic junctions of the sympathetic and parasympathetic nervous systems	ACh	Choline ester
	Nicotine	Tertiary amine
Inhibitors of axonic transmission		
Specifically block Na$^+$ conductance	Tetrodotoxin	Guanidine derivative, hemilactal
	Saxitoxin	Guanidine derivative, carbamate
	Aphanazomenon toxin	Strong N base
Affect Na$^+$ and K$^+$ fluxes	Cocaine	Tertiary amine, ester
	Procaine	Primary aromatic amine, tertiary amine, ester
	DDT	Chlorinated hydrocarbon
Inhibitors of excitatory neuromuscular synaptic transmission		
Block ACh at receptor sites of somatic nerves; do not depolarize	Tubocurarine	Quaternary N base
Block ACh at receptor sites of somatic nerves; depolarize	Succinyldicholine (at higher levels)	Choline ester
	Decamethionium	Quaternary N base
Block ACh at receptor sites of parasympathetic nerves	Atropine	Tertiary amine, ester
Inhibit ACh synthesis; block choline uptake into synthesizing particles	Hemicholinium compounds	Quaternary N base
Inhibit ACh synthesis by blocking choline acetyltransferase	4-(1-Naphthylvinyl)-pyridine	Tertiary amine
Inhibit release of ACh from biosynthetic vesicles	Botulinum toxin	Protein
Inhibit AChE	Eserine (physostigmine)	Tertiary amine, carbamate
	Organophosphates	
	Neostigmine	Quaternary N base
	Pyridostigmine	Quaternary N base
	Edrophonium	Quaternary N base
	Ambenonium	Quaternary N base
	Gymnodinium breve toxin	Neutral substance

[a] Abbreviations: ACh, acetylcholine; AChE, acetylcholine sterase.
[b] For a more detailed account, see O'Brien (1969).

larger acyl groups, such as benzilcholine [VIII] (Ariens and Simonis, 1967). The naturally occurring choline esters, such as those occurring in ox spleen

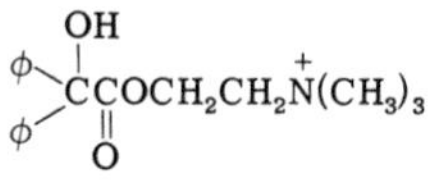

$$\phi\underset{\phi}{\overset{OH}{\underset{|}{\underset{\|}{C}}}}COCH_2CH_2\overset{+}{N}(CH_3)_3$$

[VIII]

(Banister *et al.*, 1953) and in marine organisms (see below), appear to include mainly those with definite cholinergic activity.

C. Occurrence of Choline and Related Substances in Algae and Other Marine Organisms

A number of choline derivatives have been found in various marine organisms. These include pahutoxin [IX] from a Hawaiian boxfish (Boylan and Scheuer, 1967), a glycolipid [X] from a Japanese oyster (Nakazawa, 1959), urocanylcholine (murexine) [XI] from mollusks (Erspamer and Benati, 1953a; Whittaker and Michaelson, 1954), acrylylcholine [XII] from mollusks (Whittaker, 1960), senecioylcholine [XIII] from mollusks (Keyl *et al.*, 1957; Whittaker, 1960) and from the southern oyster drill *Thias floridana* (Whittaker, 1957), and acetylcholine [XIV] from a starfish (Pentreath and Cottrell, 1968) and from *Torpedo* (Bull *et al.*, 1969). Mathias *et al.* (1958) have reported in both sea anemones and the Portuguese man-of-war the presence (in addition to histamine and serotonin) of several unidentified substances that behave pharmacologically and chemically as

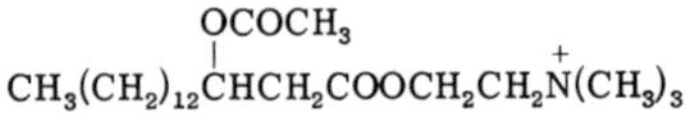

$$\underset{\overset{|}{OCOCH_3}}{CH_3(CH_2)_{12}CHCH_2COOCH_2CH_2\overset{+}{N}(CH_3)_3} \qquad (CH_3)_2CH(CH_2)_3CH=CH(CH_2)_2COOCH_2CH_2\overset{+}{N}(CH_3)_3$$

[IX]   [X]

CH=CHCOOCH$_2$CH$_2\overset{+}{N}$(CH$_3$)$_3$ (on imidazole ring N—N/H)

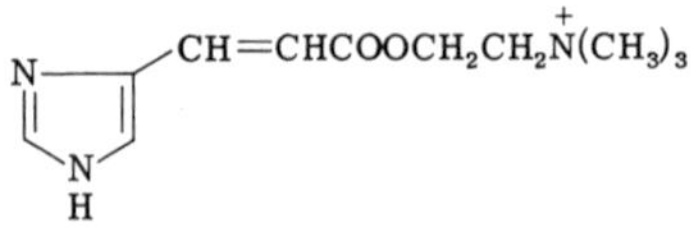

[XI]   CH$_2$=CHCOOCH$_2$CH$_2\overset{+}{N}$(CH$_3$)$_3$

                                         [XII]

$(CH_3)_2C=CHCOOCH_2CH_2\overset{+}{N}(CH_3)_3$ $CH_3COOCH_2CH_2\overset{+}{N}(CH_3)_3$

[XIII]   [XIV]

choline derivatives. Choline itself has been found in the ovaries of the shell-fish *Callistra brevisiphonata* at levels of 0.1–0.5% of their dry weight, and is believed to be responsible for the poisoning resulting from the ingestion of this shellfish (Asano, 1954). The choline is presumed to arise in the shellfish from the action of esterases on choline esters and not from the degradation of phosphatidylcholine.

Choline occurs widely among the algae (Table II). Undoubtedly, part of this choline occurs in the form of the common phospholipid, phospha-

TABLE II

CHOLINE CONTENT OF ALGAE[a]

Division	Order	Alga	Choline chloride (% of dry weight)
Cyanophyta (blue-green)	Nostocales	*Aphanazomenon flos aquae*	0.015
	Nostocales	*Lyngbya* sp.	<0.001
	Nostocales	*Phormidium luridum*	<0.001
	Nostocales	*Plectonema boryanum*	<0.001
Rhodophyta (red)	Bangiales	*Porphyra umbilicales*	0.05
	Cryptomeniales	*Euthora cristata*	0.02
	Gigartinales	*Chondrus crispus*	0.12
	Gigartinales	*Cystoclonium purpureum*	0.03
	Rhodymeniales	*Halosaccion ramentaceum*	0.08
	Ceramiales	*Ceramium rubrum*	0.01
	Ceramiales	*Phycodrys rubens*	0.10
	Ceramiales	*Polysiphonia elongata*	0.02
Pyrrophyta (dinoflagellates)	Gymnodiniales	*Amphidinium carteri*	0.39
Phaeophyta (brown)	Chordariales	*Chordaria flagelliformis*	0.04
	Desmarestiales	*Desmarestia aculeata*	0.04
	Laminariales	*Laminaria agardhii*	0.04
	Laminariales	*Laminaria digitata*	0.07
	Fucales	*Ascophyllum nodosum*	<0.001
	Fucales	*Fucus edentatus*	0.003
	Fucales	*Fucus evanescens*	0.005
	Fucales	*Fucus vesiculosis*	<0.001
	Fucales	*Fucus vesiculosis* var. spiralis	0.004
Euglenophyta	Euglenales	*Euglena gracilis*	0.08
Chlorophyta (green)	Chlorococcales	*Chlorella pyrenoidosa*	0.18
	Ulotrichales	*Ulva lactuca*	0.002

[a] Ikawa *et al.* (1968) and R. F. Taylor and M. Ikawa (unpublished).

tidylcholine. This has been shown to be the case with the green algae
Scenedesmus (Benson and Maruo, 1958) and *Chlorella* (Benson and Strickland, 1960; Nichols *et al.*, 1965; Nichols and Wood, 1968); the bacillario-
phyta (diatoms) *Nitzchia closterium* (*Cylindrotheca fusiformis*), *Nitzschia
angularis*, *Nitzschia thermalis*, *Cyclotella cryptica*, *Phaeodactylum tricornu-
tum*, and *Navicula pelliculosa* (Kates and Volcani, 1966); and the euglenid
Euglena gracilis (Hulanicka *et al.*, 1964). Of interest and perhaps of significance is the absence of choline in the blue-green and brown algae (Fucales)
examined. The absence of choline in the blue-green algae is consistent with
findings that phosphatidylcholine is absent in *Anacystis nidulans*, *Anabaena
cylindrica*, *Anabaena flos aquae*, *Anabaena variabilis*, and *Chlorogloea
fritschii* (Nichols *et al.*, 1965; Nichols and Wood, 1968), and with the fact
that choline-containing lipids do not, as a rule, occur in bacteria (Ikawa,
1967). Bacteria and blue-green algae are fundamentally related in that they
are both prokaryotic organisms, whereas the remainder of the living world
(other algal divisions, fungi, higher plants, and animals) are eukaryotic
organisms.

Aside from the phospholipid-bound choline, not a great deal is known as
yet about the occurrence of other forms of choline in algae. Lindberg
(1955b) showed the presence of choline *O*-sulfate [VI] as well as taurine
[XV], *N*-methyltaurine [XVI], and *N*,*N*-dimethyltaurine [XVII] in the
red alga *Gelidium cartilagineum*, and postulated a biosynthetic pathway
from the methylated taurines through *N*,*N*,*N*-trimethyltaurine [XVIII]
to choline *O*-sulfate. Taurine [XV] and *N*-methyltaurine [XVI] have also
been shown to occur in the red algae *Ptilota pectinata* and *Porphyra um-
bilicalis* (Lindberg, 1955b), and *N*,*N*-dimethyltaurine [XVII] occurs in
the red alga *Furcellaria fastigiata* (Lindberg, 1955a). Some unusual taurine
derivatives have been reported in red algae, such as 2-L-amino-3-hydroxy-
1-propane sulfonic acid [XIX] from *Polysiphonia fastigiata* (Wickberg,

1957) and *N*-(D-2,3-dihydroxy-*n*-propyl)taurine [XX] from *Gigartina
leptorhynchos* (Wickberg, 1956). The zwitterionic forms of these taurine
derivatives may be similar enough in structure to choline *O*-sulfate to act
in a similar or antagonistic fashion to the latter compound.

$$\overset{+}{\underset{|}{\text{NH}_3}}$$
$$\text{HOCH}_2\text{CHCH}_2\text{SO}_3^-$$

[XIX]

$$\overset{\text{OH}}{\underset{|}{}}$$
$$\text{HOCH}_2\text{CHCH}_2\overset{+}{\text{NH}}_2\text{CH}_2\text{CH}_2\text{SO}_3^-$$

[XX]

Evidence in the literature for the occurrence of neurophysiologically active choline compounds in algae is, to date, very scanty. The algae are, however, a source of very toxic substances that do affect neurophysiological systems. Many of these toxins are derived from strong bases other than choline. The most extensively studied of these is saxitoxin, an agent that is responsible for paralytic shellfish poisoning, which is produced by the dinoflagellate *Gonyaulax catenella* (Schantz *et al.*, 1966) and which accumulates in the California mussel and in the Alaska butter clam causing them to become poisonous. The blue-green alga *Aphanazomenon flos aquae*, which has been responsible for toxic blooms during the summers in some of the lakes of New Hampshire, produces a toxin that resembles saxitoxin in its physiological action (Sawyer *et al.*, 1968) and chemical properties (Jackim and Gentile, 1968). Further mention will be made of the toxin of *A. flos aquae* and its highly cationic nature in Section II,E of this chapter. Ciguatoxin is a Dragendorff reagent-positive substance that has been isolated from the moray eel (Scheuer *et al.*, 1967). It is believed to be of algal origin and to be transmitted along the food chain (Randall, 1958). Tetrodotoxin is a highly poisonous guanidine derivative isolated from Japanese puffer fish (see Scheuer, 1964) and the California newt (Mosher *et al.*, 1964). The origin of tetrodotoxin is, however, still uncertain, and views range from its being a normal metabolite, perhaps a hormone, to its origin through the ingestion of the poison or a precursor by the fish from the food chain (since it has been suggested that blue-green algae may be the primary source of the toxin) (Halstead, 1967).

This chapter is concerned primarily with the occurrence of pharmacologically active derivatives of choline and other cationic nitrogenous substances in algae. Considerable attention is given to paper chromatographic methods for the identification and detection of choline and some of its derivatives and for the detection of certain other nitrogen bases. Methods for the estimation of choline are also discussed with some emphasis placed on the microbiological assay for choline using a choline-requiring mutant of *Neurospora crassa*. The high choline content of the dinoflagellate *Amphidinium carteri* (see Table II) has prompted us to investigate the nature of the choline compounds in this organism. Some work is also reported on the strongly basic toxin of the blue-green alga *Aphanazomenon flos aquae*.

II. Experimental Procedures

A. Paper, Thin-Layer, and Column Chromatography of Choline and Related Compounds

1. PAPER CHROMATOGRAPHY

Paper chromatography is perhaps the oldest and still the best method for the identification of choline compounds. Ideally, an unknown choline compound can be identified with this method by its cochromatography with known standards in a number of solvent systems.

There are too many reported solvent systems used in the paper chromatography of choline compounds to mention here in their entirety. Since most of these systems were concerned with a limited type of choline compound, e.g., only esters, only sulfate, etc., a wider range of choline and related compounds were run in most of the solvent systems reported in the literature. The results reported here, however, are limited to those systems that appeared to be the most versatile, i.e., those systems capable of sepa-

TABLE III

Compound	R_f value in system[a,b]									
	1	2	3	4	5	6	7	8	9	10
Choline chloride	0.52	0.60	0.47	0.25	0.30	0.57	0.52	0.17	0.16	0.41
Acetylcholine chloride	0.60	0.63	0.57	0.33	0.37	0.64	0.57	0.25	0.30	0.49
Acetyl-β-methylcholine bromide	0.71	0.74	0.66	0.48	0.47	0.69	0.68	0.54	0.45	0.60
Propionylcholine chloride	0.68	0.70	0.66	0.48	0.48	0.73	0.65	0.38	0.42	0.59
Butyrylcholine chloride	0.75	0.77	0.73	0.57	0.56	0.78	0.72	0.46	0.55	0.67
Succinyldicholine dichloride	0.25	0.54	0.21	0.06	0.15	0.34	0.38	0.04	0.03	0.11
Choline O-phosphate	0.09	0	0.07	0.02	0.17	0.17	0.06	0	0	0.03
Choline O-sulfate	0.14	0.21	0.12	0.06	0.18	0.35	0.36	0.12	0.07	0.07
Ethanolamine	0.47	0.64	0.36	0.40	0.39	0.57	0.71	0.79	0.66	0.39T
N-Methylethanolamine	0.56	0.77	0.45	0.41	0.43	0.62	0.79	0.80	0.86	0.43T
N,N-Dimethylethanol-amine	0.60	0.81	0.48	0.37	0.40	0.64	0.82	0.82	0.84	0.43T

[a] See Table V for solvent systems.

[b] Abbreviations: T, tailing.

rating all the major types of choline derivatives studied as well as the related ethanolamines.

Standard samples (50 mg/ml in 50% ethanol) used include choline chloride; acetyl-, propionyl-, and butyrylcholine chloride; acetyl-β-methylcholine bromide; succinyldicholine dichloride; choline O-phosphate; choline O-sulfate; and ethanolamine, N-methylethanolamine, and N,N-dimethylethanolamine. Whatman No. 1 paper (35 × 20 cm) was used in all cases. The paper was spotted with known and unknown samples, rolled into a cylinder and stapled, placed in a covered cylindrical glass tank at 22°–25°C, and the chromatogram was run ascending until the solvent front was within 1–2 cm of the top of the paper. After drying, the choline compounds and ethanolamines were located first by exposing the paper to iodine vapors, which detected all the standards (with the occasional exception of choline O-sulfate and choline O-phosphate), and then by spraying the paper with Dragendorff's reagent (see below), which detected the choline derivatives as yellow to orange-pink spots.

R_f VALUES OF CHOLINE AND RELATED COMPOUNDS ON PAPER CHROMATOGRAPHY

					R_f value in system[a,b]								
11	12	13	14	15	16	17	18	19	20	21	22	23	24
0.27	0.61	0.74	0.28	0.47	0.48	0.52	0.43	0.40	0.33	0.51	0.48	0.30	0.38
0.47	0.72	0.80	0.32	0.54	0.49	0.55	0.48	0.46	0.41	0.59	0.57	0.37	0.46
0.61	0.77	0.88	0.51	0.67	0.61	0.67	0.61	0.58	0.53	0.68	0.69	0.52	0.57
0.59	0.76	0.87	0.44	0.62	0.58	0.63	0.60	0.56	0.53	0.67	0.67	0.51	0.59
0.69	0.79	0.91	0.51	0.69	0.65	0.69	0.69	0.65	0.60	0.72	0.76	0.62	0.70
0.07	0.60T	0.72	0.10	0.22	0.18	0.26	0.15	0.13	0.07	0.27	0.19	0.05	0.27
0	0.48	0.55	0	0	0	0	0	0.05	0	0.13	0.06	0	0.04
0.12	0.58	0.60	0.20	0.37	0.39	0.41	0.17	0.13	0.05	0.18	0.12	0.03	0.12
0.40	0.30	0.63	0.40	0.63	0.53	0.60	0.50	0.44	0.36	0.45	0.38T	0.52T	0.34
0.43	0.47	0.73	0.59	0.71	0.69	0.73	0.64	0.53	0.41	0.55	0.43T	0.60T	0.39
0.41	0.63	0.79	0.77	0.78	0.85	0.86	0.74	0.52	0.60	0.60	0.48T	0.61T	0.35

The solvent systems that worked best almost always contained an alcohol and an acid as well as water. However, there were systems employing pyridine or ammonium hydroxide which worked equally as well as the acidic systems, contrary to the claims of some workers that bases such as ammonium hydroxide will cause hydrolysis of choline esters in chromatographic systems (Whittaker and Wijesundera, 1952; Augustinsson and Grahn, 1953).

Although Whatman No. 1 paper was used in all cases, it was used not only per se, but also after modification by treatment with potassium chloride. This treatment involved drawing the correctly cut paper through a solution of 1 N KCl and allowing it to dry before use (Bremer and Greenberg, 1959; Bremer *et al.*, 1960). The solvent to be used with the treated paper was also modified by saturation with solid potassium chloride in the chromatography tank for at least 1 hour before the run was made. It was found that the use of this treated paper resulted in less tailing and more compact spots for the applied samples as well as usually lower R_f values than the same system with untreated paper. However, in some cases, the paper was undesirable due to the appearance of two solvent fronts, while in other cases equally good results were obtained in the same system with both treated and untreated paper.

The R_f values of a number of choline derivatives and related substances are reported in Tables III and IV. Table V describes the solvent systems for which the data are reported in Tables III and IV. While Table III reports our work with the standard samples mentioned above, Table IV is a compilation of our results and those of a number of other workers, and includes R_f values of extensive series of choline-related compounds studied by these workers. It is interesting to note that in almost all the systems reported an increase in the chain length of a choline ester by one carbon unit results in an increase of 0.05–0.10 in R_f value (Banister *et al.*, 1953), while isomeric esters such as propionylcholine and acetyl-β-methylcholine have very similar R_f values (Whittaker and Wijesundera, 1952). Succinyldicholine, as expected, runs far behind most of the other choline esters due to its two quaternary nitrogen groups. Choline O-sulfate and choline O-phosphate also have consistently low R_f values due to their highly ionic character. The ethanolamines show a trend of increasing R_f values as they become increasingly methylated.

Although the R_f values reported in Tables III and IV may be used as guidelines for the identification of choline unknowns, it must be borne in mind that these values may differ, within limits, from others reported for the same compounds due to differences in conditions, paper, etc. Rigid standardization of the chromatographic procedure used is the only guar-

TABLE IV

COMPILED R_f VALUES OF CHOLINE AND RELATED COMPOUNDS ON FOUR PAPER
CHROMATOGRAPHIC SYSTEMS

Compound	R_f value in system[a,b]			
	25	26	27	28
Choline chloride	0.37	0.46	0.09	0.15
Acetylcholine chloride	0.46	0.54	0.14	0.21
Acetyl-β-methylcholine bromide	0.54	0.61	0.22	0.30
Propionylcholine chloride	0.57	0.61	0.22	0.31
n-Butyrylcholine chloride	0.66	0.69	0.28	0.40
2-Methylbutyrylcholine bromide	0.73	0.80	0.36	—
n-Valerylcholine bromide	0.69	0.78	0.31	0.55
iso-Valerylcholine chloride	0.78	0.82	0.38	—
n-Caproylcholine bromide	0.68	0.79	0.36	—
Succinyldicholine dichloride	0.22	0.29	0	0.02
Benzoylcholine chloride	0.71	0.69	0.28	0.30
Crotonylcholine bromide	0.50	0.71	0.20	—
n-Pentenoylcholine bromide	0.71	0.71	0.35	—
β,β-Dimethylacrylylcholine bromide	0.70	0.71	0.35	—
Urocanylcholine bromide	—	0.54	0.06	—
Imidazolylpropionylcholine iodide	0.37	0.29	0.15	—
Indolylacetylcholine bromide	0.63T	0.73T	0.2T	—
Indolylpropionylcholine bromide	0.60	0.73	0.26	—
Nicotinoylcholine perchlorate	0.35	0.58	0.10	—
Betaine	0.46	—	—	—
Carbaminoylcholine chloride	0.30	—	—	—
Choline O-sulfate	0.21	0.32	0	0.03
Choline O-phosphate	0.10	0.15	0	0
Ethanolamine	0.45	0.52	0.34	0.46
N-Methylethanolamine	0.50	0.56	0.59	0.57
N,N-Dimethylethanolamine	0.48	0.53	0.81	0.66

[a] See Table V for solvent systems and references.
[b] Abbreviations: T, tailing.

antee for complete agreement of results and identification of unknowns.
Therefore, the use of reference standards to correct for these differences
is necessary.

2. THIN-LAYER CHROMATOGRAPHY

Thin-layer chromatography (TLC) of choline and related compounds
has not been used to the great extent that paper chromatography has due
to the high polarity and low R_f values of these compounds on most sup-

TABLE V

PAPER CHROMATOGRAPHIC SOLVENT SYSTEMS

Number	Solvent system (v/v)	Reference
1	Ethanol:acetic acid:water (90:5:5)[a]	Goldfine (1962)
2	Ethanol:NH₄OH:water (90:5:5)[a]	Goldfine (1962)
3	n-Propanol:formic acid:water (8:1:1)[a]	Whittaker and Wijesundera (1952)
4	t-Butanol:acetic acid:water (70:15:15)[a]	———
5	n-Butanol:acetic acid:water (4:1:5)	Kuehl *et al.* (1955)
6	t-Butanol:formic acid:water (70:15:15)	de Flines (1955)
7	n-Propanol:water (7:3)	de Flines (1955)
8	Acetone:water (9:1)	Harada and Spencer (1960)
9	Acetone:water (9:1)[a]	———
10	n-Propanol:acetic acid:water (8:1:1)[a]	———
11	Acetone:acetic acid:water (8:1:1)[a]	———
12	Phenol:n-butanol:water:formic acid (50:50:10:3)	Bremer and Greenberg (1959)
13	n-Propanol:formic acid:water (6:3:1)	Bremer *et al.* (1960)
14	n-Butanol:pyridine:water (6:4:3)	Brundish and Baddiley (1968)
15	t-Butanol:pyridine:water (6:4:3)	———
16	n-Propanol:pyridine:water (6:4:3)	———
17	2-Propanol:pyridine:water (6:4:3)	———
18	2-Propanol:pyridine:water (6:4:3)[a]	———
19	2-Propanol:acetic acid:water (8:1:1)	———
20	2-Propanol:acetic acid:water (8:1:1)[a]	———
21	2-Propanol:formic acid:water (8:1:1)	———
22	2-Propanol:formic acid:water (8:1:1)[a]	———
23	n-Propanol:water (9:1)[a]	Whittaker and Wijesundera (1952)
24	n-Propanol:1 *M* acetic acid (3:1)[a]	———
25	n-Butanol:ethanol:acetic acid:water (8:2:1:3)	Augustinsson and Grahn (1953); Keyl *et al.* (1957)
26	n-Propanol:1 *M* acetic acid (3:1)	Keyl *et al.* (1957)
27	n-Butanol, saturated with water	Whittaker and Wijesundera (1952); Banister *et al.* (1953); Keyl *et al.* (1957)
28	n-Butanol:n-propanol:water (60:30:15)	Whittaker and Wijesundera (1952); Banister *et al.* (1953)

[a] System used with KCl paper and KCl-saturated solvent.

ports. The advantages of TLC, however, for the identification of unknown choline compounds are great since the method can detect much smaller amounts of the compounds and can also separate mixtures of unknown compounds to a greater degree than paper chromatography due to the absence of overt tailing and spreading of the compounds often encountered in paper chromatographic systems.

Once again, our studies concerning TLC systems for choline substances were aimed at the use of both literature-reported and original solvent and support systems that are versatile enough to separate the major types of choline derivatives as well as the ethanolamines. In order to standardize our methods, prepared 20-cm² 0.25-mm silica gel and aluminum oxide plates (Brinkmann) were used. The plates were stored in a desiccator until use and were used without any preceeding activation at elevated temperatures. The plates were spotted with unknowns and the same standard samples used for paper chromatography, and were placed in covered rectangular glass TLC chambers. The chambers had been lined with Whatman 3MM paper and had been equilibrated with the solvent to be used for at least 1 hour. After the solvent had ascended to within 1–2 cm of the top, the plates were removed, dried, and subjected to iodine vapors and Dragendorff's reagent as described above. In addition, silica gel plates were sprayed with 50% sulfuric acid and charred as a further check of spot location.

Table VI lists the R_f values found for our standard samples in the various solvent and support systems described in Table VII. It is interesting to note that as in paper chromatography an increase in chain length of choline esters results in increasing R_f values. Similarly, the isomeric esters, propionylcholine, and acetyl-β-methylcholine again have consistently close R_f values, while succinyldicholine has the lowest R_f values of all the choline esters due to its diionic nature. As expected, choline O-sulfate and and choline O-phosphate have low R_f values due to their high polarities, while the ethanolamines again increase in R_f value with increasing methylation. It must be cautioned that the R_f values reported must only be used as guidelines, since they will vary for the same system depending on conditions and may vary greatly if different supports are used or if the plates are prepared differently, e.g., poured alumina or silica gel plates instead of prepared plates. Identification of an unknown necessitates cochromatography with known standards.

3. Column Chromatography

The problems inherent in the paper and thin-layer chromatography of choline compounds are also apparent in column chromatography, i.e.,

TABLE VI

Thin-Layer Chromatography R_f Values of Choline and Related Compounds

Compound	R_f value in system[a,b]											
	1[c]	2	3[c]	4[c]	5[c]	6	7[c]	8	9	10	11	12
Choline chloride	0.47	0.51	0.45	0.55	0.55	0.73	0.76	0.65	0.46	0.27	0.48	0.24
Acetylcholine chloride	0.53	0.56	0.52	0.62	0.63	0.78	0.85	0.76	0.53	0.31	0.55	0.26
Acetyl-β-methylcholine bromide	0.59	0.69	0.63	0.76	0.75	0.84	0.93	0.82	0.61	0.35	0.62	0.29
Propionylcholine chloride	0.55	0.61	0.56	0.70	0.68	0.79	0.89	0.80	0.57	0.36	0.59	0.31
Butyrylcholine chloride	0.60	0.63	0.62	0.69	0.67	0.81	0.92	0.81	0.62	0.38	0.63	0.35
Succinyldicholine dichloride	0.18	0.58	0.31	0.56	0.64	0.80	0.77	0.72	0.31T	0.10	0.36	0.11
Choline O-phosphate	0.07	0.03	0.06	0	0	0	0.07	0.03	0.14	0.04	0.12	0.13
Choline O-sulfate	0.17	0.31	0.20	0	0.21	0	0.54	0.55	0.38	0.31	0.37	0.22
Ethanolamine	0.09	0.32	0.29	0.42	0.41	0.73	0.57	0.40	0.40	0.33	0.41	0.35
N-Methylethanolamine	0.16	0.44	0.41	0.46	0.43	0.76	0.74	0.56	0.44	0.37	0.49	0.36
N,N-Dimethylethanolamine	0.45	0.47	0.49	0.73	0.65	0.85	0.87	0.70	0.47	0.40	0.55	0.36

[a] See Table VII for systems.
[b] Abbreviations: T, tailing.
[c] R_f values in first phase.

TABLE VII

THIN-LAYER CHROMATOGRAPHY SYSTEMS

Number	Solvent system (v/v)	Support	Reference
1	n-Butanol:water:formic acid (60:35:15)	Alumina	Stahl (1969)
2	n-Butanol:water:acetic acid (66:17:17)	Alumina	Stahl (1969)
3	n-Butanol:water:acetic acid (40:50:10)	Alumina	Stahl (1969)
4	Methanol:CCl$_4$:acetic acid (28:12:1)	Alumina	Sullivan and Brady (1965)
5	Methanol:HCl (95:5)	Alumina	Reissmann and Wieske (1967)
6	Ethanol:7% ammonia (2:1)	Alumina	Reissmann and Wieske (1967)
7	n-Butanol:water:acetic acid (4:1:1)	Alumina	Taylor (1964)
8	Phenol:t-butanol:formic acid:water (50:50:3:10)	Alumina	————
9	n-Propanol:phenol:water:acetic acid (40:40:10:10)	Silica gel	————
10	n-Propanol : pyridine : water : acetic acid (6:4:3:1)	Silica gel	————
11	Phenol:2-propanol:formic acid:water (50:50:3:10)	Silica gel	————
12	Ethanol:water:acetic acid (4:1:1)	Silica gel	————

the very polar nature of choline derivatives, such as succinyldicholine, choline O-sulfate, and choline O-phosphate, make recovery of these compounds difficult once they are absorbed on a column.

Cation exchange columns have been used with some success for the separation of individual classes of choline derivatives and related substances. One of the original applications involved the use of the carboxylate resin Amberlite XE-97 (the fine mesh version of Amberlite IRC-50) for the separation of choline esters with elution by 0.1 M NaH$_2$PO$_4$ (pH 4–4.5) and 0.1 N HCl (Gardiner and Whittaker, 1954). This method was subsequently used for the separation of the choline esters, senecioylcholine, acrylylcholine, and urocanylcholine, found in marine gastropods (Whittaker and Michaelson, 1954; Keyl et al., Whittaker, 1960). The first two esters were eluted with the phosphate buffer, while the third required elution with HCl due to its ability to act as a divalent cation. Urocanylcholine has also been isolated by the use of a nonionic neutral cellulose column developed with n-butanol saturated with 1 N HCl (Erspamer and

Benati, 1953a). Similar use of a neutral cellulose column has been applied to the separation of muscarine from choline (Balenovic and Stefanac, 1956). These latter workers also used a Dowex 50-X8 cation exchange column for preparative scale chromatography in which elution with 2.5 N HCl caused choline to elute from the column before muscarine.

The separation of the choline-related ethanolamines has also been accomplished by column chromatography. The system used involves a Dowex 50 (H$^+$) column with 1.5 N HCl as eluent (Pilgeram *et al.*, 1953; Bremer *et al.*, 1960; Goldfine, 1962). In this system, the ethanolamines are eluted before choline, and are then further separated into ethanolamine and its two methyl derivatives on a second Dowex 50 column.

Since our own experiences have been centered on more polar choline derivatives such as choline *O*-sulfate and choline *O*-phosphate, our use of column chromatography has been limited due to the adherence of these compounds to most resins. We have employed both Rexyn 102 (H$^+$), a carboxylic cation exchanger, and AG 50W-X4 (Biorad Laboratories), a sulfonic acid cation exchanger. Elution for both types of columns (2.5 × 30 cm) involved 500-ml volumes of a series of increasingly more acidic solutions from 0.05 M acetic acid to 1 N HCl. On both columns, classes of choline compounds were separated, but not individual compounds. For example, on the Rexyn 102 column, choline eluted first and then its esters with 0.05–0.1 M acetic acid, while choline *O*-sulfate required elution with 0.5 N HCl. With the sulfonic acid resin, no choline compounds were eluted until 0.1 N HCl was used, and at this pH the stability of the choline esters and other derivatives is in question. The combination of the acid lability of choline compounds, together with the difficulty of separating the choline compounds from the buffer salts they are eluted with on columns such as the Amberlite XE-97 mentioned above, make large scale preparation of these compounds by some other means, e.g., preparative paper chromatography, more desirable.

B. Detection and Analytical Methods for Choline and Related Substances

1. Reagents for the Detection of Choline and Related Substances

Due to their rather unique chemical structures, choline and guanidine compounds as well as other related strong bases may be detected on chromatograms by a variety of reagents, a number of which are listed in Table VIII. In all cases, it is recommended that the reagents be sprayed onto the chromatograms to ensure that no shifting of spots will occur, which is possible if the chromatogram is drawn through a trough.

TABLE VIII

REAGENTS FOR THE DETECTION OF CHOLINE, GUANIDINE, AND OTHER RELATED BASES ON PAPER AND THIN-LAYER CHROMATOGRAMS

Reagent name	Specificity	Color of spot	Reference
Dragendorff	Choline and other quaternary bases; various alkaloids	Yellow to orange-red	p. 467[a]; p. 873, No. 97[b]
Iodoplatinate	Choline derivatives, p. 498[b]	Blue, pink	p. 519[a]; p. 883[b]
Dipicrylamine	Choline and its esters (nonspecific)	Red	p. 872[b]
Jaffe (picric acid–alkali)	Creatine and similar compounds	Red, orange	p. 292[a]; p. 894[b]
Iodine	Nonspecific	Yellow, brown	p. 519[a]; p. 882[b]
Hydroxylamine–ferric chloride	Choline esters (nonspecific)	Purple	p. 880[a]; [c]
Weber (pentacyanoaquoferriate [PCF]; Ferricyanide–nitroprusside [FCNPl])	Mono- and N,N-disubstituted guanidines; Hydroxyguanidine[d]	Red, orange	p. 291[a]; p. 891[b]
Diacetyl (α-naphthol diacetyl)	Guanidine, mono- and disubstituted guanidines; Hydroxyguanidine[d]	Pink, purple	p. 291[a]
Sakaguchi (8-hydroxyquinoline hypobromite)	Monosubstituted guanidines	Green; Red, orange	p. 290[a]; p. 881[b]

[a] Smith (1969).
[b] Stahl (1969).
[c] Whittaker and Wijesundera (1952).
[d] Kalyankar et al. (1958).

Once a choline compound has been located with a reagent such as Dragendorff's, further information concerning its identity may be gained by treating another chromatogram with a group-specific reagent spray. For example, treatment of a previously determined Dragendorff-positive spot with Hanes-Isherwood reagent (Stahl, 1969, p. 886) would ascertain identity of choline *O*-phosphate if a blue spot resulted, and the use of the hydroxylamine–ferric chloride reagent on a known Dragendorff-positive spot would indicate the presence of a choline ester.

2. CHEMICAL ANALYSIS AND DETERMINATION OF CHOLINE AND RELATED COMPOUNDS

The chemical method most extensively used for the analysis of choline compounds in extracts from natural sources involves precipitation of these compounds as their reineckate salts. Essentially, the method involves direct precipitation of extracted choline or choline derivative upon treatment with an aqueous solution of ammonium reineckate (for detailed methods, see Banister *et al.*, 1953; Asano, 1954; Engel *et al.*, 1954; Dittmer and Wells, 1969; Griffith and Nyc, 1971a). The resulting precipitate may be used directly as a derivative, and its melting point can be compared with those of known choline reineckates or mixtures of reineckates, or it may be dissolved in acetone and used for the direct colorimetric determination (at 520–530 nm) of the total choline in the extracted tissue (e.g., see Thaxton and Bowie, 1968). The acetone solution may also be freed of the reineckate by adding saturated aqueous silver sulfate. Silver reineckate precipitates from the solution, and the solution may then be subjected to choline chromatographic analysis.

A useful general method for the estimation of esters has been used for the estimation of choline esters and involves the hydroxylamine–ferric chloride reaction (Hestrin, 1949). Choline esters react with the reagent to give purple solutions that may be estimated colorimetrically for choline content at 540 nm. The method is nonspecific for ester chain length, and must be carried out in the absence of any noncholine esters. Our studies with this method have also shown that a negative test is given by choline and choline *O*-sulfate.

A more recent method described for the detection of choline esters involves the fluorometric determination of the salicylhydrazone produced upon the treatment of esters first with hydrazine and then with salicylaldehyde (Fellman, 1969). Thus far, this method has proved successful with acetyl-, propionyl-, and butyrylcholine.

There are many other specific precipitation reactions for choline extracted from natural sources. These will not be mentioned here since they have not been applied to choline derivatives. For accounts of the periodate, phosphotungstic acid, dipicrylamine, gold chloride, and other precipitation reactions, the reader is referred to other sources (Engel *et al.*, 1954; Dittmer and Wells, 1969; Griffith and Nyc, 1971a,b).

3. Gas Chromatography of Choline and Related Compounds

Gas chromatography of choline compounds has not been highly successful due to the highly ionic nature and low volatility of these compounds. There are, however, two general methods that have had limited success in the identification and quantitative determination of choline compounds by gas chromatography.

The first method involves the conversion of cholines to volatile derivatives or hydrolysis products. A primary application of this method is directed specifically at acetyl- and propionylcholine, and involves hydrolysis of the choline esters to liberate acetic or propionic acids and subsequent reduction of the acids to their respective alcohols (Stavinoha *et al.*, 1964). The alcohols are quantitated on a 20% Carbowax 6000 on Chromosorb W column. A later modification of this method involves a direct quantitation of the acetic acid produced from acetylcholine hydrolysis on a Porapak Q-S column (Cranmer, 1968). However, both of these methods are limited to the estimation of the acyl component of choline esters, and are thus not applicable to many other choline derivatives.

Another method involving derivative formation which is not dependent upon the acyl group of choline esters involves the N-demethylation of choline compounds with sodium benzenethiolate (Jenden *et al.*, 1967; 1968). In this method, quaternary ammonium compounds are converted to their corresponding tertiary amines by benzenethiolate ion, and the resulting amines are chromatographed on a 1% phenyldiethanolamine succinate on Polypak 1 column. Although this method shows promise in the estimation of submicrogram quantities of choline esters (see Jenden *et al.*, 1970), its rather long and arduous procedure and the possibility that quantitation will be lost due to impurities in the reaction mixture attacking the choline ester groups (see Shama *et al.*, 1966; Vaughn and Baumann, 1962) make its simplification and a more extensive study with other choline compounds necessary.

The second type of method that has been reported for the gas chromatography of choline involves a pyrolysis reaction of the cholines with subsequent direct sweeping of the pyrolysis products onto a 20% Carbowax 6000 on Chromosorb W or onto a 6% SE-30 on Anakrom ABS column (Szilagyi *et al.*, 1968). Although this method cannot be applied directly to choline compounds in tissue extracts without their prior purification, it is relatively straightforward and shows great promise in the future for the determination and quantitation of choline compounds.

Much remains to be accomplished in the field of choline gas chromatography. Thus far, no method has been applied to choline compounds other than choline and its esters. This is understandable since compounds such as choline O-sulfate and choline O-phosphate, as well as esters such as succinyldicholine, are even less volatile than the esters studied thus far. Further research is needed to develop systems applicable to all choline derivatives and, ideally, systems enabling the direct determination of choline compounds per se.

4. SPECTRAL ANALYSIS OF CHOLINE COMPOUNDS

Spectral analysis of choline compounds is possible by all the usual methods of spectroscopy provided a suitable system can be devised for these compounds which takes into account their highly ionic and hygroscopic properties.

Infrared spectroscopy may be used on either solutions or dry samples of choline compounds or their prepared derivatives. In the former method, choline and its esters are dissolved in absolute ethanol and placed in a fixed path sodium chloride cell for the spectra. This method has been utilized in studies of the 2000–1600-cm^{-1} region of the spectra of acetylcholine and related compounds to postulate a cyclic conformation for acetylcholine (Fellman and Fujita, 1962). Those choline compounds not very soluble in ethanol, e.g., choline O-sulfate and choline O-phosphate, may be prepared for spectroscopy as KBr pellets or in a Nujol mull (see (see Erspamer and Benati, 1953b). However, if the choline compound is very hygroscopic, a derivative of the compound may first be prepared and then made into a KBr pellet (see Whittaker, 1959) or Nujol mull for spectroscopy. The comparably taken spectra of known choline compounds can then be used in the identification of unknown compound spectra.

Ultraviolet spectroscopy is not of great use in choline determinations except for a few cases where unsaturation exists in choline derivatives. Urocanylcholine [XI] has been found to have λ_{max} of 285 nm at pH 4.5 with ϵ_{max} of 1.67×10^4 (Pasini et al., 1952; Erspamer and Benati, 1953b), and the aurichloride of β,β-dimethylacrylylcholine [XIII] exhibits the typical absorption band of an α,β-unsaturated carbonyl compound at 223 nm. Utilization of the visible spectrum for choline determinations has already been mentioned with respect to the reineckate and hydroxylamine reactions.

Mass spectroscopy of cholines has been limited to one method that involves a combined gas chromatographic–mass spectrometric system for the identification of N-demethylated choline esters produced by the sodium benzenethiolate method described above under gas chromatography (Hammer *et al.*, 1968). Again, as with gas chromatography, volatility is the limiting factor in mass spectrometry, and volatile derivatives of the choline compounds must be developed before this method can be of use.

C. Bioassay Systems for Choline and Related Substances

1. *Neurospora crassa* ASSAY

One of the most sensitive methods for the determination of choline in natural substances and tissues is a bioassay using a mutant strain of *Neurospora crassa* which requires an exogenous source of choline or a choline derivative for growth. This method is sensitive for low microgram amounts of choline compounds.

The algal cells to be assayed for total choline content are lyophilized, and 150-mg samples are hydrolyzed by refluxing with 30 ml of 3 N HCl for 18–24 hours. The hydrolyzates are concentrated *in vacuo* to dryness, and the flasks containing the resulting residues are placed in a vacuum desiccator containing a dish of sodium hydroxide pellets to remove the last traces of acid. The residues are dissolved in approximately 10 ml of water; the resulting solutions are neutralized with sodium hydroxide; and the final volumes are adjusted to 25.0 ml. Aliquots of 5.0 ml of these solutions are passed through a Permutit (Fisher) column (100 × 6 mm containing about 1 g Permutit) (Horowitz and Beadle, 1943), which absorbs the choline in the sample, but not the interfering methionine. After washing the column with 5.0 ml of 0.3% NaCl, the choline is eluted from the column with 10.0 ml of 5% NaCl. Aliquots of this eluent are then assayed with the choline-requiring mutant of *N. crassa* (in our studies, strain 485 from the Fungal Genetics Stock Center, Dartmouth College, Hanover, N. H.) and Choline Assay Medium (Difco) (Horowitz and Beadle, 1943). After growth of the organism, the dry weight of the mycelia in the flasks containing aliquots of the unknown sample is related to a concurrently run choline chloride standard growth curve to determine the amount of choline in the sample. Results are expressed as choline chloride in the unknown sample.

The assay described has shown that the mutant of *N. crassa* used will respond equally well, on a molar basis, to known standards of choline, choline *O*-sulfate, succinyldicholine, *N,N*-dimethylethanolamine, and *N*-methylethanolamine, to a lesser extent to choline *O*-phosphate, acetyl-, propionyl-, and butyrylcholine, and not significantly to acetyl-β-methylcholine and ethanolamine (see Figs. 1 and 2). In addition, other workers

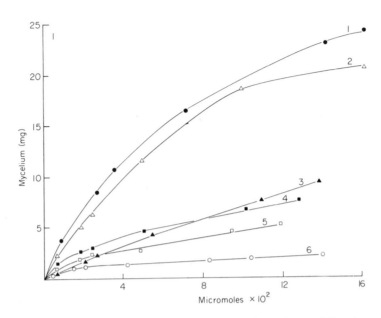

FIG. 1. Milligrams of mycelium of *N. crassa* resulting from adding increasing concentrations of choline esters to choline-free media. 1, Choline chloride; 2, succinyldicholine dichloride; 3, acetylcholine chloride; 4, propionylcholine chloride; 5, butyrylcholine chloride; 6, acetyl-β-methylcholine bromide.

have found that no response is elicited in the assay by betaine, creatine, sarcosine, neurine, N,N-diethylethanolamine, dimethylamine, trimethylamine, and tetramethylammonium chloride (Griffith and Nye, 1971b). This relatively specific response of the organism to choline compounds has been used in conjunction with chromatographic methods where specific areas of preparative-scale paper chromatograms have been eluted and assayed for choline (Ikawa and Chakravarti, 1970). A positive growth response in the assay establishes the cholinelike nature of the substance eluted from the chromatogram. Further identification of the compound is then achieved by the use of cochromatography with known standards by paper and thin-layer chromatography, by specific chemical tests as described above, and by physiological bioassay systems (see below). An example of this chromatogram–bioassay technique is described below with respect to *Amphidinium carteri*.

2. PHYSIOLOGICAL ASSAY SYSTEMS

In addition to the *N. crassa* assay system, cholinelike compounds may also be recognized by their action on both isolated biological tissue preparations and whole animals. The isolated preparations have been mostly used for the assay and identification of naturally occurring choline derivatives, especially esters, while whole animals as well as isolated preparations have been used extensively for studies concerned with the nature of the action of both natural and synthetic choline derivatives.

The isolated preparations most used for choline assays include frog rectus abdominis muscle (see Chang and Gaddam, 1933; Banister *et al.*, 1953), guinea pig ileum (see Banister *et al.*, 1953; Bisset *et al.*, 1960), the longitudinal muscle of the leech *Hirudo medicinalis* (see MacIntosh and Perry, 1950; Bisset *et al.*, 1960), and various heart preparations, notably that of the shellfish *Mercenaria* (*Venus*) *mercenaria* (Welsh and Taub, 1948). These preparations have been used for both the qualitative and quantitative assay of choline compounds. The relative activities of a number of choline esters to the activity of acetylcholine differ measurably when assayed on different preparations, e. g., propionyl- and butyrylcholine are more active than acetylcholine on frog rectus muscle, but less active on guinea pig ileum (Banister *et al.*, 1953). Studies with the heart of *M. mer-*

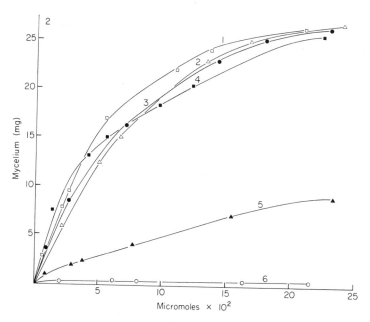

Fig. 2. Milligrams of mycelium of *N. crassa* resulting from adding increasing concentrations of choline derivatives and ethanolamines to choline-free media. 1, Choline *O*-sulfate; 2, *N*-methylethanolamine; 3, choline chloride; 4, *N*,*N*-dimethylethanolamine; 5, choline *O*-phosphate; 6, ethanolamine.

cenaria have shown that choline and its short chain esters all affect the heart with the same acetylcholine-like action, but require quantitatively different concentrations to produce this activity, while substitution of ethyl for methyl groups on the quaternary nitrogen of choline and acetylcholine results in the complete loss of acetylcholine-like activity (Welsh and Taub, 1948).

Both isolated tissue preparations and whole animals such as conscious chicks and anesthetized cats have been used for studies concerned primarily with the mechanism of action of choline and its natural and synthetic derivatives rather than with the identity of the compounds. Such studies have revealed that choline analogs with methyl groups on the quaternary nitrogen exhibit typical depolarizing action on the motor nerve end plates, while those analogs with larger substituent groups on the quaternary nitrogen exhibit an anticholinergic curarelike action on these motor nerves (Bowman and Rand, 1962; Bowman *et al.*, 1967; Brimblecombe and Roswell, 1969).

D. Studies on Amphidinium carteri

Members of the genus *Amphidinium*, dinoflagellates in the family Gymnodiniidae, have, as yet, only been implicated as possessing toxic properties. The supernates from cultures containing 1.5×10^6 flagellates per milliliter of *Amphidinium klebsii* and *Amphidinium rhynchocephalum* have been reported to cause fish kills in 15–25 minutes (McLaughlin and Provasoli, 1957), while *Amphidinium carteri* has been reported to release an acetylcholine analog that may act as a protective agent against zooplankton (Wangersky and Guillard, 1960).

Our own experiences with *A. carteri* began with observations that fish kills would occur in culture supernates. This fact, together with the indication that the fish toxic factor(s) might be cholinelike in nature, led us to assay dry cells of the organism grown in modified seawater media (see Sasner, Chapter V) for choline using the *N. crassa* assay. The assay revealed that *A. carteri* cells contained from 0.36 to 0.41% dry weight of choline chloride equivalent. Since the assay is relatively specific for choline and its derivatives, it appeared that for algae (see Table II) *A. carteri* contained large amounts of choline or of some choline derivatives, and further studies were undertaken to characterize the derivatives. Attempts were also made to extract choline factors from culture supernates for further characterization. However, the low molecular weight, dialyzable nature of the choline factors together with the solubility of the factors being restricted to aqueous and ethanolic solutions have made extraction of the factors away from the large amounts of salts in the media as yet unsuccessful. Thus, our work with the choline factors has been limited to extraction of salt-free harvested cells, and assumes that any unbound choline derivatives that can be extracted from the whole cells may also be released by the cells into the media in late culture phases to act as possible toxic factors.

The *Neurospora* assay as described above estimates only total choline content of a tissue or organism, since the sample is acid hydrolyzed prior to the assay. Thus, choline bound in nonpharmacologically active forms, such as phospholipids, is estimated along with pharmacologically active forms of choline. Thus, to separate any active choline compounds from lipid-bound choline compounds in *A. carteri*, 1.0-g quantities of dry cells are extracted with 250 ml of 95% ethanol for 24 hours on a mechanical stirrer. The resulting alcoholic extract of the cells is centrifuged, and the cell debris is extracted with 250 ml of 90% ethanol. The two ethanolic supernates, which contain any freely occurring choline compounds as well as most of the lipid-bound choline and the pigments of the cells, are combined and evaporated to dryness *in vacuo*. The resulting residue is suspended in 100 ml of distilled water and partitioned against 100 ml of *n*-butanol in a separatory funnel. After standing for approximately 12 hours, the clear, slightly yellow lower aqueous phase is drawn off and repartitioned with 50 ml of fresh *n*-butanol. The two upper phase butanol solutions are combined and washed with 50 ml of distilled water to ensure that all of the water-soluble components of the extract are removed from the butanol solution. This water wash is then combined with the aqueous phase of the partition, the combined aqueous solution is evaporated to dryness *in vacuo*, and the resulting residue is dissolved in 1–2 ml of water and analyzed as described below. The cell debris and the butanol partition phases are combined, evaporated to dryness *in vacuo*, acid hydrolyzed, and assayed for total choline content with *Neurospora*. The results of this latter assay reveal that the water-insoluble and bound forms of choline account for only 0.07–0.10% of the dry weight of the original *A. carteri* cells. Thus, 0.26–0.34% of the dry weight *A. carteri* cells is comprised of water-soluble choline factors that can elicit a positive *Neurospora* response (see below for further proof) and that are extracted by ethanol from whole cells.

The ethanolic extract of *A. carteri* was studied by chromatographic and chemical methods. The results of paper and thin-layer chromatography of the extract are shown in Tables IX and X. The extract separated into three iodine- and Dragendorff-positive components in a number of systems. This three-component separation was further verified by spraying silica gel plates of the separated components with 50% sulfuric acid and then

TABLE IX

<small>Paper Chromatography of Ethanolic Extracts
of *A. carteri* Dry Cells</small>

| System | R_f value of spot | | |
number[a]	Slowest	Middle	Fastest
1	0.14[b]	0.27	0.41
4	0.05[b]	0.12	0.17
5	0.12	0.17[b]	0.23
6	0.17	0.35[b]	0.49
7	0.18	0.29	0.36[b]
8	0.0	0.13[b]	0.38
10	0.06[b]	0.14	0.29
11	0.0	0.12[b]	0.22
13	0.34	0.59[b]	0.68
14	0.05	0.09	0.20[b]
15	0.09	0.22	0.38[b]
16	0.15	0.37[b]	0.40
17	0.11	0.23	0.41[b]
18	0.05	0.17[b]	0.47
19	0.12[b]	0.24	0.47
20	0.0	0.05[b]	0.34
21	0.13	0.18[b]	0.36
22	0.11[b]	0.35	0.53
23	0.03[b]	0.07	0.22
24	0.02	0.12[b]	0.28
25	0.05	0.17	0.21[b]

[a] See Table V.
[b] Cochromatographed with choline *O*-sulfate.

by charring. After this treatment, only the same three spots corresponding to the Dragendorff-positive spots were detected. Of the three components in the extract, one component cochromatographed in all systems with known choline *O*-sulfate, while the other two components occasionally cochromatographed with known compounds, but not consistently enough to warrant identification. In any case, it appears that if one or both of these latter two unidentified components is a choline ester (see below), it is more polar than esters such as acetyl-, propionyl-, acetyl-β-methyl-, and butyrylcholine. It should be noted that the three compounds did not always chromatograph in the same relative order, i. e., choline *O*-sulfate changes its relative position from one solvent system to another. Such radical changes in R_f values and in the order of movement with changes in solvent systems is in agreement with other observations concerning characteristics of choline compound chromatography (Engel *et al.*, 1954).

As a chemical test for the presence of choline esters in the ethanolic extract of *A. carteri* cells, the extract was tested with the hydroxylamine reaction (Hestrin, 1949). A positive purple color reaction resulted, indicating that one or both of the two unknown Dragendorff-positive components of the extract were esters since the known component, choline *O*-sulfate, gave a negative test with the reaction.

To correlate the separation of the ethanolic extract components with choline activity, both *Neurospora* and physiological assays were carried out on the components. Preparative paper chromatography was used to separate the components of the ethanolic extract of 1 g of *A. carteri* cells. The extract was spotted onto 40- × 50-cm sheets of Whatman No. 1 paper and run in covered glass tanks with 400 ml of an appropriate solvent for 20 hours. Two systems were used, paper chromatography systems 1 and 17 (see Table V), the former a KCl-treated system and the latter a non-KCl system. After the runs, thin vertical strips were cut from the chromatograms and sprayed with Dragendorff's reagent to locate the choline compounds. These strips were then realigned with their respective chromatograms, and each chromatogram was sectioned to separate the areas corresponding to the Dragendorff-positive spots on the developed strip. The sectioned chromatograms were cut apart, and each section was cut into

TABLE X

THIN-LAYER CHROMATOGRAPHY OF ETHANOLIC EXTRACTS OF *A. carteri* DRY CELLS

System number[a]	R_f value of spot		
	Slowest	Middle	Fastest
4	0.0[b]	0.04	0.33
5	0.0	0.21[b]	0.53
6	0.0[b]	0.30	0.73
7	0.04	0.11	0.53[b]
8	0.14	0.32	0.55[b]
9	0.04	0.15	0.38[b]
10	0.16	0.30[b]	0.42
11	0.0	0.08	0.37[b]
12	0.13	0.22[b]	0.45

[a] See Table VII.

[b] Cochromatographed with choline *O*-sulfate.

pieces and eluted with water. The resulting solutions were separated from the chromatogram paper, evaporated to dryness *in vacuo*, and the residues were dissolved in a known volume of distilled water (about 10.0–12.0 ml). Aliquots of these final solutions, each corresponding to a specific area on the chromatogram, were then assayed unhydrolyzed in the *Neurospora* assay. The resulting choline activities of the chromatogram sections are shown in Figs. 3 and 4 for the two chromatography systems used. As can be seen in these figures, the Dragendorff-positive areas of the chromatograms correspond exactly to the areas of choline activity. Note the choline *O*-sulfate is the slowest (No. 1) spot in Fig. 3 and the fastest (No. 3) spot in Fig. 4, and that the middle (No. 2) spot appears to be the same component in both chromatogram systems on the basis of its relative activity. This chromatogram assay procedure conclusively demonstrates that three nonlipoidal choline derivatives occur in *A. carteri*.

As further proof of the choline activity of at least one of the two unknown ethanol extract components, the middle (No. 2) spot of chromatographic system 1 (Fig. 3) was eluted from a chromatogram, freed of KCl by repeated precipitation of the salt from absolute ethanol, and assayed

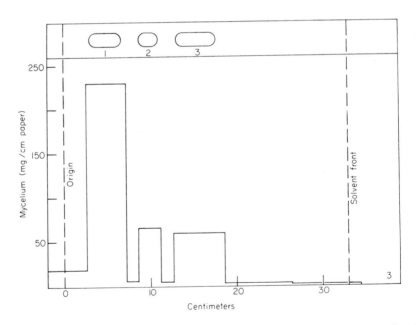

FIG. 3. Preparative paper chromatography and *N. crassa* assay of the unhydrolyzed ethanolic extract of *A. carteri* cells in solvent system 1; ethanol:acetic acid:water (90:5:5, v/v) with KCl-treated paper and solvent.

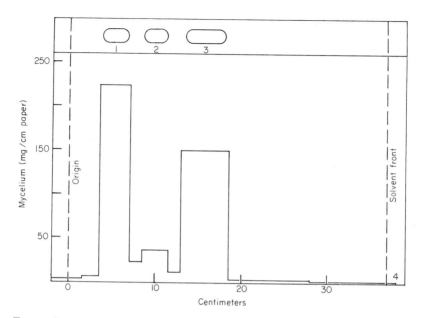

Fig. 4. Preparative paper chromatography and *N. crassa* assay of the unhydrolyzed ethanolic extract of *A. carteri* cells in solvent system 17; 2-propanol:pyridine:water (6:4:3, v/v), no KCl treatment.

physiologically on a number of heart systems. The component exhibited typical acetylcholine-like activity on these preparations, although it was not as active as acetylcholine on a weight for weight basis (see Sasner, Chapter V for these physiological tests). This finding of an acetylcholine-like activity, but requirement for greater concentrations of material for such activity, indicates that the middle (No. 2) component in paper chromatographic system 1 is some type of choline ester. Further studies are in progress in an attempt to identify this and the other choline-containing component of the ethanolic extract.

Thus it can be concluded that *A. carteri* contains three choline derivatives, one of which is choline *O*-sulfate and another which behaves physiologically, chemically, and nutritionally like a choline ester. These choline derivatives may be responsible for the reported and observed toxicity of *A. carteri* to marine organisms.

E. Studies on Aphanazomenon flos aquae

Studies have been conducted in this laboratory (M. Alam and M. Ikawa, unpublished) on toxic *A. flos aquae* cells collected by centrifugation from natural essentially unialgal blooms that occurred in Kezar Lake, North Sutton, New Hampshire. The toxin, isolated in a chromatographically pure state, is a strongly basic substance. It reacts with ninhydrin to give a purple color, and it reacts positively in the Weber and diacetyl, and negatively in the Jaffe and Sakaguchi tests. In certain respects, therefore, it appears to differ from saxitoxin, which does not give a purple color with ninhydrin, reacts negatively in the Sakaguchi test, positively in the Jaffe and Weber tests (Mold *et al.*, 1957), and positively in the diacetyl test. Saxitoxin and *Aphanazomenon* toxin also appeared to behave differently on thin-layer chromatography. Purified *Aphanazomenon* toxin blocks nerve conduction without appearing to affect the transmembrane resting potential, and therefore resembles saxitoxin and tetrodotoxin in its action (see Sasner, Chapter V).

III. Discussion

When one considers the toxic and pharmacologically active naturally occurring compounds described in the plant world, one finds that, over the years, very large numbers have been derived from high plant sources. These include numerous alkaloids, heterocyclic oxygen compounds, and aromatic benzenoid compounds. In more recent times, after an outbreak of turkey fatalities of epidemic proportions which occurred in England in 1960 and which was traced to peanut meal contaminated with aflatoxin, a fungal metabolite, concentrated efforts by a number of investigators have revealed a whole spectrum of toxic products from fungi (see, for example, Lillehoj *et al.*, 1970). In comparison, the amount of definitive chemical work done to date on toxic substances of algal origin is indeed very limited. At the present time, most of the toxic algal species are described as members of the cyanophyta (blue-green algae), the pyrrophyta (dinoflagellates), and the chrysophyta (golden brown algae). These are microscopic algae, as opposed to macroscopic algae (seaweeds), and some of the difficulties involved in the chemical study of toxins from these algae are due to the heroic efforts required to culture these microorganisms on a sufficiently large scale to permit chemical isolation of their toxins [see Gorham (1964) for an illustration of the magnitude of the operation used in the isolation of the toxin microcystin from laboratory cultures of the blue-green alga, *Microcystis aeruginosa*]. In the culturing of these microscopic algae, yields, at best, generally do not even approach yields realizable in the culturing of bacterial cells, because the algae require much longer incubation times, and their cells number per unit volume are considerably less. In some instances, advantage has been taken of natural algal blooms for toxin isolation. Thus, natural blooms of the dinoflagellate *Gymnodinium breve* (Martin and Chatterjee, 1970) and of the blue-green alga *Aphanazomenon flos aquae* (M. Alam and M. Ikawa, unpublished) have been utilized for this purpose. In some instances, where a toxin is transvected along a food chain, advantage has been taken of the relatively high toxin concentrations that have accumulated in the transvecting organisms for chemical isolation work. This has been especially true in the study of saxitoxin, the toxin of *Gonyaulax catanella*, which is accumulated by the California mussel and Alaska butter clam (Schantz *et al.*, 1957; Casselman *et al.*, 1960).

We can only speculate why, if a reason does exist, so many of the microscopic algae are toxin-producing organisms. The fact that many of these toxins are neurotoxins that have profound physiological effects on higher animals make them an interesting and potentially important group of substances from the standpoint of how they might aid in the elucidation of biochemical and physiological cellular process as well as how they might be developed into pharmacologically useful drugs (see Chapter I).

Although the results are still fragmentary, studies presented here on *Amphidinium carteri* suggest that choline derivatives may assume an important role in algal toxigenicity. Of the three water-soluble choline derivatives demonstrated in this dinoflagellate, one has been identified as choline *O*-sulfate, while the remaining two have, as yet, not been identified. That at least one of these unidentified compounds has a cholinergic activity in physiological systems makes it of considerable interest. Whether other dinoflagellates and other less-studied algae also have high choline contents comparable to *A. carteri* is still open to speculation. A more extensive survey of the total choline content of these algae would aid in clearing up this point. We have been working on this particular aspect of algal chemistry.

The fact that blue-green algae appear to contain very little or no choline in any form in their cells would exclude choline compounds as being the toxic agents of toxigenic blue-green algae. However, studies on *Aphanazomenon flos aquae* have shown that other strongly basic nitrogenous compounds can be involved in toxicity. Since these compounds are also highly cationic nonvolatile water-soluble substances, methods used in the study of choline compounds are also applicable in their study.

What would greatly expedite the study of derivatives of choline and other strong nitrogenous bases would be a breakthrough in methodology. A simple and direct method with high resolving power, accuracy, and sensitivity is needed for the identification and estimation of these types of compounds. The nonvolatility, highly cationic nature, and lack of a suitable quantitative color reaction for these compounds, in general, has hampered adapting the high sensitivity and resolving capacities of gas and column chromatography to these compounds. At present, paper and thin-layer chromatography are the methods of choice for the identification of these compounds, but these methods leave much to be desired as far as quantitative determinations are concerned. High speed, high pressure liquid chromatographic systems have now been developed to the point where they are highly sensitive and capable of high resolution. The development of this type of system, which is capable of analyzing substances not amenable to gas chromatography, offers hope in the future for the convenient identification and quantitative determination of choline and related compounds.

ACKNOWLEDGMENTS

This work was supported in part by Grant EC-00294 from the United States Public Health Service.

REFERENCES

Ariens, E. J., and Simonis, A. M. (1967). Cholinergic and anticholinergic drugs, do they act on common receptors? *Ann. N. Y. Acad. Sci.* **144**, 842–868.

Asano, M. (1954). Occurrence of choline in the shellfish *Callista brevisiphonata* Carpenter. *Tohoku J. Agr. Res.* **4**, 239–250.

Augustinsson, K., and Grahn, M. (1953). The separation of choline esters by paper chromatography. *Acta Chem. Scand.* **7**, 906–912.

Balenovic, K., and Stefanac, Z. (1956). Separation of quaternary bases from *Amanita muscaria* L. on cross-linked sulphonated polystyrene resins. *Chem. Ind.* (*London*) p. 23.

Banister, J., Whittaker, V. P., and Wijesundera, S. (1953). The occurrence of homologs of acetylcholine in ox spleen. *J. Physiol.* (*London*) **121**, 55–71.

Bellenger, N., Nissen, P., Wood, T. C., and Segel, I. H. (1968). Specificity and control of choline *O*-sulfate transport in filamentous fungi. *J. Bacteriol.* **96**, 1574–1585.

Benson, A. A., and Maruo, B. (1958). Plant phospholipids. I. Identification of the phosphatidyl glycerols. *Biochim. Biophys. Acta* **27**, 189–195.

Benson, A. A., and Strickland, E. H. (1960). Plant phospholipids. III. Identification of diphosphatidyl glycerol. *Biochim. Biophys. Acta* **41**, 328–333.

Bisset, G. W., Frazer, J. F. D., Rothschild, M., and Schachter, M. (1960). A pharmacologically active choline ester and other substances in the garden tiger moth, *Arctia caja* (L.). *Proc. Roy. Soc., Ser. B* **152**, 255–262.

Bowman, W. C., and Rand, M. J. (1962). The neuromuscular blocking action of substances related to choline. *Int. J. Neuropharmacol.* **1**, 129–132.

Bowman, W. C., Hemsworth, B. A., and Rand, M. J. (1967). Effects of analogs of choline on neuromuscular transmission. *Ann. N. Y. Acad. Sci.* **144**, 471–482.

Boylan, D. B., and Scheuer, P. J. (1967). Pahutoxin, a fish poison. *Science* **155**, 52–56.

Bremer, J., and Greenberg, D. M. (1959). Mono- and dimethylethanolamine isolated from rat-liver phospholipids. *Biochim. Biophys. Acta* **35**, 287–288.

Bremer, J., Figard, P. H., and Greenberg, D. M. (1960). The biosynthesis of choline and its relation to phospholipid metabolism. *Biochim. Biophys. Acta* **43**, 477–488.

Brimblecombe, R. W., and Roswell, D. G. (1969). A comparison of the pharmacological activities of tertiary bases and their quaternary ammonium derivatives. *Int. J. Neuropharmacol.* **8**, 131–141.

Brundish, D. E., and Baddiley, J. (1968). Pneumococcal C-substance, a ribitol teichoic acid containing choline phosphate. *Biochem. J.* **110**, 573–582.

Bull, G., Hebb, C., and Morris, D. (1969). Synthesis of acetylcholine in the electric organ of *Torpedo*. *Comp. Biochem. Physiol.* **28**, 11–28.

Casselman, A. A., Greenhalgh, R., Brownhill, H. H., and Bannard, R. A. (1960). Clam poison. I. The paper chromatographic purification of clam poison dihydrochloride. *Can. J. Chem.* **38**, 1277–1290.

Chang, C. H., and Gaddam, H. J. (1933). Choline esters in tissue extracts. *J. Physiol. (London)* **79**, 255–285.

Cranmer, M. F. (1968). Estimation of the acetylcholine levels in brain tissue by gas chromatography of acetic acid. *Life Sci.* **7** (*pt. 1*), 995–1000.

de Flines, J. (1955). The occurrence of a sulfuric acid ester of choline in the mycelium of a strain of *P. chrysogenum*. *J. Amer. Chem. Soc.* **77**, 1676–1677.

Dittmer, J. C., and Wells, M. A. (1969). Quantitative and qualitative analysis of lipids and lipid components. *In* "Methods in Enzymology" (J. M. Lowenstein, ed.), Vol. 14, pp. 482–530. Academic Press, New York.

Engel, R. W., Salmon, W. D., and Ackerman, C. J. (1954). Chemical estimation of choline. *Methods Biochem. Anal.* **1**, 265–286.

Erspamer, V., and Benati, O. (1953a). Identification of murexine as β-[imidazolyl-(4)]-acrylcholine. *Science* **117**, 161–162.

Erspamer, V., and Benati, O. (1953b). Isolierung des Murexins aus Hypobranchialdrüsenextrakten von Murex trunculus und seine Identifizierung als β-[Imidazolyl-4(5)]-acryl-cholin. *Biochem. Z.* **324**, 66–73.

Fellman, J. H. (1969). A chemical method for the determination of acetylcholine: Its application in a study of presynaptic release and a choline acetyltransferase assay. *J. Neurochem.* **16**, 135–146.

Fellman, J. H., and Fujita, T. S. (1962). The conformation of acetylcholine. *Biochim. Biophys. Acta* **56**, 227–231.

Gardiner, J. E., and Whittaker, V. P. (1954). The identification of propionylcholine as a constituent of ox spleen. *Biochem. J.* **58**, 24–29.

Goldfine, H. (1962). The characterization and biosynthesis of an *N*-methylethanolamine phospholipid from *Clostridium butyricum*. *Biochim. Biophys. Acta* **59**, 504–506.

Gorham, P. R. (1964). Toxic algae. *In* "Algae and Man" (C. D. F. Jackson, ed.), pp. 307–336. Plenum, New York.

Griffith, W. H., and Nyc, J. F. (1971a). Choline. II. Chemistry. *Vitamins* **3**, 3–15.

Griffith, W. H., and Nyc, J. F. (1971b). Choline. VII. Estimation. *Vitamins* **3**, 70–75.

Halstead, B. W. (1967). "Poisonous and Venomous Marine Animals of the World," Vol. 2, p. 711. US Govt. Printing Office, Washington, D. C.

Hammer, C. G., Hanin, I., Holmstedt, B., Kitz, R. J., Jenden, D. J., and Karlen, B. (1968). Identification of acetylcholine in fresh rat brain by combined gas chromatography–mass spectrometry. *Nature (London)* **220**, 915–917.

Harada, T., and Spencer, B. (1960). Choline sulfate in fungi. *J. Gen. Microbiol.* **22,** 520–527.

Hestrin, S. (1949). The reaction of acetylcholine and other carboxylic acid derivatives with hydroxylamine and its analytical application. *J. Biol. Chem.* **180,** 249–261.

Horowitz, N. H., and Beadle, G. W. (1943). A microbiological method for the determination of choline by use of a mutant of *Neurospora. J. Biol. Chem.* **150,** 325–333.

Hulanicka, D., Erwin, J., and Bloch, K. (1964). Lipid metabolism of *Euglena gracilis. J. Biol. Chem.* **239,** 2778–2787.

Ikawa, M. (1967). Bacterial phosphatides and natural relationships. *Bacteriol. Rev.* **31,** 54–64.

Ikawa, M., and Chakravarti, A. (1970). Occurrence of choline in *Lactobacillus plantarum. Bacteriol. Proc.* pp. 152.

Ikawa, M., Borowski, P. T., and Chakravarti, A. (1968). Choline and inositol distribution in algae and fungi. *Appl. Microbiol.* **16,** 620–623.

Jackim, E., and Gentile, J. (1968). Toxins of a blue-green alga: Similarity to saxitoxin. *Science* **162,** 915–916.

Jenden, D. J., Lamb, S. I., and Hanin, I. (1967). Identification and microestimation of choline esters by gas chromatography. *Fed. Proc., Fed. Amer. Soc. Exp. Biol.* **26,** 296.

Jenden, D. J., Hanin, I., and Lamb, S. I. (1968). Gas chromatographic microestimation of acetylcholine and related compounds. *Anal. Chem.* **40,** 125–128.

Jenden, D. J., Campbell, B., and Roch, M. (1970). Gas chromatographic estimation of choline esters in tissues: A modified procedure for submicrogram quantities. *Anal. Biochem.* **35,** 209–211.

Kalyankar, G. D., Ikawa, M., and Snell, E. E. (1958). The enzymatic cleavage of canavanine to homoserine and hydroxyguanidine. *J. Biol. Chem.* **233,** 1175–1178.

Kates, M., and Volcani, B. E. (1966). Lipid components of diatoms. *Biochim. Biophys. Acta* **116,** 264–278.

Keyl, M. S., Michaelson, I. A., and Whittaker, V. P. (1957). Physiologically active choline esters in certain marine gastropods and other invertebrates. *J. Physiol. (London)* **139,** 434–454.

Kuehl, J. J., Jr., Lebel, N., and Richter, J. W. (1955). Isolation and characterization studies on muscarine. *J. Amer. Chem. Soc.* **77,** 6663–6665.

Lillehoj, E. B., Ciegler, A., and Detroy, R. W. (1970). Fungal toxins. *Essays Toxicol.* **2,** 1–136.

Lindberg, B. (1955a). Low molecular weight carbohydrates in algae. X. Investigation of *Furcellaria fastigiata. Acta Chem. Scand.* **9,** 1093–1096.

Lindberg, B. (1955b). Methylated taurines and choline sulphate in red algae. *Acta Chem. Scand.* **9,** 1323–1326.

MacIntosh, F. C., and Perry, W. M. L. (1950). Biological estimation of acetylcholine. *Methods Med. Res.* **3,** 78–92.

McLaughlin, J. J. A., and Provasoli, L. (1957). Nutritional requirements and toxicity of two marine *Amphidinium. J. Protozool.* **4,** Suppl., 7.

Maizel, J. V., Benson, A. A., and Tolbert, N. A. (1956). Identification of phosphoryl choline as an important constituent of plant saps. *Plant Physiol.* **31,** 407–408.

Martin, D. F., and Chatterjee, A. B. (1970). Some chemical and physical properties of two toxins from the red-tide organism, *Gymnodinium breve. U.S., Fish Wildl. Serv., Fish. Bull.* **68,** 433–443.

Mathias, A. P., Ross, D. M., and Schacter, M. (1958). Distribution of histamine, 5-hydroxytryptamine, tetramethylammonium and other substances in coelenterates possessing nematocysts. *J. Physiol. (London)* 142, 56P–57P.

Mold, J. D., Bowden, J. P., Stanger, D. W., Maurer, J. E., Lynch, J. M., Wyler, R. S., Schantz, E. J., and Riegel, B. (1957). Paralytic shellfish poison. VII. Evidence for the purity of the poison isolated from toxic clams and mussels. *J. Amer. Chem. Soc.* 79, 5235–5238.

Mosher, H. S., Fuhrman, F. A., Buchwald, H. D., and Fischer, H. G. (1964). Taricha-toxin-tetrodotoxin: A potent neurotoxin. *Science* 144, 1100–1110.

Nakazawa, Y. (1959). Studies on the new glycolipide in oyster. V. The nitrogenous components and structure of the glycolipide. *J. Biochem. (Tokyo)* 46, 1579–1585.

Nichols, B. W., and Wood, B. J. B. (1968). A new glycolipid specific to nitrogen-fixing blue-green algae. *Nature (London)* 217, 767–768.

Nichols, B. W., Harris, R. V., and James, A. T. (1965). The lipid metabolism of blue-green algae. *Biochem. Biophys. Res. Commun.* 20, 256–262.

Nissen, P., and Benson, A. A. (1961). Choline sulfate in higher plants. *Science* 134, 1759.

Nissen, P., and Benson, A. A. (1964). Active transport of choline sulfate by barley roots. *Plant Physiol.* 39, 586–589.

O'Brien, R. D. (1969). Poisons as tools in studying the nervous system. *Essays Toxicol.* 1, 1–59.

Pasini, C., Vercellone, A., and Erspamer, V. (1952). Synthèse des murexins (β[imidazoyl-4(5)]-acryl-cholin). *Justus Liebigs Ann. Chem.* 578, 6–10.

Pentreath, V. W., and Cottrell, G. A. (1968). Acetyl choline and cholinesterase in the radial nerve of *Asterias rubens*. *Comp. Biochem. Physiol.* 27, 775–785.

Pilgeram, L. O., Gal, E. M., Sassenrath, E. N., and Greenberg, D. M. (1953). Metabolic studies with ethanolamine-1,2-C^{14}. *J. Biol. Chem.* 204, 367–377.

Randall, J. E. (1958). A review of ciguatera, tropical fish poison, with a tentative explanation of its cause. *Bull. Mar. Sci. Gulf Carib.* 8, 236–267.

Reissmann, W., and Wieske, T. (1967). Detection of N-methylated ethanolamines in phosphatide hydrolyzates by thin-layer chromatography. *Anal. Biochem.* 19, 46–49.

Sawyer, P. J., Gentile, J. H., and Sasner, Jr., J. J. (1968). Demonstration of a toxin from *Aphanizomenon flos-aquae* (L). Ralfs. *Can. J. Microbiol.* 14, 1199–1204.

Schantz, E. J., Mold, J. D., Stanger, D. W., Shavel, J., Riel, F. J., Bowden, J. P., Lynch, J. M., Wyler, R. S., Riegel, B., and Sommer, H. (1957). Paralytic shellfish poison. VI. A procedure for the isolation and purification of the poison from toxic clam and mussel tissues. *J. Amer. Chem. Soc.* 79, 5230–5235.

Schantz, E. J., Lynch, J. M., Vayvada, G., Matsumoto, K., and Rapoport, H. (1966). The purification and characterization of the poison produced by *Gonyaulax catanella* in axenic culture. *Biochemistry* 5, 1191–1195.

Scheuer, P. J. (1964). The chemistry of toxins isolated from some marine organisms. *Fortschr. Chem. Org. Naturst.* 22, 265–278.

Scheuer, P. J., Takahashi, W., Tsutsumi, J., and Yoshida, T. (1967). Ciguatoxin: Isolation and chemical nature. *Science* 155, 1267–1268.

Shama, M., Deno, N. C., and Remar, J. F. (1966). The selective demethylation of quaternary ammonium salts. *Tetrahedron Lett.* pp. 1375–1379.

Smith, I., ed. (1969). "Chromatographic and Electrophoretic Techniques," 3rd ed., Vol. I. Wiley, New York.

Stahl, E., ed. (1969). "Thin-Layer Chromatography, A Laboratory Handbook." Springer-Verlag, Berlin and New York.

Stavinoha, W. B., Ryan, L. C., and Treat, E. L. (1964). Estimation of acetylcholine by gas chromatography. *Life Sci.* 3, 689–693.

Sullivan, G., and Brady, L. R. (1965). Thin-layer chromatographic separation of betaine, choline and muscarine. *Lloydia* 28, 68–70.

Szilagyi, P. I. A., Schmidt, D. E., and Green, J. P. (1968). Microanalytical determination of acetylcholine, other choline esters and choline by pyrolysis–gas chromatography. *Anal. Chem.* 40, 2009–2013.

Taylor, E. H. (1964). Thin-layer chromatography of choline and derivatives. *Lloydia* 27, 96–99.

Thaxton, V. L., and Bowie, W. C. (1968). A method for the determination of lecithin in plasma as choline. *Clin. Chim. Acta* 21, 171–174.

Tomasz, A. (1967). Choline in the cell wall of a bacterium: Novel type of polymer-linked choline in *Pneumococcus. Science* 157, 694–697.

Vaughan, W. R., and Baumann, J. B. (1962). Reactions of alkyl carboxylic esters with mercaptides. *J. Org. Chem.* 27, 739–744.

Wangersky, P. J., and Guillard, R. R. L. (1960). Low molecular weight organic base from the dinoflagellate *Amphidinium carteri. Nature* (*London*) 185, 689–690.

Welsh, J. H., and Taub, R. (1948). The action of choline and related compounds on the heart of *Venus mercenaria. Biol. Bull.* 95, 346–353.

Whittaker, V. P. (1957). β,β-Dimethylacrylcholine, a new naturally occurring physiologically active ester of choline. *Biochem. J.* 66, 35P.

Whittaker, V. P. (1959). The identity of natural and synthetic β,β-dimethylacrylylcholine. *Biochem. J.* 71, 32–34.

Whittaker, V. P. (1960). Pharmacologically active choline esters in marine gastropods. *Ann. N.Y. Acad. Sci.* 90, 695–705.

Whittaker, V. P., and Michaelson, I. A. (1954). Studies on urocanylcholine. *Biol. Bull.* 107, 304.

Whittaker, V. P., and Wijesundera, S. (1952). The separation of esters of choline by paper chromatography. *Biochem. J.* 51, 348–351.

Wickberg, B. (1956). Isolation of N-(D-2,3-dihydroxy-N-propyl)-taurine from *Gigartina leptorhynchos. Acta Chem. Scand.* 10, 1097 -1099.

Wickberg, B. (1957). Isolation of 2-L-amino-3-hydroxyl-1-propane sulfonic acid from *Polysiphonia fastigiata. Acta Chem. Scand.* 11, 506–511.

CHAPTER VIII

Pharmacology and Mode of Action of Prymnesin

ZVI PASTER

I. Introduction

Toxigenic algae often become a serious public problem when they are associated with mass animal mortality. In most of the reported cases, intoxications were associated with a massive bloom of one of the known toxigenic algae. Relatively little is known about the natural conditions, physical, or biological factors which cause such outbreaks. Human intoxications are fortunately not too numerous. Most documented cases have been associated with consumption of toxic clams and mussels ("paralytic shellfish poisoning," Halstead, 1965), which are capable of concentrating in their internal organs a large number of the toxic algae cells without being themselves affected.

Most of the known toxic algae are dinoflagellates. *Prymnesium parvum* Carter is a toxic marine phytoflagellate of the order Chrysomonadinae. It is widely distributed in seawater, rock pools, estuaries, and brackish water (Otterstrøm and Steemann-Nielsen, 1940; Reich and Aschner, 1947; Droop, 1954). The flagellate has become the subject of extensive research since 1947, when *P. parvum* outbreaks endangered the commercial fish breeding industry of Israel (Reich and Aschner, 1947). In 1954, the organism was isolated and grown in axenic culture. The isolation was done independently by Droop in Scotland from rock pools and in Israel by Reich and Aschner from brackish water.

In nature, the toxin produced by *P. parvum* kills only gill-breathing forms of animals, such as fish or tadpoles, while lung-breathing species, such as adult frogs, are unaffected. On the other hand, various laboratory vertebrate species such as frogs, cats, and rabbits can be killed or paralyzed by intravenous or intraperitoneal injections of either a crude or a pure preparation of the toxin. In addition to its lethal action on fish (ichthyotoxicity) and on other laboratory animals, *Prymnesium parvum* toxin exhibits other biological activities. It has a lytic effect on erythrocytes, Ehrlich ascites cells, human amnion cells, Chang liver cells, mouse peritoneal macrophages, as well as on bacteria (Dafni and Shilo, 1966; Shilo and Rosenberger, 1960; Paster, 1968a,b; Ulitzur and Shilo, 1970b). *Prymnesium parvum* toxin affects smooth muscle (isolated guinea pig ileum) by inducing a contraction that is later followed by a decreased sensitivity to acetylcholine and various other smooth muscle stimulants (Bergmann *et al.*, 1964). *Prymnesium parvum* toxin blocks neuromuscular transmission without affecting the nerve or the muscle. An effect was also observed on the electrical activity of the heart muscle (Parnas and Abbott, 1965). *Prymnesium parvum* toxin seems to be a mixture of several active compounds that are synthesized by the organism through its life cycle, and are released mainly after the death and disintegration of the algae.

The name "prymnesin" was first used by Yariv and Hestrin (1961) to describe the extracellular toxic material collected from water samples rich in *P. parvum*.

II. Requirements for Growth and Toxin Production

Prymnesium parvum is a photosynthetic organism and therefore can be found in nature in well-illuminated places, such as in the upper layers of

TABLE I

Artificial Nutritional Media for Growth of *Prymnesium parvum*[a,b]

Constituents	Quantity per liter
NaCl	10.00 g
$MgSO_4 \cdot 7 H_2O$	3.00 g
KCl	0.80 g
$CaCl_2 \cdot 2 H_2O$	0.10 g
H_3BO_3	0.01 g
$NaNO_3$	0.20 g
Na_2HPO_4	0.05 g
Tris buffer	1.00 g
$MnCl_2 \cdot 4 H_2O$	5×10^{-3} g
$FeCl_3 \cdot 6 H_2O$	1×10^{-3} g
$Na_2MoO_4 \cdot 2 H_2O$	1×10^{-3} g
$ZnSO_4 \cdot 7 H_2O$	0.15×10^{-3} g
$CoCl_2 \cdot 6 H_2O$	3×10^{-6} g
Thiamine HCl	10×10^{-6} g
Vitamin B_{12}	0.1×10^{-6} g
Glycerol	$0.5 M$
DL-Alanine	$0.05 M$

[a] From Paster (1968b).
[b] The pH of the media was brought to 8.2–8.4 before sterilization.

water. A significant correlation was found between the number of organisms in the water and the degree of toxicity. However, high cell concentrations in nature did not always cause a massive mortality (Reich and Aschner, 1947). A rapid loss of toxicity occurred without a corresponding decrease in the number of organisms, and this was ascribed to the presence of a high number of bacteria in nontoxic *P. parvum* water blooms (Reich and Aschner, 1947). Suspensions of *Proteus vulgaris* and *Bacillus subtilis* decreased the potency of *P. parvum* culture filtrates by at least 50% in 1 hour (Shilo and Aschner, 1953).

The isolation of *P. parvum* by Droop (1954) and Reich and Kahn (1954) enabled the study of the nutritional requirements and conditions for toxin production of this organism. There were several attempts to obtain mass cultures by using artificial seawater (Droop, 1954; McLaughlin, 1958; Yariv and Hestrin, 1961; Paster *et al.*, 1966). Excellent growth of *P. parvum* and toxin production were observed by Paster (1968b) using the media shown in Table I. The NaCl concentration for optimal growth and toxin production was between 0.3 and 5%. Growth was possible in ranges between 6 and 12% NaCl, but only with a concomitant loss of toxicity (McLaughlin, 1958).

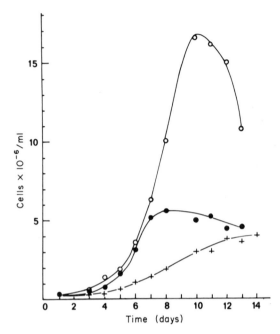

Fɪɢ. 1. Growth curves of *Prymnesium parvum* under continuous illumination at 20°C. +, Inorganic salts with vitamins B_1 and B_{12} only; ●, inorganic salts, vitamin B_1, and B_{12}, and 0.5 M glycerol; ○, inorganic salts, vitamins, glycerol, and ᴅʟ-alanine. (From Paster, 1968a.)

Thiamine and vitamin B_{12} were found to be essential for growth. Full growth was made possible by using 10 μg of thiamine per liter of media (McLaughlin, 1958). In addition to being an essential factor for *P. parvum* (Droop, 1954; Rahat and Reich, 1963a), vitamin B_{12} was found to accelerate its growth in light and darkness (Rahat and Jahn, 1965). Vitamin B_{12} could be replaced only by a few related "incomplete" analogs, i.e., only those devoid of one or both benzimidazole methyl groups. None of these replacements was found to be as good as vitamin B_{12} itself (Rahat and Reich, 1963b). As a nitrogen source, *P. parvum* can use a wide variety of nitrogen-containing compounds such as nitrates, ammonia, arginine, asparagine, methionine, histidine, alanine, glycine, serine, proline, leucine, isoleucine, tyrosine, aspartic acid, and glutamic acid (McLaughlin, 1958; Rahat and Reich, 1963a,b; Rahat and Jahn, 1965). *Prymnesium parvum* is unique in being able to use both ethionine and methionine as nitrogen sources although ethionine is toxic to other algae (Johnson *et al.*, 1957).

D-Alanine was the most suitable amino acid for supporting mass toxic cultures in the laboratory (Paster *et al.*, 1966) (Fig. 1).

Since *P. parvum* toxin is light sensitive (Reich and Parnas, 1962), the toxin is harvested after 12 hours of darkness (McLaughlin, 1958; Rahat and Reich, 1963a). There were several unsuccessful attempts to grow *P. parvum* in the dark (McLaughlin, 1958), and *P. parvum* was considered to be an obligate phototroph. In 1965, Rahat and Jahn found that of a wide variety of carbon compounds only glycerol at the optimal concentration of 0.5 *M* could support growth of *P. parvum* cells in total darkness. The addition of glycerol enhanced cell growth even under well-illuminated conditions (Paster, 1968b; Padilla, 1970). Glycerol enhanced growth rate and toxin synthesis within 24 hours of its addition to the cells (Padilla, 1970). The ichthyotoxic and hemolytic activities of the cultures grown in the dark were greater than in the light-grown cultures (Rahat and Jahn, 1965; Paster *et al.*, 1966), presumably as a result of photoinactivation of the toxin in the light-grown cultures.

While *P. parvum* can grow in up to 12% NaCl, toxicity is greater in low concentrations of artificial seawater than in higher ones. The highest toxicity is obtained in 5% seawater and the lowest in 30% seawater. Shilo and Rosenberger (1960) have found that maximum toxin production can be obtained in 2% salinity. Padilla (1970) has found that the highest hemolytic content is in cells grown at 2.28% salinity. The addition of calcium (0.2 m*M* $CaCl_2$) to the media increased the toxicity of *P. parvum* cultures (Reich and Rotberg, 1958). Thus, salinity of the growth media is a very critical factor in determining the toxicity of *P. parvum* in ponds or cultures. Absence of extracellular ichthyotoxic activity in cultures grown in media with salinity higher than 30% seawater (Reich and Rotberg, 1958) is not a result of reduction in toxin production, since *P. parvum* grown in 30% seawater contain large amounts of intracellular ichthyotoxin (Parnas *et al.*, 1963). Ulitzur and Shilo (1964) showed that NaCl concentration of the test solution had a direct effect on the ichthyotoxic activity and that in 15% seawater there was already a 98% loss of toxicity. In experiments with streptomycin and Ca^{2+} as cofactor, increasing amounts of NaCl up to 3 mg/ml caused a progressive inhibition of the ichthyotoxicity. *Prymnesium parvum* cells harvested from media low in phosphates were found to be ten to twenty times as toxic as cells grown in media enriched with inorganic phosphates (Shilo, 1967).

Cultures grown under constant illumination showed no extracellular ichthyotoxicity, but did show hemolytic activity (Reich and Parnas, 1962). This is presumably because photoinactivation of the extracellular ichthyotoxic activity is more rapid than that of the hemolytic activity (Reich *et al.*, 1965). Light intensity is a very critical ecological factor in *P. parvum* blooms. In water pools, where and when *P. parvum* is found, the highest population is usually found at depths of 40–60 cm, which apparently constitutes the layer of toxin formation. The upper layers of the water, which are exposed to intense sunlight, are poor in *P. parvum* cells or toxic activity (Parnas and Spiegelstein, 1963). While Shilo (1967) claims that light is absolutely essential for toxin synthesis, Rahat and Kushnir (1971) showed that cultures grown in total darkness are still toxic.

Intracellular toxin can be detected in cultures as early as the seventh day of growth. Extracellular toxin, on the other hand, is detectable no earlier than the tenth day. An attempt to localize the cellular site of prymnesin production by testing its hemolytic action resulted in a membrane fraction containing 20% of the hemolytic activity. This fraction was separated by density gradient centrifugation and consisted mainly of membranous vesicles and lipid granules (Padilla, 1970).

III. Purification of Prymnesin

There were several attempts to purify prymnesin, the first of which was by Yariv (1958). It was subsequently concentrated from culture filtrates and pond water using adsorption on $Mg(OH)_2$ precipitates (Yariv and Hestrin, 1961). Yariv obtained a dry, stable powder with an activity of up to 1300 hemolytic units and 400 ichthyotoxic units per milligram. Further purification was achieved by treatment with acetone and methanol, which increased activity about fivefold. Since the amount of prymnesin present in the culture media or water samples is very small, large quantities of media should be used in order to obtain enough toxin. Shilo and Rosenberger (1960) extracted the toxin from dry cells concentrated by centrifugation. They used acetone for removal of pigments and methanol for extracting the toxin, which resulted in an extract containing up to 40,000 hemolytic units per mg.

Based on Shilo and Rosenberger's findings, Paster (1968b) purified prymnesin (presumably one of the active compounds in prymnesin) and elucidated its chemical structure. Cells were concentrated by centrifugation. The pigments were removed with acetone washes, and crude prymnesin was extracted with methanol. The toxin in the methanolic solution was precipitated by the addition of three volumes of diethyl ether at 4°C. The precipitate was dissolved in water and fractionated on Sephadex G–100. The active fractions were combined, and the toxin was extracted into *n*-butanol. The butanol phase that contained the pure prymnesin was collected and dried *in vacuo*. This preparation gave a single peak in elec-

TABLE II

CHEMICAL AND BIOLOGICAL PROPERTIES OF PRYMNESIN[a]

Elementary analysis:C, 42.5%; H, 6.95%; [O (calculated), 50.55%]; N, P, and S, zero
Molecular weight (calculated):23000 ± 1800[b]
Lipid constituents:About 30%; C 14 − C 16 − C 18:0 − C 18:1 = 2:8:2:1 moles
Sugar constituents:About 70%; glucose:galactose:mannose = 2:1:1 moles
Biological activity:LD_{50} for *Gambusia affinis* (IP) = 1.8 ± 0.4 μg/300 mg body weight[c]
　　　　　　　　LD_{50} for mice (IP) = 1.4 ± 0.3 mg/kg
　　　　　　　　H_{50} (rabbit erythrocytes) = 25 ng/ml
　　　　　　　　I_{50} (guinea pig ileum) = 30 ng/ml

---

[a] From Paster (1968a).

[b] Calculated from sedimentation velocity.

[c] The LD_{50} is given for the average weight of minnows used because the lethal dose per gram changed with the size and weight of the fish.

trophoresis and in ultracentrifugation (Paster, 1968b). The chemical and biological properties of prymnesin are summarized in Table II.

A somewhat different method for purification of prymnesin was described by Ulitzur and Shilo (1970a). The toxin was extracted from the cells with chloroform–methanol 7:3 (by volume) after acetone washing. The chloroform–methanol extract was subjected to silicic acid chromatography, and the toxin was eluted with chloroform–methanol 1:1 (by volume). The toxic fraction obtained was dissolved in chloroform–methanol 9:1 and stored overnight at −10°C. The precipitate obtained was collected by filtering through glass fiber filter paper (Whatman CF/A) and dissolved in methanol. The toxic material was again precipitated by three volumes of diethyl ether at −10°C, and the precipitate was then suspended in 25% *n*-butanol in water. The upper butanolic phase that contained the toxin was removed. Another washing was done, and the toxin from the combined upper layers was again precipitated with diethyl ether. This precipitate was dissolved in a mixture of chloroform–methanol–water 8:4:3, and was collected from the lower phase. The toxin obtained was named "Toxin B" and contained 3000 hemolytic units per microgram. Toxin B obtained by Ulitzur and Shilo was found to be a mixture of at least six hemolytic fractions, and was chemically different from the toxin purified by Paster (1968a) (see Section XI). Tritium-labeled toxin was obtained by growing *P. parvum* cells in culture enriched with [³H]glycerol. The toxin was extracted into methanol and was further purified by gel filtration chromatography using Sephadex LH-20 and methanol as eluent (Martin and Padilla, 1971).

IV. The Hemolytic Effect

Yariv (1958) was the first to report that prymnesin possessed hemolytic activity in addition to its ichthyotoxic activity. By far the most convenient and sensitive method of assaying prymnesin is still by measuring its hemolytic activity. Rabbit erythrocytes are most commly used (Reich *et al.*, 1965; Paster *et al*, 1967; Paster, 1968a), although other types of erythrocytes have also been used (Yariv and Hestrin, 1961). Thus, hemolysis has been used as a rapid method for determination of specific activity of prymnesin during the purification procedure. The amounts of prymnesin needed for hemolytic assay were 100 times less than those needed for ichthyctoxic assay. A full discussion of prymnesin-induced hemolysis is given in the following Chapter (Chapter IX). Summarized below are related investigations performed in my laboratory.

A. Hemolytic Assay

Blood is freshly withdrawn from a rabbit heart into a capped Erlenmeyer flask and shaken for 3 minutes with glass beads to prevent coagulation. The blood is centrifuged to separate erythrocytes from the whole serum. The erythrocytes are washed with saline at pH 7 until the supernatant is discarded, and erythrocytes are diluted to 5% suspension in phosphate-buffered saline (Na_2HPO_4 0.028 M, adjusted to pH 7 by addition of 0.084 M KH_2PO_4; this mixture is mixed with an equal volume of 0.286 M NaCl). One milliliter of the appropriate toxin dilution in saline is added to 4 ml of washed erythrocyte suspension (final concentration 1%), and the mixture is incubated at 37°C for 30 minutes. The supernatant resulting from centrifugation is diluted with 2.5 volumes of 0.1% Na_2CO_3, and the optical density is measured at 540 nm. By using different dilutions of toxin, the concentration producing 50% hemolysis (H_{50}) is calculated. One hemolytic unit is defined as the amount of toxin that causes 50% hemolysis at the above conditions (Reich *et al.*, 1965; Paster, 1968a). The hemolytic assays of different workers involve the use of different incubation times, different methods of dilution, diluents of different compositions and pH, or erythrocyte suspensions from different sources (Yariv and Hestrin, 1961; Shilo and Rosenberger, 1960; Paster, 1968a; Padilla, 1970; Martin and Padilla, 1971). Such factors probably explain the range of values obtained for a hemolytic unit of prymnesin.

B. Kinetics and Mechanism of Hemolysis

Although the hemolytic activity of prymnesin was demonstrated by using the extracellular toxin (Yariv and Hestrin, 1961), it was later con-

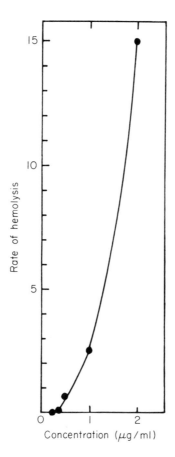

Fɪɢ. 2. Rate of hemolysis as a function of prymnesin concentration. The rate was calculated from the slope of hemolysis curve at 37°C with 1% rabbit erythrocyte suspension. (From Paster, 1968b.)

firmed that neither the hemolytic nor the ichthyotoxic activities of prymnesin are solely extracellular, for they may be extracted from the cells in amounts larger than those present in supernatant. Purified prymnesin usually retains its hemolytic and ichthyotoxic activities.

The time course of hemolysis induced by prymnesin has a typical sigmoid curve. The rate of hemolysis is a function of the toxin concentration, and increases exponentially with the toxin concentration (Fig. 2). The hemolytic reaction is characterized by a prelytic period that is followed by rapid hemolysis until the maximal effect is reached (Paster, 1968a; Martin and Padilla, 1971). The lower the toxin concentration, the longer is

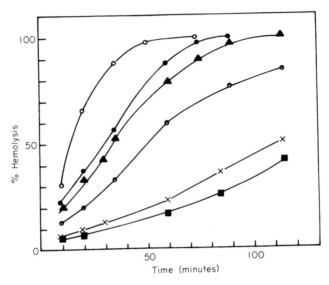

F_IG_. 3. The effect of different inorganic and organic cations on rate of hemolysis induced by 0.3 μg/ml prymnesin. One percent erythrocyte suspension was incubated in the above isotonic solutions of electrolytes. pH was 7.4 and temperature 37°C.   O, Choline HCl; ●, KCl; ▲, NaCl; ◓, benzyltrimethylammonium chloride; ×, CaCl₂; ■, MgCl₂. (From Paster, 1968b.)

the prelytic period and the slower the hemolysis rate. There is a critical toxin concentration below which the hemolysis will not occur. The critical concentration was found to be 0.25 μg/ml/1% erythrocyte suspension (Paster, 1968a). Based on its molecular weight, it has been calculated that 5000 molecules of prymnesin are needed for every erythrocyte in order to initiate hemolysis. The prelytic period can be prolonged without causing any visible hemolysis if the erythrocytes are incubated at temperatures lower than 8°C. Incubation at 4°C does not interfere with the reaction between the toxin and the erythrocytes, since washing the erythrocytes, which are exposed to prymnesin with fresh saline, and reincubation at 37°C induce almost the same hemolysis as is expected when the erythrocytes are incubated directly with the toxin at 37°C (Paster, 1968b). However, a hemolytic reaction that has already been induced by prymnesin at 37°C cannot be stopped by rapid cooling of the system to 4°C, although there is a slight decrease in the rate of the hemolytic reaction compared to the one at 37°C.

Both the prelytic and lytic phases are temperature dependent reactions. A linear relationship is obtained from the Arrhenius plot of the rates of both phases. An activation energy of 10 kcal/mole/degree for the range of 20°–42°C is obtained for the lytic phase (Paster, 1968b) and 19 kcal/mole/degree for the range of 15°–25.5°C for the prelytic phase (Martin and Padilla, 1971).

The hemolytic reaction by prymnesin was found to be totally dependent upon the presence of electrolytes in the incubation medium. Replacing the phosphate-buffered saline with isotonic sucrose (0.27 M) prevents the hemolytic reaction, while partial replacement of the saline with sucrose slows down the hemolytic reaction. The rate of hemolysis is also dependent on the type of ions present, as seen in Fig. 3. On the other hand, lipid compounds such as cholesterol, lecithin, and cephalin in very small quan-

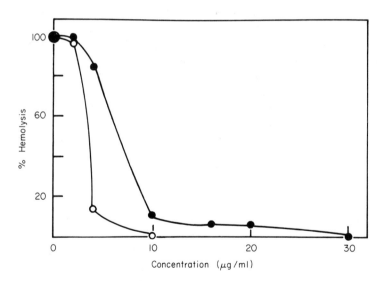

Fig. 4. Inhibition of the hemolytic effect of 0.2 μg/ml pure prymnesin by cholesterol (●) and lecithin (○).

tities inhibit the hemolytic effect of prymnesin (Paster, 1968b; Martin and Padilla, 1971). Cephalin and lecithin are more effective inhibitors than cholesterol. The inhibitor concentration required to produce 50% inhibition is 30 and 55 μM for cephalin and cholesterol, respectively (Martin and Padilla, 1971), while 20 $\mu g/ml$ of lecithin and 40 $\mu g/ml/\mu g$ prymnesin of cholesterol are needed to produce 50% inhibition (Paster, 1968b) (Fig. 4). While no hemolysis can be observed when erythrocytes are suspended in isotonic sucrose and exposed to prymnesin, washing the treated erythrocytes and resuspension in isotonic electrolyte solution results in release of hemoglobin. These results indicate that during the prelytic period prymnesin reacts with the erythrocyte membrane and only later is this followed by release of hemoglobin. The binding of prymnesin to the erythrocyte membrane during the prelytic phase is demonstrated by using erythrocyte ghosts (Paster, 1968b; Martin and Padilla, 1971).

The advantage of exposing red cell ghosts to the toxin is that the reaction between the membrane and the toxin can be tested without interference of any hemolytic reaction. Prymnesin and erythrocyte ghosts are incubated for different time periods; the ghosts are removed by centrifugation; and fresh red blood cells are added to the supernatant. The hemolysis that results estimates the nonattached toxin left in the medium. When a 6% erythrocyte ghost suspension is incubated with 0.7 μg of prymnesin at 4°C, 14 minutes are needed to adsorb 50% of the available prymnesin from the supernatant (the low temperature was chosen to prevent toxin inactivation) (Paster, 1968b). In 0.5-minute exposure at 25.5°C, 40% of the toxin appears to be removed from the supernatant (Martin and Padilla, 1971), while 12 minutes are needed at 4°C (Paster, 1968b).

A radiochemical study with ³H-labeled prymnesin was carried out in order to study the extent of binding of prymnesin to erythrocytes and ghost membranes. The fraction of toxin associated with cells, either erythrocytes or ghosts, is quite similar (Martin and Padilla, 1971). This suggests the same number of sites and similar binding mechanisms of the toxin in both cases.

The hemolysis by prymnesin results from interaction between the toxin molecules and the cell membrane components during the prelytic period, leading to an irreversible change in the membrane and the subsequent leaking of hemoglobin from the cell. In the prelytic period of hemolysis, while the adsorption of prymnesin on the erythrocyte takes place, subtle changes might be expected, and this is probably, the rate-limiting process. This phase is inhibited by cholesterol or lecithin (Paster, 1968a). The second phase, during which hemoglobin leaks out of the damaged cell, does not require the presence of toxin in the incubation medium. This phase can be inhibited by osmotic stabilizers, such as isotonic sucrose, or by lowering the temperature. The relatively low concentrations of lecithin, cholesterol, and cephalin required for inhibition of hemolysis indicate that this inhibition is not due to osmotic stabilization. The results point to a competitive inhibition reaction between the inhibitor and prymnesin; they compete for the same target site. The lysis inhibition occurs via a decrease in effective concentration of hemolysin—by formation of a prymnesin–inhibitor complex (Paster, 1968b; Martin and Padilla, 1971). Since cholesterol and lecithin are natural components of the red blood cell membrane, these molecules can be assumed to be the attaching site of the toxin molecules.

V. Effect on Smooth Muscle

Prymnesin exhibits a broad spectrum of effects on isolated preparations such as nerves and muscles. A very peculiar action is observed on the smooth muscle of guinea pig ileum. First, the toxin evokes contractions, followed by a reversal of the acetylcholine-induced contraction (Bergmann *et al.*, 1964). Addition of 20–50 ng/ml of prymnesin to the bathing solution of the guinea pig ileum causes a slow and prolonged contraction lasting 4–5 minutes, followed by a slow decline, at which time the response to acetylcholine is greatly inhibited. Repeated washing gradually restores the response to acetylcholine (Fig. 5). The antispasmodic

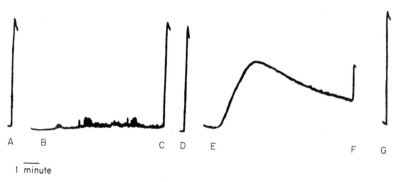

A   B   C   D   E   F   G

1 minute

Fɪɢ. 5. The effect of active prymnesin and photoinactive prymnesin on the guinea pig ileum. A, Acetylcholine 20 ng/ml; B, 100 ng/ml of prymnesin after 4 hours of illumination; C, 20 ng/ml of acetylcholine without washing the inactive prymnesin; D, acetylcholine after washing the toxin; E, 100 ng/ml of active prymnesin; F, 20 ng/ml of acetylcholine without washing; G, 18 minutes after repeated washing there is a full recovery to acetylcholine. Calibration time mark, 1 minute. (From Bergmann *et al.*, 1964.)

effect of prymnesin is a function of time and toxin concentrations. Complete insensitivity to acetylcholine is reached about 5 minutes after the exposure to prymnesin, while 40 ng/ml are needed to achieve 50% inhibition of the acetylcholine effect on the ileum muscle. Exposing the ileum muscle to prymnesin causes the muscle to be less sensitive to other smooth muscle stimulants, such as histamine, nicotine, bradykinin, and 5-hydroxytryptamine (Bergmann et al., 1964). On the other hand, morphine in a concentration of 20–60 ng/ml reduces the height of contraction induced by prymnesin by about one-half. Morphine, at the same time, has little effect on the contraction induced by acetylcholine. This fact may lead to the assumption that the results observed on the ileum muscle are mainly due to the ganglionic effect of prymnesin. The two effects of prymnesin on the ileum muscle can be selectively inactivated by illumination or high temperature. The antagonistic effect on the various smooth muscle stimulants is abolished after 60 minutes of illumination by visible light, while the contractile effect is abolished only after 4 hours of illumination.

Prymnesin has no effect on rat uterus musculature, whether taken from a pregnant or nonpregnant animal. Concentrations 100 times higher than those that affect the ileum produce neither of the two effects on the uterus.

VI. Effects on the Central Nervous System

Intravenous injection of prymnesin into a frog produces paralysis within several minutes, which then results in death. Injection of prymnesin into a cat produces a sharp drop in blood pressure and a cessation of respiration (Parnas et al., 1963). It was further shown that sublethal doses injected into a frog abolish the polysynaptic reflexes before they affect the monosynaptic ones. Contralateral reflexes desappear earlier than the ipsilateral ones, while there is no effect on the body musculature per se, which remains sensitive to direct stimulation.

One has to accept these results with caution. First, there is not enough information available. Second, further examination of the neurotoxic acrivity of prymnesin shows that motor paralysis observed in intoxication is not due to blockage of impulses along the nerve trunk, but, rather, it is the result of the toxin action on the nerve end, or the myoneural junction (Parnas and Abbott, 1965).

VII. Effects on the Neuromuscular Junction

The isolated frog sartorius muscle with its sciatic nerve is affected by small quantities of prymnesin. When this preparation is immersed in

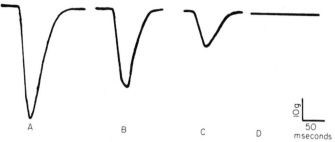

FIG. 6. Effect of prymnesin on isometric twitches of frog sartorius muscle. The response is to indirect stimulations, each pulse was for 0.05 msecond. A, Control; B, C, D, responses at 2-, 5-, and 10-minute intervals after addition of 300 μg/ml prymnesin. Calibration marks, 50 mseconds and 10 g; temperature, 20°C. (From Parnas and Abbott, 1965.)

physiological saline solution with prymnesin, the muscle shows a decline in its mechanical response to indirect stimulation (Fig. 6). When nerve stimulation is fully blocked, the muscle still responds to direct stimulation, and, at the same time, the sciatic nerve itself still propagates action potentials. Even with toxin concentrations ten times higher than those needed to block the mechanical response, the nerve still conducts action potentials for at least 1 hour. These results clearly indicate that the myoneural junction is the site of prymnesin action (Fig. 7). End plate potentials, which are recorded from the same preparation, are abolished 15 minutes

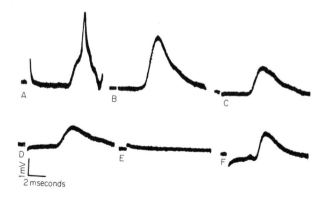

FIG. 7. End plate potentials in frog sartorius recorded externally with glass micropipette. A, Curare (10⁻⁶ g/ml) was added, end plate potential with a spike; B, end plate potential only, after addition of 1.5 × 10⁻⁵ g/ml curare; C, D, E, recordings 2, 10, and 15 minutes after the addition of 1 mg/ml prymnesin; F, after washing for 30 minutes. Calibration marks, 1 mV and 2 mseconds. (From Parnas and Abbott, 1965.)

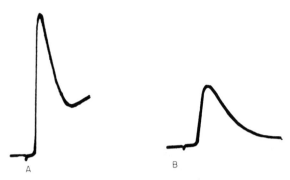

A   B

Fig. 8. Action potentials in crayfish DEAM fiber recorded with internal glass micropipette in response to nerve stimulations. A, Control; B, 2 minutes after adding 0.5 μg/ml of prymnesin. (From Parnas and Abbott, 1965).

after the addition of pyrmnesin to the bathing solution. Prymnesin has a synergistic effect with curare and interferes with the response of the postsynaptic membrane to externally applied acetylcholine (Parnas and Abbott, 1965). It seems that pyrmnesin acts on the postsynaptic membrane of the end plate, rather than on the presynaptic membrane.

The deep extensor abdominal medialis muscles (DEAM) of the crayfish, *Orconectes virilis*, and of the lobster, *Homarus americanus*, were used by Parnas and Abbott to investigate the neurotoxic mechanism of prymnesin. These preparations were found to be most sensitive to prymnesin, at least several hundred times more so than the frog sartorius preparations (Fig. 8). The majority of crustacean neuromuscular junctions appear not to be cholinergic (Florey, 1963; Takeuchi and Takeuchi, 1964). It is worthwhile noting that the addition of prymnesin to DEAM of the crayfish or the lobster (2 μg/ml) blocks the muscle action potential evoked by indirect stimulation. This block is completed in 5 minutes, while the nerve or the muscle still responds to direct stimulation. In spite of the different chemical transmitters used in the frog sartorius muscle and the crustacean DEAM, prymnesin affects both preparations in the same manner, namely, by blocking the postsynaptic membrane.

VIII. Effects on Heart Muscle

Prymnesin has a very peculiar effect on the activity of frog heart *in vivo*. Intravenous injections of 5–10 μg of prymnesin per gram body weight causes the heart to stop in diastole. This effect is usually preceded by marked depolarization of the heart muscle and by shortening of the typical action potential plateau. There is no explanation of this effect of prymnesin on the frog heart, especially when this effect is not antagonized by atropine or morphine. It has been speculated that prymnesin produces its effect through altering the permeability of the frog muscle membrane to Ca^{2+} ions (Shilo, 1967).

IX. Cytotoxic Effects

In addition to red blood cells, various mammalian cells and bacteria undergo morphological changes when exposed to prymnesin. These changes usually result in cell lysis. The mammalian cells tested were Ehrlich ascites cells (Dafni and Shilo, 1966; Dafni, 1969), HeLa cells, normal liver, and amnion cells in tissue culture (Shilo and Rosenberger, 1960). Addition of prymnesin to Ehrlich ascites cells produces a series of morphological changes, such as an increase in cell volume, accompanied by focal pouchings that grow into pseudopod-like extrusions. These effects are followed by permeability changes. There is abnormal uptake of trypan blue and increased leakage of intracellular potassium and later of various macromolecules such as DNA, RNA, and proteins. The cytotoxic effect of prymnesin is dependent on pH and temperature. The primary events resulting from exposure of Ehrlich ascites cells to prymnesin are rapid swelling and leakage of potassium ions. Lowering the pH from 7.4 to 6.4, or the temperature from 37°C to 27°C, inhibits cell lysis, while raising the temperature to 37°C or the pH to 7.4 induces cell lysis. On the other hand, lowering the temperature or the pH while the reaction is in progress slows the reaction dramatically. The damage inflicted on these cells by prymnesin is irreversible, although the lysis itself can be delayed by changing environmental conditions such as pH and temperature.

Recently, Ulitzur and Shilo (1970b) have reported a lytic effect of prymnesin on bacteria. Although *Escherichia coli* (ML 35) and *Pseudomonas fluorescens* bacteria are resistant to prymnesin, their spheroplasts are very sensitive to it. Protoplasts of *Micrococus lysodeikticus* and *Bacillus subtilis* are affected by prymnesin as well. The most susceptible organism tested was *Mycoplasma laidlawii*, which was found to be at least 500 times more sensitive than *E. coli* spheroplasts (Ulitzur and Shilo, 1970b). Unlike other bacteria, except for certain saprophytic species, the mycoplasmas have no cell wall, a fact that may explain the high susceptibility of *M. laidlawii* to prymnesin. Other bacteria tested become susceptible to prymnesin only after treatment with lysozyme–EDTA or when they are grown in the presence of penicillin, which destroys part or their entire cell wall. (These experiments will be discussed in greater detail in the next chapter.)

X. Inactivation of Prymnesin

Prymnesin is a very labile compound (Shilo and Rosenberger, 1960; Parnas *et al.*, 1962; Reich *et al.*, 1965). In 1939, Otterstrøm and Steemann-Nielsen reported that boiling water containing a high number of *P. parvum* organisms abolishes ichthyotoxic activity. Later it was reported by Yariv and Hestrin (1961) that a 15-minute incubation at 98°C at pH 4 is sufficient to destroy all the hemolytic and ichthyotoxic activities. On the other hand, no loss of activity was observed when the toxin was incubated in a sealed ampul under the same incubation conditions. The pH has a marked effect on the stability of prymnesin. Twenty-four hours in alkaline conditions (pH 8) at room temperature eliminates the biological activities of prymnesin. Shilo and Rosenberger (1960) claimed that exposure of prymnesin to alkaline conditions (0.5 N NaOH) inactivates its hemolytic and cytotoxic activities without affecting its ichthyotoxic one. Reich *et al.* (1965) and Z. Paster (unpublished) showed that incubation for 2 hours under alkaline conditions in borax buffer (pH 10) produces 50% inactivation of the ichthyotoxic and hemolytic effect and 90% inactivation of the antispasmodic one. Prymnesin is much more stable under acidic conditions (pH 5) and at low temperature. Prymnesin dissolved in organic solvents is more stable than aqueous solutions. It is recommended that prymnesin be stored in a dry, desiccated form since it is a very hygroscopic compound (Z. Paster, unpublished).

Prymnesin solution in water or in organic solvents undergoes rapid inactivation when exposed to UV or visible light (Parnas *et al.*, 1962). When prymnesin is extracted directly from the cells, no loss in culture toxicity is observed even after 24 hours under illumination—a fact that suggests that the intracellular toxin is protected, presumably by being bound to a protecting compound or by storage in special vesicles (Padilla, 1970).

The photoinactivation of prymnesin takes place either by visible light ranging from 400 nm to 510 nm, or by UV irradiation (225 nm). This photoinactivation is not affected by the presence of cell pigments. The same inactivation rate occurs whether the illumination is carried out in an atmosphere of pure oxygen or pure nitrogen (Parnas *et al.*, 1962). Addition of 1% glutathione has no effect on the rate or degree of photoinactivation. The photoinactivation of prymnesin is characterized by changes in its absorption spectrum. Under UV irradiation, the general pattern of the absorption spectrum is retained, but the absorption intensity is diminished. On the other hand, under visible light the peak absorption gradually shifts from 260 nm to 240 nm. It is interesting that the biological activity is completely destroyed long before the spectral changes come to an end. Reich *et al.* (1965) showed that while the ichthyotoxic and hemolytic activities decline at a comparable rate as a result of visible light illumination or UV irradiation the antispasmodic activity disappears much faster. One-half to one-third of the hemolytic and ichthyotoxic activities are retained after 2 hours of irradiation, while only one-quarter to one-tenth of the antispasmodic activity is preserved. The rate of destruction under the conditions tested, namely temperature, pH, UV, and visible light, enables us to distinguish the antispasmodic activity in prymnesin from its hemolytic and ichthyotoxic ones.

XI. The Relation between Structure and Activity

Two precedures for purification of prymnesin are in use (Paster, 1968a; Ulitzur and Shilo, 1970a). Both methods are based on differential extraction with organic solvents, precipitation in a mixture of organic solvents, column chromatography, and partition between diphasic solvents. Although the products obtained by the two methods are qualitatively identical—they show the same biological activities as the crude preparation— their chemical structure is different. Since prymnesin shows several biological activities, this raises the question of whether the different toxic activities are different expressions of the same compound, depending upon the biological system in use, or a mixture of different toxic ompounds. The data available support the second alternative, although these active compounds, while being chemically different, exert their actions through the same mechanism. This mechanism consists of nonspecific damage to various biological membranes. The expression of this damage depends on the type of biological system used.

The differential inactivation of the various toxic activities shown by Reich *et al.* (1965) adds further support to the assumption that prymnesin is a mixture of active compounds. The separation of two hemolysins was first indicated by Yariv and Hestrin (1961). Shilo and Rosenberger (1960) were able to show that the ratio between the hemolytic and ichthyotoxic activity may vary under different growth conditions. Most surprising is the fact that two different chemical compounds were purified from *P. parvum*: a glycolipid (Paster, 1968a,b) and a lipoprotein–carbohydrate molecule (Ulitzur and Shilo, 1970a), both of which retain all the activities of the original extract. Both compounds possess almost the same physical properties, such as solubility in organic solvents, foaming activity, and detergentlike properties, which result from their nonpolar lipid moiety and their polar, carbohydrate or proteinaceous moiety. Toxin B, as it was

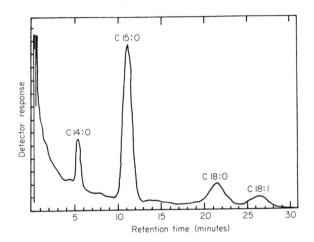

FIG. 9. Gas chromatogram of the methyl esters of the fatty acids from prymnesin obtained after hydrolysis. The chromatography was carried out at 170°C, stationary phase was 19% ethyleneglycol succinate in Gas chrom P., 100–200 mesh. C 14:0, Myristic acid; C 15:0, palmitic acid; C 18:0, stearic acid; C 18:1, oleic acid. (From Paster, 1968a.)

named by Ulitzur and Shilo (1970a), is a mixture of six separate toxic compounds. This mixture contains 22% protein, 10–12% hexoses, 0.47% inorganic phosphate, and twelve as yet unidentified fatty acids. Among a variety of enzymes tested, only papain destroys the hemolytic activity without affecting the ichthyotoxic one (Ulitzur and Shilo, 1970a).

Studies made in our laboratory have shown that prymnesin is a high molecular weight glycolipid. This toxic glycolipid retains all of the original biological activities (see Table II). It gives a single peak in analytical ultracentrifugation and appears as a single component in an electrophoretic system. It molecular weight, as calculated from ultracentrifugation, is 23,000 ± 1800. The skeleton of its structure is a polysaccharide, containing nearly 100 hexose molecules, composed of glucose, mannose, and galactose in a ratio of 2:1:1. In this polysaccharide, twenty-six hydroxyl groups are esterified by four long chain fatty acids, myristic, stearic, palmitic, and oleic acid in a ratio of 2:8:2:1 (Fig. 9). Elementary analysis shows the presence of carbon, hydrogen, and oxygen only and the absence of phosphorous, nitrogen, and sulfur (Paster, 1968b). The various biological activities related to prymnesin probably result from an interaction with the cell membrane. One may further speculate that the attachment of prymnesin to the biological membrane takes place where molecules such as lecithin and cholesterol are found, and, as a result, a rearrangement is imposed on the membrane, and it becomes very permeable and leaky. (See the next chapter for a discussion of this toxin–membrane interaction.)

In nature, prymnesin is toxic mainly to gill-breathing species such as fish, mollusks, arthropods, and also to the gill-breathing stage of amphibians. The mechanism of intoxication works by altering the natural gill membrane permeability. Fish immersed in water containing a sublethal concentration of prymnesin show an increased uptake of ^{125}I, trypan blue and ^{131}I-labeled human serum (Ulitzur and Shilo, 1966). Fish sensitivity to prymnesin can be increased if synergistic compounds are added to the test solution. The synergists tested are calcium or magnesium ions and streptomycin (Yariv and Hestrin, 1961) or polyamines such as spermine (Ulitzur and Shilo, 1964). It is apparent that this synergism does indeed exist, since the individual compounds are by themselves toxic to fish, and, by exposing the fish to these synergists, the gill membrane permeability is altered, and even sublethal doses of prymnesin are toxic. It is interesting that while in nature prymnesin acts through the gill membrane intraperitoneal injection of much smaller amounts of the toxin to *Gambusia affinis* minnows will produce the same effects. The synergistic action of calcium, however, does not take place when prymnesin is injected into the fish (Bergmann *et al.*, 1963).

In conclusion, the broad spectrum of prymnesin activity results from its detergentlike structure, and all the effects related to this compound are a result of the changes that prymnesin induces in a variety of biological membranes. The precise mechanism by which prymnesin affects these membranes is still unclear. The assumption that the blocking action of prymnesin on excitable membranes may not involve sodium conductance, but rather calcium movement, can make prymnesin an outstanding tool for neurophysiological research. The potential medical and scientific value of prymnesin seems to lie in its cytotoxic and neuromuscular blocking activities, which have not yet been sufficiently explored.

REFERENCES

Bergmann, F., Parnas, I., and Reich, K. (1963). Observations on the mechanism of action and on quantitative assay of ichthyotoxic from *Prymnesium parvum* Carter. *Toxicol. Appl. Pharmacol.* **5**, 637–649.

Bergmann, F., Parnas, I., and Reich, K. (1964). Dual action of the toxin of *Prymnesium parvum* Carter on the guinea pig ileum. *Brit. J. Pharmacol.* **22**, 47–55.

Dafni, Z. (1969). Primary effect of *Prymnesium parvum* toxin *J. Protozool.* **16**, Suppl., 138.

Dafni, Z., and Shilo, M. (1966). The cytotoxic principles of the phytoflagellate *Prynesium parvum*. *J. Cell Biol.* **28**, 461–471.

Droop, M. R. (1954). A note on the isolation of a small marine algae and flagellatas in pure culture. *J. Mar. Biol. Ass. U.K.* **33,** 511–514.

Florey, E. (1963). Acetylocholine in invertebrate nervous system. *Can. J. Biochem. Physiol.* **41,** 2619–2626.

Halstead, B. W. (1965). "Poisonous and Venomous Marine Animals of the World," Vol. 1, pp. 161–179. US Govt. Printing Office, Washington D.C.

Johnson, B. C., Holdworth, E. S., Porter, L. W. G., and Kon, S. K. (1957). Vitamin B_{12} and the methyl group synthesis. *Brit. J. Nutr.* **11,** 313–323.

McLaughlin, J. J. A. (1958). Euryhaline Chrysomonads: Nutrition and toxigonesis of *Prymnesium parvum* with notes on *Isochrysis galbana* and *Monochrysis lutery*. *J. Protozool.* **5,** 75–81.

Martin, D. F., and Padilla, G. M. (1971). Hemolysis induced by *Prymnesium parvum* toxin kinetics and binding. *Biochim. Biophys. Acta* **241,** 213–225.

Otterstrøm, C. V., and Steemann-Nielsen, E. (1940). Two cases of extensive mortality in fishes caused by the flagellate *Prymnesium parvum* Carter. *Rep. Dan. Biol. Sta.* **44** (non vidi).

Padilla, G. M. (1970). Growth and toxigenesis of the chrysomonad *Prymnesium parvum* as a function of salinity. *J. Protozool.* **17,** 456–462.

Parnas, I., and Abbott, B. C. (1965). Physiological activity of the ichthyotoxin from *Prymnesium parvum*. *Toxicon* **3,** 133–145.

Parnas, I., and Spiegelstein, M. (1963). Photoinactivation of ichthyotoxin of *Prymnesium parvum* in cultures and fish ponds. *Fish. Fish Breed., Isr.* **1,** 13–17.

Parnas, I., Reich, K., and Bergmann, F. (1962). Photoinactivation of ichthyotoxin from axenic cultures of *Prymnesium parvum* Carter. *Appl. Microbiol.* **10,** 237–239.

Parnas, I., Bergmann, F., and Reich, K. (1963). Pharmacological effects of ichthyotoxin of *Prymnesium parvum*. *Bull. Res. Counc. Isr., Sect. E* **10,** 225.

Paster, Z. (1968a). Prymnesin; the toxin of *Prymnesium parvum* Carter. *Rev. Int. Oceanogr. Med.* **10,** 249–258.

Paster, Z. (1968b). "Purification and Properties of Prymnesin, the Toxin Formed by *Prymnesium parvum* (Chrysomonadinae)." Ph.D. Thesis, Hebrew University, Jerusalem, Israel.

Paster, Z., Reich, K., Bergmann, F., and Rahat, M. (1966). Studies on the growth of *Prymnesium parvum* Carter, and the formation of its toxin, (Prymnesin). *Experientia* **22,** 790–794.

Paster, Z., Reich, K., and Bergmann, F. (1967). Studies on the hemolytic effect of prymnesin. *J. Protozool.* **14,** suppl., 178.

Rahat, M., and Jahn, T. (1965). Growth of *Prymnesium parvum* in the dark; note on ichthyotoxin formation. *J. Protozool.* **12,** 246–250.

Rahat, M., and Kushnir, M. (1971). Toxin synthesis in dark and light grown cultures of *Prymnesium parvum*. In "Toxins from Plant and Animal Origin" (A. de Vries and E. Kochva, eds.), Vol. I, pp. 191–202. Gordon & Breach, New York.

Rahat, M., and Reich, K. (1963a). The B_{12} vitamin and growth of the flagellate *Prymnesium parvum* Carter. *J. Gen. Microbiol.* **31,** 195–202.

Rahat, M., and Reich, K. (1963b). The B_{12} vitamin and methionine in the metabolism of *Prymnesium parvum* (Chrysomonade). *J. Gen. Microbiol.* **31,** 203–209.

Reich, K., and Aschner, M. (1947). Mass development and control of the phytoflagellate *Prymnesium parvum*, in fish ponds in Palestine. *Palestine J. Bot., Ser.* **4,** 14–23.

Reich, K., and Kahn, J. (1954). A bacteria free culture of *Prymnesium parvum* (Chrysomonadinae). *Bull. Res. Counc. Isr., Sect. B* **4,** 144–149.

Reich, K., and Parnas, I. (1962). The effect of illumination on ichthyotoxin in axenic cultures of *Prymnesium parvum* Carter. *J. Protozool.* **9,** 38–41.

Reich, K., and Rotberg, M. (1958). Some factors influencing the formation of toxin poisonous to fish in bacteria-free cultures of *Prymnesium parvum. Bull. Res. Counc. Isr.* **74,** 199–202.

Reich, K., Bergmann, F., and Kidron, M. (1965). Studies on the homogeneity of prymnesin the toxin isolated from *Prymnesium parvum* Carter. *Toxicon* **3,** 33–39.

Shilo, M. (1967). Formation and mode of action of algal toxins. *Bacteriol. Rev.* **31,** 180–193.

Shilo, M., and Aschner, M. (1953). Factors governing the toxicity of cultures containing phytoflagellate *Prymnesium parvum* Carter. *J. Gen. Microbiol.* **8,** 333–343.

Shilo, M., and Rosenberger, R. (1960). Studies on the toxic principle formed by the chrysomonad, *Prymnesium parvum* Carter. *Ann. N.Y. Acad. Sci.* **90,** 866–876.

Takeuchi, A., and Takeuchi, N. (1964). The effect on crayfish muscle of iontophoretically applied glutamate. *J. Physiol. (London)* **170,** 296–317.

Ulitzur, S., and Shilo, M. (1964). A sensitive assay system for determination of the ichthyotoxicity of *Prymnesium parvum. J. Gen. Microbiol.* **36,** 161–169.

Ulitzur, S., and Shilo, M. (1966). Mode of action of *Prymnesium parvum* ichthyotoxin. *J. Protozool.* **13,** 332–336.

Ulitzur, S., and Shilo, M. (1970a). Procedure for purification and separation of *Prymnesium parvum* toxins. *Biochim. Biophys. Acta* **201,** 350–363.

Ulitzur, S., and Shilo, M. (1970b). Effects of *Prymnesium parvum* toxins, cetyltrimetylamonium bromide and sodium dodecylsulphate on bacteria. *J. Gen. Microbiol.* **62,** 363–370.

Yariv, J. (1958). "Toxicity of *Prymnesium* Cultures." Ph.D. Thesis, Hebrew University, Jerusalem, Israel.

Yariv, J., and Hestrin, S. (1961). Toxicity of the extracellular phase of *Prymnesium parvum* cultures. *J. Gen. Microbiol.* **24,** 165–175.

CHAPTER IX

Interactions of Prymnesin with Erythrocyte Membranes

GEORGE M. PADILLA AND DEAN F. MARTIN

I. Introduction

As discussed in the previous chapter and in recent reviews, the toxic principles derived from *Prymnesium parvum* have distinct toxicological activities that can be easily demonstrated phenomenologically, but that cannot as yet be ascribed to fully identified chemical species (Shilo, 1967, 1971). On this basis alone, there are differing interpretations of the available experimental data, especially if one takes the view that specific toxicities should not be ascribed to preparations that have not been chemically identified. This is hardly a fruitful approach. It tends to negate or diminish the importance of selected investigations; it more likely reflects the prejudices of the reviewer without offering new insights into the fundamental problem in marine pharmacognosy—the development of specific bioactive compounds. Therefore, we think it is useful to consider in some detail the extent to which the toxin prymnesin can be a probe of cellular function and the kinds of experiments which may be designed to specify its interaction with a specific cellular element—the cell membrane—the major locus of its pharmacological effect.

A. Prymnesin

Although the initial impetus for the study of *P. parvum* toxins arose from the need to clearly delineate the factors that govern toxigenesis in the field and laboratory (see Chapter VIII, Section III, and Shilo, 1971), investigators were soon examining the specific toxin–membrane interactions in an attempt to separate the various toxic principles, while determining their specific mode of action. This work is briefly summarized below.

B. Ichthyotoxin

Ulitzur and Shilo (1964, 1966) conducted a detailed series of investigations on the ichthyotoxin fraction. They studied the uptake of trypan blue and radioactive-labeled human serum albumin, and found that increased uptake of both substances is largely dependent on the presence of ichthyotoxin as well as various cationic substances such as spermine, 3,3-diaminodipropylamine (DADPA), or magnesium chloride. They also showed that polyamines are most effective as synergists for the expression of ichthyotoxicity. However, the presence of 0.3% NaCl in the ichthyotoxin–synergist media (a given mixture of toxin and synergist) markedly suppressed the uptake of trypan blue. The effect of ichthyotoxin pretreatment on the sensitivity of the gills toward various fish poisons such as spermine, EDTA, and holothurin was also investigated (Ulitzur and Shilo, 1964). While such a pretreatment increased the sensitivity ten to forty times, the damage to the gills induced by brief exposure to ichthyotoxin was reversible. Thus, they concluded that intoxication of gill-breathing animals takes place in two stages: (1) a reversible damage leading to the loss

TABLE I

EFFECT OF DIFFERENT SYNERGIST CONCENTRATIONS ON ICHTHYOTOXICITY
AND IN ICHTHYOTOXIN PRETREATMENT ON TRYPAN BLUE UPTAKE,
[125]I UPTAKE, AND SENSITIVITY TO TOXICANT (DADPA)[a]

Parameter	DADPA concentration (M)		
	0	2×10^{-4}	4×10^{-4}
[125]I uptake (cpm/fish)	920	1500 ± 200	2500 ± 270
Effect of DADPA (% mortality)	0	50	100
Trypan blue gill staining	None	Partial	Complete
Ichthyotoxicity on fish with 10 ITU (% mortality)	0	50	100

[a] From Ulitzur and Shilo (1966).

of selective membrane permeability; such damage is expressed only under specific conditions required for ichthyotoxic activity such as the presence of cationic synergists and a suitable pH (pH 9); and (2) fish mortality results from the sensitization of the fish to any number of toxicants present in the surrounding medium. These substances, though not toxic when placed directly upon the gills (in the absence of prymnesin), can now penetrate the membrane, enter the systemic circulation, and cause paralysis and death.

An example of this effect is shown in Table I (Ulitzur and Shilo, 1966). In this experiment, the fish were pretreated for 20 minutes in tris buffer (0.02 M at pH 9, 25°C) containing 10 ichthyotoxin units [an ichthyotoxin unit (ITU) is defined as the minimal amount that kills all the fish tested within 3 hours] and different synergist concentrations as shown in the Table. Dye uptake was determined by immersing the fish briefly in a 1% solution of trypan blue. The gills were examined microscopically for the degree of staining. Radioiodine (^{125}I) uptake was expressed in counts per minute per fish. The sensitivity of the fish to 3 $\times$ 10^{-3} M DADPA in 0.02 M tris buffer (pH 9) was determined as percent mortality after 8 hours of immersion at 25°C.

As shown in Table I, without any addition of DADPA (second column), fish will take up approximately 920 cpm of ^{125}I per fish. There was no mortality with DADPA or 10 ITU of prymnesin, nor was there trypan blue uptake. At 2 $\times$ 10^{-4} M DADPA, however (third column), ^{125}I uptake increased to 1500 cpm per fish, and 50% of the fish died upon exposure to DADPA or ichthyotoxin. The gills were partially stained. Doubling the

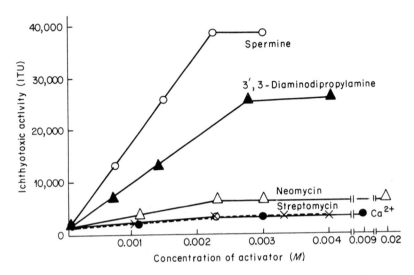

FIG. 1. Effect of certain cationic activators on the ichthyotoxic activity of *Prymnesium parvum*. The relative ichthyotoxicity was determined in 0.02 M tris buffer (pH 9) at 22°C. (From Shilo, 1971. Courtesy of the author and Academic Press.)

concentration of DADPA to 4×10^{-4} M increased radioiodine uptake almost twofold. A 100% mortality with both DADPA and ichthyotoxin was evident, and the gills were completely stained. No further changes were seen at concentrations of DADPA up to 3.2×10^{-3} M.

It is this phenomenon, described as "cation activation" by Shilo (1971), which is of considerable interest. Figure 1 summarizes the relationship between toxicity and presence of certain cationic activators (Shilo, 1971). Calcium and streptomycin have a slight synergistic effect on ichthyotoxicity, with neomycin being slightly more effective. DADPA and spermine are potent activators. Spermine induces almost a fourfold increase in ichthyotoxicity. As noted above, DADPA in this concentration range induced a twofold increase in the permeability of the gills to radioiodine (Ulitzur and Shilo, 1966). Since the fish are also sensitive to this compound (when exposed for as long as 8 hours), it is difficult to separate the two effects. Shilo (1971) suggests that the toxin and cationic activators act as a complex, with a resultant increase in ichthyotoxicity.

The complex could interact with charged groups on the toxin molecules, reducing the degree of ionization and making them more reactive with the membrane. This possibility is supported by earlier work of Shilo (1967) who showed that radioactive spermidine binds strongly to purified prymnesin. [See Shilo (1971) for further discussion.]

C. Cytotoxin

Shilo and Rosenberger (1960) were the first to show that prymnesin is toxic to tissue culture cells. They found that the sensitive cell lines include Ehrlich ascites cells, HeLa cells, human amnion cells, and the Chang strain of liver cells. A common feature of the cytotoxic action was the induction of pseudopodia-like extrusions, ultimately resulting in the complete break-down of the cell membrane as indicated by the uptake of trypan blue. The hemolytic and ichthyotoxic activity in various preparations of prymnesin varied from 700 to 1. This was one of the early indications that at least two different toxic factors were produced. (See Chapter VIII for further discussion.)

In a subsequent study, Dafni and Shilo (1966) examined in considerable detail the events leading to cytolysis of Ehrlich ascites tumor cells by *P. parvum* cell extracts. Four criteria were used to follow the cytotoxic action: (1) uptake by the cells of trypan blue (see Fig. 2); (2) release of intracellular macromolecules such as RNA and protein; (3) change in cell volume of the injured cells; and (4) microscopic observations of morphological changes. The morphological changes induced by the cytotoxins were similar to those described by Shilo and Rosenberger (1960). With prolonged exposure, the toxin induced the formation of vesicles to the extent that only naked cell nuclei and cell debris remained after complete breakdown of the cell membrane. The toxin was acting like a surface-active agent, possibly solubilizing portions of the cell membrane at specific sites.

The kinetics of cytolysis revealed that prior to cytolysis there is a marked increase in the median volume of the cells immediately after addition of the cytotoxin (Dafni and Shilo, 1966). This is shown in Fig. 2, which is taken from this study. These workers also showed that the time course and extent of swelling are dependent on pH and temperature, as is the loss of material from the swollen cells. For example, at pH 6.4 and at 27°C, the cells showed marked swelling without leakage of macromole-cules or uptake of the dye. At pH 7.4 and 37°C, however, the cells were readily stained and lost considerable cytoplasmic material (not shown in Fig. 2). Only when the cells reached a maximum level of swelling did they begin to lose material, at which time the cell volume decreased drastically. At a concentration of 0.1 μl prymnesin per milliliter, changes were fairly slow, but of the same order of magnitude as the effect of the ichthyotoxin on gill membranes. Between 30 and 40 minutes were required for the volume to reach a maximum (Fig. 2). A gradual disruption of the membrane integrity must be involved since another 20 minutes are required for the dye to penetrate the cells.

They also discovered that the lytic sequence can be arrested by lowering

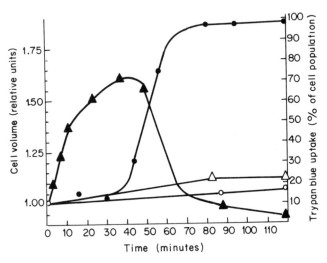

Fɪɢ. 2. The effect of *P. parvum* cytotoxin on Ehrlich ascites cell volume and trypan blue uptake. Cells were incubated up to 120 minutes at pH 7.4, 37°C. Triangles, cell volume; circles, trypan blue uptake; solid symbols, toxin-treated cells; open symbols, untreated control cells. (From Dafni and Shilo, 1966. Courtesy of the authors and Rockefeller Univ. Press.)

the pH and/or temperature, even after many of the cells had already lysed. In addition, the swelling appeared to be largely reversible up to a point close to lysis. The authors suggested that the sequence of lysis elicited by prymnesin is similar to that seen in immune cytolysis (Dafni and Shilo, 1966). In a subsequent report, Dafni (1969) made use of the fact that at a lower pH (pH 6.4) only swelling is observed. She found that within the first 3–10 minutes 80–90% of the potassium leaks out of the cells and apparently exchanges with external sodium. No change in the cell volume was seen at this point. Further incubation resulted in a continual entry of external sodium, but at a slower rate. Since the potassium content did not change, a gradual swelling ensued. The author suggested that the primary effect of *P. parvum* cytotoxin is due to a nonspecific disruption of the membrane permeability which appears to be pH independent (Dafni and Giberman, 1972).

A recent study was conducted by Ulitzur and Shilo (1970a) on the effect of *P. parvum* toxins on several bacteria and mycoplasma organisms. They found that intact cells are unaffected by the toxin at a concentration of 3.3 μg/ml. [They used the intracellular fraction, "Toxin B," purified by the method of Ulitzur and Shilo (1970b).] This concentration of toxin is 100 times greater than was needed to lyse spheroplasts of *Escherichia coli.* The authors suggested that intact bacteria may be resistant to *P. parvum* toxins primarily because the cell wall prevents entry of the toxin and thus nullifies its attack upon the bacteria membranes. Thus, removal of the cell wall by EDTA–lysozyme treatment increases the sensitivity to the toxin. Figure 3 summarizes some of these experiments (Shilo, 1971).

The toxin was also used on protoplasts of *Bacillus subtilis* as well as on a strain of *Mycoplasma.* With these cells, a wide range of sensitivities was found with the micrococcus being the most sensitive (50% were lysed by concentrations as small as 0.05 ng/ml). The mycoplasma organisms were, in turn, 500 times more sensitive than the *E. coli* spheroplasts. As with tissue culture cells, the lytic activity of the toxins increased when the pH was raised from 6 to 8. Mycoplasma organisms were also protected against the lytic activity of *P. parvum* toxins by spermine (0.001 *M*) by approximately fifteenfold. Finally, treatment of *E. coli* with EDTA rendered the cells sensitive to attack by *P. parvum* toxins. A similar lysis was induced

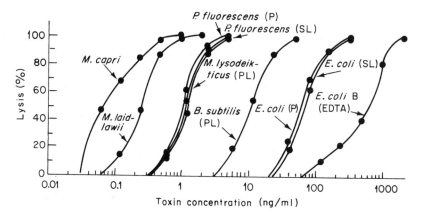

Fig. 3. The lytic activity of *Prymnesium* Toxin B on intact *Escherichia coli* B, spheroplasts of *E. coli* and *Pseudomonas fluorescens*, protoplasts of *Bacillus subtilis* and *Micrococcus lysodeikticus*, and *Mycoplasma capri* and *M. laidlawii*. *Escherichia coli* and *P. fluorescens* spheroplasts were suspended in a solution of 0.3 *M* sucrose in 0.06 *M* tris buffer (pH 8). *Bacillus subtilis* and *M. lysodeikticus* were suspended in a solution of 1 *M* sucrose and 0.005 *M* sodium chloride in 0.01 *M* tris buffer (pH 8). The *Mycoplasma* cells were suspended in a solution of 0.04 *M* sucrose and 0.25 *M* sodium chloride in 0.002 *M* tris buffer (pH 8). Intact *E. coli* B cells were suspended in 0.3 *M* sucrose solution in 0.06 *M* tris buffer (pH 8) containing 2×10^{-4} *M* EDTA. The degree of lysis was determined by the change in optical density of the solution after 60 minutes at 35°C. PL, Protoplast prepared with lysozyme; SL, spheroplast prepared by lysozyme–EDTA method (Repaske, 1958); P, spheroplasts prepared with penicillin. (From Shilo, 1971. Courtesy of the author and Academic Press.)

in *E. coli* cells in the presence of EDTA and detergents such as sodium dodecyl sulfate and cetyltrimethylammonium bromide.

The authors concluded that the *P. parvum* toxin preparation has a strong affinity for biological membranes, possibly due to the unique chemical structure of the toxins. On the basis of published chemical analyses (Paster, 1968; see also Chapter VIII) and isolation by various purification schemes (column chromatography, thin-layer chromatography, gel electrophoresis, etc.), the toxin appears to contain lipid and polar moieties. In this respect it is comparable to synthetic detergents and lysophospholipids. The difference is that *P. parvum* toxin is at least 3000 times more active than digitonin or isolecithin in hemolytic potency (Ulitzur and Shilo, 1970a).

D. Hemolysin

The wide variety of cellular activities dependent on membrane function and the methods that have been developed to measure them (e.g., determination of ion transport by isotopic techniques, measurement of ionic conductances, antibody–antigen interaction at the cell surface, contact inhibition, etc.) have relegated the technique of hemolysis to a secondary position as an analytical method. Because of its inherent simplicity, it has been mainly used as a means of assessing the strength and purity of toxins derived from *P. parvum*. Yet, as stated by Ponder (1948), "the red cell was the first animal cell on which extensive and systematic studies of permeability were made, and a new method was no sooner borrowed from the exact scientist than it was tried out on the mammalian red cell." About 20 years later, this may again be the case, since hemolysis offers many opportunities to gain insight into structure–function relationships of cell membranes.

In 1965, Reich *et al.* examined the hemolytic action induced by *P. parvum* toxins. They found that hemolysis begins with a delay of about 15 minutes, and the maximal lytic effect is reached after about 40 minutes. The rate of hemolysis (mainly reflecting a shortening of the "latent" period) was dependent on the concentration of toxin adsorbed on the red cells and, therefore, proportional to the external concentration. These investigators also found that even a short exposure to the toxin is sufficient for binding. This was demonstrated by exposing sequential batches of erythrocytes to the toxin and then by measuring the hemolytic activity remaining in the supernatant fluid by exposing fresh cells to it. Up to 80% of the toxin could be removed by four separate brief exposures of red blood cells without their undergoing hemolysis.

Bergmann and Kidron (1966) further examined the relationship between toxin binding and hemolysis with rabbit erythrocytes and Ehrlich ascites cells. They found that bacterial β-hemolysin added at a concentration that did not induce hemolysis in rabbit erythrocytes was readily adsorbed by the cells, and induced a "prelytic" change in them so that the lag phase of subsequent osmotic lysis was reduced progressively from approximately 150 to 40 seconds (i.e., when the cells were pretreated up to 20 minutes with 0.05 IU/ml of β-hemolysin). Beyond 20 minutes, there was no further reduction in the prelytic phase. Exposure of red blood cells for 30 seconds to 3 μg/ml of prymnesin also shortened the latency of osmotic hemolysis from 3 minutes to about 1.5 minutes or to 0.5 minute if the period of pretreatment was extended to 3 minutes. Pretreatment of rabbit erythrocytes with β-hemolysin had a synergistic effect on prymnesin-induced hemolysis by increasing the level from approximately 6% (control) to 53%. They also found that very small quantities of lytic agent can be detected and that once the binding has taken place washing does not remove it from the cells. The value of this approach is that the combination of two hemolytic processes uncovers latent disruptive effects of lytic agents, and they can be evaluated quantitatively. In these studies, the synergistic effect of β-hemolysin and prymnesin was mainly analyzed with respect to the reduction of the latent (or prelytic*) phase of hemolysis and subsequent loss of hemoglobin (expressed as the titer of hemolysis). The initial effect of β-hemolysin was presumed to be due to an enzymic interaction with the sphingomyelin (or related components) of the membrane. Since erythrocytes from different animals have different types and proportions of phospholipids, differential effects can be obtained with a given lytic agent. Yet, differential sensitivity can also result from a change in arrangement of the phospholipids within the membrane, or from the increased exposure to the lytic agent as the cell is osmotically deformed during the prelytic phase and the early stages of hemolysis. Thus, there was an obvious need to examine more closely the effect of *P. parvum* toxins on the kinetics of hemolysis and to relate this phenomenon to specific membrane functions in erythrocytes. The methods and experimental protocols used in these studies will be described in some detail below.

II. Methodology

A. Materials

1. ISOTONIC BUFFER

Isotonic buffer (10 mM phosphate-buffered saline solution, pH 5.5) has been commonly used to study the hemolytic activity of various lysins.

---

* Prelytic is equivalent to prolytic.

Another common buffer, Ringers blood buffer, has also been used. This buffer can be prepared by mixing 100 ml of 10× buffer (final millimolar concentrations: NaCl, 143; KCl, 5; $MgSO_4$, 1; $CaCl_2$, 2) and 10 ml of sodium phosphate buffer (2.5 M, pH 7.5) and by diluting to 1 liter.

2. Blood

Heparinized rabbit blood stored at 4°C is suspended in isotonic buffer. Erythrocytes are collected by centrifugation in a clinical centrifuge (2 minutes at 1800 rpm) and are washed twice with blood buffer. For determination of the hemolytic activity for kinetic studies, a standard erythrocyte suspension is prepared by dilution to an absorbance of 1.00 unit at 540 nm. Under these conditions, the electronic cell count of the standard suspension is about 10^7 cells per milliliter. When completely lysed, the standard cell suspension should have an absorbance of about 0.18–0.20 units at 540 nm.

3. *Prymnesium parvum* Toxin

The toxin can be isolated from *P. parvum* cultures grown in artificial seawater media (10‰) maintained at 25°C under constant illumination (Padilla, 1970). The seawater (or an artificial seawater mixture such as Instant Ocean, Wycliffe, Ohio) is enriched with liver fusion (Oxoid, Inc., 300 mg/liter), glycerol (0.25 M), and vitamins B_1 and B_{12} (0.02 and 0.01 μg/liter, respectively). After 5–7 days of growth at a density of 10^7 cells per milliliter, cells are collected by centrifugation (5000 g, 10 minutes), ground in a tissue grinder, and pigment is extracted with acetone. The acetone and insoluble residue are extracted several times with methanol to obtain the toxin. The combined methanolic extracts are purified by gel filtration chromatography using Sephadex LH-20 in methanol at a rate of 0.5 ml/minute. Fractions (4 ml/tube) are collected, tested for hemolytic activity, and suitable fractions are combined. Standard aliquots are maintained at −20°C for comparative studies.

4. Labeled Prymnesin

Toxins may be obtained from cultures enriched with suitable radioactive precursor materials. For example, artificial or natural seawater (500 ml) is inoculated with 10–20 ml of glycerol-free *P. parvum* stock culture. The inoculated culture is then treated with 40 ml of presterilized (e.g., by filtration through 0.22-μm porosity Millipore filters) 3.44 M glycerol containing 500 μCi of [2-³H]glycerol (200 mCi/mM, New England Nuclear Corp.). Cells are harvested; the toxin is isolated and purified as described above.

B. Techniques of Hemolysis

1. HEMOLYTIC UNITS

Hemolytic activity can be determined in two ways: as extent of hemolysis or by kinetic determination. The first method is commonly used to determine the number of hemolytic units present. A hemolytic unit is defined as the amount of toxin in 0.1 ml of methanol that causes 50% hemolysis of 2.9 ml of standard erythrocyte suspension after a defined time at a defined temperature. The defined conditions do vary from worker to worker, e.g., Padilla and co-workers (Padilla, 1970; Martin and Padilla, 1971a; Rauckman and Padilla, 1970) determined hemolytic activity at room temperature, exposure of 10 minutes, and pH 5.5, the pH at which hemolytic activity was found to be maximal for rat erythrocytes (Padilla, 1970). Reich *et al.* (1965) used a mixture of 5 ml of phosphate-buffered saline (PBS) (pH 7.0) and 1 ml of the appropriate toxin dilution; they added saline-washed rabbit erythrocytes to give a 7% suspension. The mixture is incubated at 37°C for 45 minutes. After centrifugation (4000 rpm for 2 minutes), the supernatant is diluted with 2.5 volumes of bicarbonate buffer, and the absorbance is read at 540 nm (PBS buffer: 0.028 M Na_2HPO_4, adjusted to pH 7.0 by addition of 0.084 M KH_2PO_4; the mixture is diluted with an equal volume of 0.286 M NaCl; bicarbonate buffer: 0.1% Na_2CO_3, 3 volumes; 0.1% $NaHCO_3$, 1 volume). With 0.5 μg/ml of toxin, there is approximately a 15-minute lag period, and 50% hemolysis is reached after approximately 23 minutes. (See Chapter VIII for an alternate method of analysis.)

In a subsequent investigation, Bergmann and Kidron (1966) used the Fragiligraph (Elron, Inc., Haifa, Israel) as described by Danon (1963). The instrument contains a semipermeable cell into which 0.075 ml of a buffered suspension of cells (usually 1:10 dilution) is added. The cell is placed in a test tube containing distilled water, and the curve of hemolysis, based on increasing transparency of the suspension, is automatically recorded. Such a fragility curve is obtained in less than 10 minutes.

2. DETERMINATION OF KINETICS

The second way in which the hemolytic potency of toxins can be assayed is by establishing the rates of hemolysis colorimetrically at 540 nm using a double beam spectrophotometer (e.g., Beckman DB-G), equipped with a thermostated cell compartment and a strip-chart recorder. The reference cell is filled with blood buffer, and the sample cell is filled with 2.9 ml of standard red blood cell suspension that is allowed to reach the reaction temperature before being mixed thoroughly with 0.1 ml of methanolic toxin

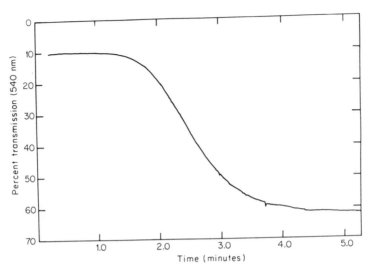

Fɪɢ. 4. Typical rate plot of hemolysis of rabbit erythrocytes using 2.5 hemolytic units (HD$_{50}$) of prymnesin. (From Martin and Padilla, 1971a. By permission of Elsevier Publishing Co.)

solution. Kinetic data (absorbance as a function of time) are obtained from the strip-chart recorder—directly, if it is equipped with a linear-log attachment, or indirectly as percent transmittance (Fig. 4), being converted by means of calibration of absorbance values (Martin and Padilla, 1971b). Useful kinetic parameters can be obtained directly from a plot by calcu-

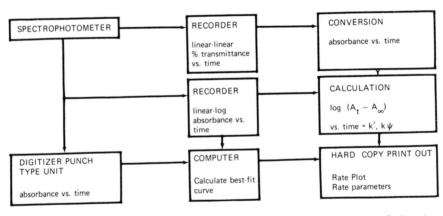

Fɪɢ. 5. Block diagram summarizing methodology for calculation of hemolytic rate constants. (From Martin *et al.*, 1972a. Courtesy of Academic Press.)

lating by conventional means, or they can be obtained as computer-derived constants from a spectrophotometer equipped with a digitizing unit (Fig. 5 shows a block diagram of operation). The effect of inhibitors is measured in essentially the same way, except that a methanolic solution of toxin (0.05 ml) and inhibitor (0.05 ml) is added with mixing to 2.9 ml of red blood cell suspension.

C. Kinetic Analysis

Three groups of parameters can be derived from the conventional colorimetric kinetic determinations. These include qualitative parameters, first-order kinetic parameters, and computer-derived parameters.

1. QUALITATIVE PARAMETERS

From the plot obtained (absorbance as a function of time, Fig. 6), we see that the changes associated with hemolysis can be divided into three phases: *a prelytic period*, the initial phase preceding the onset of lysis during

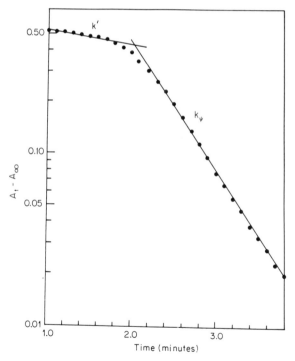

FIG. 6. First-order rate plot of prymnesin-induced hemolysis using data obtained from Fig. 4. (From Martin and Padilla, 1971a. By permission of Elsevier Publishing Co.)

which there is very little change or perhaps a slight increase in absorbance associated with cell swelling; *the lytic phase,* characterized by rapid change followed by the *final phase,* an absorbance-independent phase. The first phase can be characterized in general terms as the length of time of the prelytic period, t_p, which has been used previously (Martin and Padilla, 1971a), and the final phase can be characterized by the value of A_∞, the absorbance of the final solution. In a general way, t_p varies inversely with the concentration of hemolysin, and is also directly related to the concentration of inhibitor present (Martin *et al.,* 1971) The value of A_∞ is typically about 0.2 for the conditions defined earlier, but the value is also a function of the concentration of inhibitor present and will increase, indicating incomplete reactions with increasing concentrations of inhibitor. In addition, the reciprocal of the length of the prelytic phase, t_p^{-1}, has been directly related to concentration of certain inhibitors. These values, reflecting as they do the general phases of the course of the onset of hemolysis, are useful and have the advantage that they may be obtained from a direct chart reading. A third parameter might be suggested: the slope of the kinetic phase, expressed by ΔA divided by Δt. It appears, however, that obtaining kinetic data as first-order rate constants, for example, may be a more useful practice.

2. First-Order Kinetic Constants

The prelytic and lytic periods can be characterized in a more satisfactory manner by calculating specific rate constants. Consecutive pseudo first-order rate constants, k' and k_ψ are obtained from conventional first-order rate plots (Fig. 6). It is somewhat difficult to obtain accurate values for the first rate constant that appears to be associated with toxin binding and cell swelling during the prelytic period just prior to the onset of the lytic phase. The accuracy is limited by the number of points available for any satisfactory estimate at least at room temperature and by the need for an accurate measurement of A_∞, the final absorbance of the first process. The specific rate constant associated with the second process, k_ψ, can be obtained with good precision, and usually good first-order rate plots can be obtained for more than 95% of the reaction. The constants are calculated from the linear portion of the rate plot, $-\log_e(A_t - A_\infty)$, as a function of time using the conventional relationship $k_\psi = m$. Here m is the slope, and A_t and A_∞ refer to the absorbance values at times t and at the completion of the reaction, respectively.

3. Computer-Derived Parameters

Though specific first-order rate constants are useful, they nevertheless require replotting the data if a linear-log recorder is not available, and

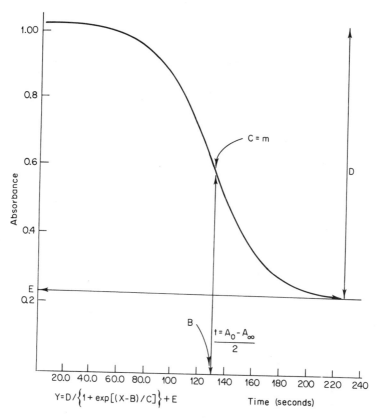

FIG. 7. Tracing of a hard copy print out of a hemolytic rate determination, absorbance (ordinate) as a function of time (abscissa, seconds), with the computer-derived parameters indicated and recorded. (See text for details.)

require, moreover, calculation of the rate constants. By means of a Digital Equipment Corporation PDP-15/40 computer equipped with a Tektronix T-4002 graphic computer terminal, it is possible to supply kinetic data (absorbance as a function of time) directly into the computer and to obtain computer-derived constants. The computer program (Martin *et al.*, 1972a) is written in Focal language (Copyright ©, Digital Equipment Corp.). The input data are presented visually, and, if satisfactory, a curve is plotted, and, if in agreement with the plotted data, a photostatic copy (Fig. 7) of the display is obtained by means of an accessory Tektronix 4601 hard copy unit. A program devised by T. Dessent was designed to calculate four parameters and to fit the rate data [Eq. (1)].

$$Y = D/\{1 + \exp[(X - B)/C]\} + E \tag{1}$$

Here, Y is equal to absorbance values, X is equal to time expressed in seconds, D is a spread factor $(A_i - A_\infty)$, where A_i is the initial absorbance observed during the prelytic period ($= 1.0$ absorbance units) and A_∞ is the final absorbance, C is equal to the slope of the lytic phase, B is equal to the midpoint time value, i.e., the value of t at which A_t is equal to D, and E is the off-set constant and is approximately equal to A_∞. In relation to the other rate parameters, C^{-1} is directly related to the pseudo first-order rate constant, k_ψ, and B is closely related to the length of the prelytic period, t_p.

D. Hypotonic Lysis

In this method, red blood cells are collected, washed free of plasma, etc., as discussed above (Section II,A,2). An aliquot from a stock suspension (usually 0.1 ml) is added to 2.9 ml of buffered saline solution to give a final cell count of $\sim 6 \times 10^7$ red blood cells per milliliter. When completely lysed and centrifuged, the supernatant should have an absorbance of 1.0 at 540 nm (Rauckman and Padilla, 1970). The hypotonic test solution is prepared with 10 mM phosphate buffer (pH 5.5) and NaCl from 82.5 to 87.5 mM so that 45–55% of the cells will lyse after a 5-minute incubation at room temperature (Seeman, 1966). Methanolic extracts of toxin, individual lipids, and lipids extracted from erythrocyte ghosts are added in a 0.1-ml aliquot to 3 ml of red blood cell suspension to give the desired concentration.

Human red blood cell ghosts are prepared by hemolysis in distilled water according to the procedure of Marchesi and Palade (1967). The lipids are extracted into isopropanol and chloroform followed by filtration to remove the solid residue. After rectification of the Folch and Reed type (Folch *et al.*, 1957; Reed *et al.*, 1960), the lipid extracts obtained are kept in chloroform at $-15°$C (Ways and Hanahan, 1964; Rose and Oklander, 1964). Chloroform is removed under vacuum prior to use, since it is highly hemolytic. The dry residue is redissolved in methanol at a concentration of 1.78 mg/ml. It contains the three major red blood cell lipids: cholesterol, lecithin (phosphatidylcholine), and cephalin (phosphatidylethanolamine). At this concentration, the final concentration in red blood cell suspension should be approximately 10^{-4} M (Rauckman and Padilla, 1970). Further dilutions of this solution can be made to give concentrations of 10^{-5}–10^{-10} M. Standard solutions of commercially available cholesterol (Aldrich Chemical Co.) and cephalin and lecithin (Nutritional Biochemicals Corp.) are prepared in methanol so that a 0.1-ml aliquot in 3 ml of suspension will give a 10^{-3}–10^{-10} M concentration. In the experiments reported here, no attempt was made to further purify these lipids. Methanol is added to all the control tubes. Hypotonic lysis is usually conducted in triplicate at each concentration.

E. Potassium Influx Rates with Red Cells

1. BUFFERS

Prepare magnesium buffer by dissolving 190 mmoles of magnesium chloride (38.6 g $MgCl_2 \cdot 6$ H_2O) in distilled water and diluting to 1 liter. Adjust the pH of the solution to 7 by adding small amounts of solid magnesium carbonate. Filter when the pH is stabilized. Prepare normal Ringer solution as described in Section II, A.

2. TECHNIQUE

Wash an aliquot of cells twice with cold magnesium buffer, and resuspend in normal Ringer buffer (Villamil and Kleeman, 1969). Samples (8.7 ml, hematocrit 0.02) are incubated in 50-ml Erlenmeyer flasks in a shaker bath at 37°C for 5 minutes. Add isotope (^{42}KCl in normal Ringer, 1 ml; 3 μCi/ml of sample) simultaneously with 0.3 ml of methanol (control) or a methanolic solution of toxin (test). Withdraw 2-ml aliquot samples after 1 minute and at appropriate times thereafter. Pipette aliquots immediately into 5 ml of magnesium chloride buffer. Decant in an ice water bath, and centrifuge within 5 minutes (10,400 g, 4 minutes). Supernatant fluid is saved for counting. Resuspend pellets twice in cold $MgCl_2$ buffer, and recentrifuge as before. Treat washed pellets with 2 ml of hemolyzing soltuion (3 mM CsCl, 18.7 mM NH_4OH, 0.003% Acatinox detergent). Determine the absorbance of hemolyzed solutions at 540 nm. Assay all solutions for activity in a γ scintillation counter. Calculate flux values, ^iM_k, Eq. (2) as mM K/liter original packed cells $\times$ hour) (cf. Hoffman, 1969).

$$^iM_K = \frac{G}{\Delta t S}\left[\frac{B}{OD_B} - \frac{A}{OD_A}\right] \tag{2}$$

Here, A and B are the γ activities (counts per minute, cpm) corrected for background for the first and second aliquot; OD refers to the corresponding absorbance values for the hemolyzed solutions; S is the activity of the supernatant (cpm) corrected for background, Δt is the time interval (in hours) between removal of the two aliquots; and G is the conversion factor (Hoffman, 1969), Eq. (3).

$$G = \frac{V_K HO\,K_o}{V_H} \tag{3}$$

Here, V_K is the volume of supernatant counted (0.002 liter); K_o is the supernatant potassium ion concentration (determined by means of atomic absorption spectroscopy); V_H is the volume (0.010 liter) used to measure OD_A and OD_B; and HO is equal to $(A_{pc} \times DF)/Hct$, where A_{pc} is the absorbance of 1.6 ml of original erythrocyte suspension diluted to 10 ml with hemolyzing solution; DF is the dilution factor; and Hct is the hematocrit for the original erythrocyte suspension.

F. Calorimetry

The calorimeter used in this work is a Beckman Model 190 Microcalorimeter modified for flow microcalorimetry with a pair of syringes, each of which can be driven by independent constant rate impellers. By adjusting gear ratios, different flow rates and thus different stoichiometries can be achieved. The design of the calorimeter is based on the heat burst method of calorimetry described by Kitzinger and Benzinger (1960).

Methanolic solutions of prymnesin are diluted with phosphate buffer (0.4 ml diluted to 10 ml). Control solutions are prepared using methanol instead of methanolic prymnesin. Blood suspensions are prepared in phosphate buffer and have hematocrits of about 40%.

TABLE II

MICROCALORIMETRY OF PRYMNESIN–BOVINE RED CELL INTERACTIONS
AT pH 6.2 AND 25°C[a]

Prymnesin concentration relative[c]	Flow rates (ml/min)		Heat of reaction (CU)[b]		
	Blood	Buffer or prymnesin	Viscous heat	Reaction and viscous heat	Net heat
1.0	0.30[d]	0.0795	32.8	41.5	8.7
1.0	0.30	0.156	44.9	53.9	9.0
1.0	0.30	0.30	68.4	76.6	8.2
1.0	0.30	0.60	122	124	2
0.75	0.156[e]	0.0395	15.8	16.0	0.2
0.75	0.156	0.0795	23.3	26.3	3.5
0.75	0.156	0.156	26.6	37.1	10.5
0.75	0.156	0.30	28.6	36.2	7.6

[a] From Binford *et al.* (1972).
[b] See Binford *et al.* (1972) for conversion from chart units, CU, to heat.
[c] Concentration, 1.0 = HD_{50} units per milliliter.
[d] Hematocrit, 38%.
[e] Hematocrit, 45%.

Microcalorimetry runs are conducted with concentrated solutions of prymnesin and blood (hematocrit, 40%). For each flow rate, two kinds of determinations are made: heat of reaction plus heat of viscous flow (using prymnesin solution and blood suspension) and heat of viscous flow (using buffer and blood suspension). Pertinent data are summarized in Table II.

III. Results

The events preceding and accompanying toxin-induced lysis are of considerable interest even though problems arose in the past because of analytical and methodological limitations. Ponder (1948) noted that in several instances a truly theoretical treatment failed because one parameter or another could not be determined directly. Since the publication of his monograph, useful experimental approaches and analytical techniques have become available that alleviate these problems to a considerable extent. For example, spectrophotometric methods have become available that permit a more adequate characterization of rates of toxin binding and lysis. Radioactively labeled toxin(s) are now available, so they can be used to indicate the extent of binding to erythrocyte and ghost membranes. Finally, with the aid of data acquisition systems and computers (see Fig. 5), useful mathematical treatments can be rendered to indicate the type of inhibitors (or activators) in these systems. As we will discuss briefly below, such mathematical analyses bring us closer to a kinetic if not an operational description of the toxin–membrane interaction.

A. Kinetic Studies

In an examination of the kinetic pattern of prymnesin-induced hemolysis, we suggested a simple model that shows a reasonable analogy with enzyme kinetics, particularly with respect to Michaelis-Menten or Lineweaver-Burk treatment (Martin and Padilla, 1971a). No doubt this is an oversimplification in view of the known molecular complexity of both prymnesin and the cell membrane. Yet the analogy is probably valid for several reasons. In the first place, the two parameters used to calculate the values of k_ψ from the usual Michaelis-Menten kinetics, Eq. (4) (Martin and Padilla, 1971a), adequately describe the lysis step.

$$k_\psi = \frac{k_\psi m \ (L, \ HD_{50})}{K_m + (L, \ HD_{50})} \tag{4}$$

Second, the values for the pseudo first-order rate constant are in excellent agreement with the experimental values in the low and intermediate concentration ranges (HD_{50} = 0.125–25.0). The agreement fails at high concentration ranges (HD_{50} = 25–1250), and the calculated values of the specific rate constant are higher than observed (Martin and Padilla, 1971a). In that study, it was suggested that the disparity could be attributable to inhibition by the hemolysin or by-products. It is interesting to note that Shilo (1971) also found that the relationship between the hemolytic activity and toxin concentration deviates from linearity above lysin concentrations of 30 μg/ml, i.e., a higher hemolytic activity is observed than is calculated. He ascribed this departure to the formation of micelles of toxin, which, in turn, undergo an undefined "phase shift." However, it is difficult to see how this would enhance the toxicity expressed as hemolytic units (HD_{50}).

Since our data did not permit a distinction between the possibility that the toxin (L) interacts with a single compound or with several active complexes (C) at suitable sites on the erythrocyte membrane (E), we extended our analysis to the interaction between hemolysin, erythrocytes, and inhibitors (I) as shown by Eq. (5).

$$E + L \underset{k_{-1}}{\overset{k_1}{\rightleftharpoons}} C; C \underset{k_{-2}}{\overset{k_2}{\rightleftharpoons}} E + P; L + I \underset{k_{-3}}{\overset{k_3}{\rightleftharpoons}} L_i; E + L_i \underset{k_{-4}}{\overset{k_4}{\rightleftharpoons}} C_i \qquad (5)$$

This investigation was a natural extension of the observation of Rauckman and Padilla (1970) who found that cholesterol interacted with prymnesin as time progressed, and cephalin, while being itself a nonspecific hemolysin at relatively high concentrations (about 10^{-5} M), exerted a protective action by a nonspecific binding to the membrane. (This aspect of the problem is further discussed in Section III,D.)

Specific rate constants were determined as a function of concentration of inhibitor added to a suspension of erythrocytes exposed to 12.5 hemolytic units (this being the intermediate range in terms of the Michaelis-Menten kinetics). The inhibited rate data were expressed in two ways: (1) as a relative rate constant, k_{rel} (the ratio of the inhibited rate constant to the uninhibited rate constant, k_ψ) and (2) as the inhibition parameter, $(1-k_{rel})/k_{rel}$ (Martin and Padilla, 1971a). The results showed that cephalin is a more active inhibitor than cholesterol at concentrations at which cephalin is not a hemolysin (0.01–0.1 mM).

In analogy with enzyme processes and assuming that a steady state probably applies to the interaction of prymnesin and the red cell membranes, a diagnostic plot was derived to express the interactions as illustrated by Eq. (5) above (Martin and Padilla, 1971a). Inhibition of lysis could occur by at least three pathways: (1) a decrease in the effective concentration of hemolysin through the formation of a toxin–inhibitor complex

TABLE III

Nature of the Interaction of Hemolysin, Erythrocytes, and Inhibitors as Indicated by a Diagnostic Plot[a]

Pathway	Relationship	Diagnostic plot
1	Decrease in effective concentration of hemolysin by formation of a lysin–inhibitor complex (L_i)	Hyperbola, concave downward
2	Formation of a complex (L_i) that interacts with erythrocytes in competition with lysin	Linear relationship
3	Competitive hemolysin displacement by inhibitor	Curve, concave upward

[a] See Fig. 8.

(L_i); (2) interaction between a complex (L_i) and the erythrocyte membrane in competition with hemolysin; and (3) competitive displacement of the hemolysin by the inhibitor. Table III summarizes the different relationships expected if the inhibition parameter is expressed as a function of inhibitor concentration.

As shown by Fig. 8, pathway 1 seems to apply to both cephalin and

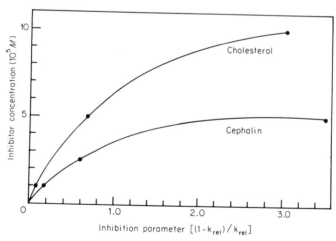

Fig. 8. Diagnostic plot, inhibitor concentration as a function of the inhibition parameter, showing the parabolic relationship indicative of the formation of inhibitor–prymnesin complex. (From Martin and Padilla, 1971a. By permission of Elsevier Publishing Co.)

cholesterol in the range studied. We should also mention that in a subsequent study (Martin *et al.*, 1972b) pathway 2 was found to be valid in the interaction between prymnesin and *Gymnodinium breve* toxin. We can anticipate that further studies of effective inhibitors and prymnesin–membrane interaction will be rewarding.

The stoichiometry of the interaction cannot, of course, be revealed by the analytical approaches described above. A Hill-type plot can, however, be used to shed some light on this aspect of the problem. Loftfield and Eigner (1969) suggested that types of enzyme inhibitions are amenable to a treatment in which the logarithm of the function of degree of inhibition shows a linear relationship with the logarithm of inhibitor concentration. This kind of analysis has not been applied to toxin–erythrocyte systems, which, as noted above, bear a formal relationship to enzyme systems, but the approach may be useful because, in many instances, the slope of the straight line of the Hill-type plot has an integral value. This value indicates that exactly one or two or more (depending upon the value of the slope) inhibitor molecules react cooperatively to inactivate (or inhibit)

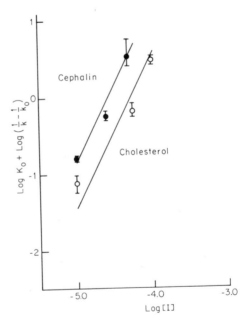

Fɪɢ. 9. Hill-type plot for lipid inhibition of prymnesin-induced hemolysis of rabbit erythrocytes. Straight lines of slope 2.0 are indicated.

the enzyme. A nonintegral value is easily visualized as a consequence of incomplete inhibition (Loftfield and Eigner, 1969). This approach is applied to the lipid–prymnesin–erythrocyte system as shown in Fig. 9. The straight line has a slope of exactly two. The previous diagnostic plot indicated that a toxin–inhibitor complex was formed, and the Hill-type plot would suggest at least two lipid molecules (cholesterol and cephalin) are associated with each effective unit of prymnesin in the active complex.

In summary, the approach in which a variety of analytical analyses are used, *viz.*, to indicate successively the interaction, nature of inhibition, and finally the stoichiometry, seems to be a most useful one. The utility and effectiveness will await further examples, but at this juncture the approach seems immensely superior to systems in which static (or end point) systems are employed.

B. Toxin Binding

It is clear that a major feature of prymnesin-induced hemolysis is the accumulation of the toxin at the erythrocyte surface during the prelytic period (Martin and Padilla, 1971a). About 40% of the labeled toxin is firmly bound to the membrane, of which 10% is loosely bound as indicated by its easy removal with methanolic washing. The fraction of prymnesin bound appears to be independent of the number of cells added. In addition, the fraction of toxin associated with the membrane remains constant regardless of whether the cells are intact or are osmotically lysed into ghosts prior to exposure to the labeled toxin. This suggests that there is no fundamental difference in the binding of prymnesin in spite of the resultant deformation of membrane structure upon lysis. In contrast, other lysins such as saponin, sodium taurocholate and glycocholate force us to consider three quantities that may be involved in the membrane interaction: (1) the amount of lysin originally added; (2) the amount determined colorimetrically during the prelytic period; and (3) the amount determined by hemolytic assay. The first two quantities appear to be about the same. The third is approximately 60% of the first quantity. The difference between the second and third amount is ascribed by Ponder (1948) to material that is chromogenic, but not hemolytic. Thus, in terms of binding, there is a significant difference between prymnesin and another marine bioactive agent, saponin.

A second way in which the binding properties of prymnesin were revealed was by exposure of erythrocytes to the antimalarial drug primaquine (Martin *et al.*, 1971). This compound was found to produce hemolytic anemia in certain susceptible patients (Beutler, 1969). It belongs to a class of compounds which seem to induce "fragmentation" of the membrane through a loss of membrane lipids, reduction in surface area, increase in spheroidicity, and decrease in deformation of cells. Primaquine itself appears to produce "internalization" of the erythrocyte membrane by invaginations followed by closures and sealing of the intracellular vacuoles in a process reminiscent of pinocytosis (Ginn *et al.*, 1969). Of interest in the present discussion is the fact that although the hemolytic rate constant (k_ψ) increases in a biphasic manner upon incubation with 1 mM primaquine, the binding of labeled prymnesin rises, at most, by about 20%. Rather, primaquine induces a gradual decrease in the median cell volume again in a biphasic manner and in parallel with the changes in the hemolytic rate constant (Martin *et al.*, 1971). The effect on the size distribution of the erythrocytes becomes manifest only if the cells are exposed to hypotonic stress. The conclusion of these studies, supported by the fact that flux rates for potassium remain unchanged, seems to be that primaquine may stabilize the cell membrane.

The binding tendencies of prymnesin are, however, affected by the pH of the solution. This can be correlated with the microcalorimetric measurements, which show that there is maximum binding in the pH range of 4.6–5.5; it will be recalled that at pH 5.5 there is maximum hemolytic activity. This suggests the existence of a high degree of association between toxin and the erythrocyte membrane (Binford *et al.*, 1972).

Not only is the method convenient, but it offers several advantages, among which are directness and rapidity of the measurement. The binding of certain hemolysins was measured indirectly in previous studies. For example, the action of *G. breve* toxin in limiting the prymnesin-induced hemolysis was expressed in terms of the hemolytic rate constants involved (Martin *et al.*, 1972b). As will be discussed below, Seeman's method also shows that prymnesin is a specific interacting lysin (Rauckman and Padilla, 1970).

Figure 10 summarizes one aspect of the results of the calorimetry binding studies. The high correlation coefficient (0.986) for the binding and the calorimetric profiles suggest that the toxin–membrane interaction may be the result of three related factors: (1) prymnesin may have a pK_D at the critical pH value of 5.5; (2) the maximum binding is related to the maximem hemolysis rate which is known to occur at pH 5.5 (Padilla, 1970); and (3) the critical pH value reflects the dissociation constant of sialic acids present on the erythrocyte membranes.

As discussed by Binford and co-workers (Binford *et al.*, 1972), it is difficult to select from these three possibilities. It is unlikely that the first factor is relevant judging from the known composition of prymnesin (it

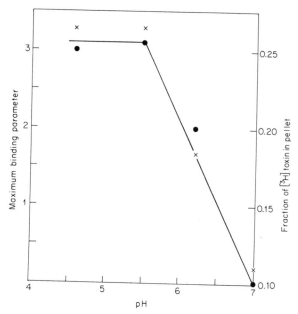

Fig. 10. Maximum binding parameter (MBP)–pH profile for tritium-labeled prymnesin and bovine erythrocytes at 25°C. The left ordinate (●) shows the MBP measured at each pH indicated. The right ordinate (X) indicates the fraction of the labeled toxin measured in the pellet. (See text for details.) (From Binford *et al.*, 1972.)

would require a reactive carboxyl group with a pK_D equivalent to acetic acid). The second possibility is partially discounted by the fact that when the calorimetric binding analysis is performed with bovine erythrocytes rather than with rat cells as previously reported (Padilla, 1970) the tendency for the cells to lyse is at a *minimum* at pH 4.6–5.5, not a *maximum*. Moreover, the hemolytic rate parameters, rather than the measurement of gross hemolysis (i.e., percent lysis after a defined incubation period), are not available for erythrocytes as a function of pH. The authors are left with the tentative conclusion that the charged molecules with which prymnesin interacts at the erythrocyte membrane are undergoing some undefined change in property at pH 5.5 (Binford *et al.*, 1972).

C. Toxin-Induced Permeability Changes

The effect of prymnesin on potassium fluxes cannot be conveniently measured because of the drastic action that this bioactive material has on the red cell membranes (Dafni and Giberman, 1972). Preliminary results

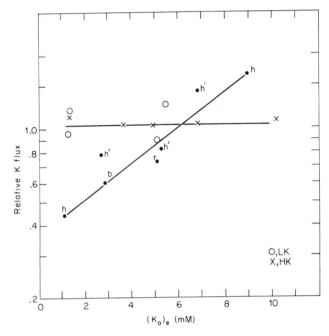

Fig. 11. Relative flux ($K_{test}/K_{control}$) as a function of external potassium concentration for erythrocyte suspensions in a normal Ringer buffer at 37°C. Test runs contain *G. breve* toxin (0.4 mg toxin/ml red blood cell suspension). Control runs contain corresponding volume of methanol. Blood types are identified: h, human; h′, second human; b, bovine; r, rabbit.

with *G. breve* toxin, however, do reveal its effect on the potassium flux of several types of red cells. The *G. breve* toxin does not induce hemolysis (Martin *et al.*, 1972b); however, the logarithm of relative flux in the presence of *G. breve* toxin (e.g., the presence of *G. breve* toxin relative to suitable control) does depend upon the external potassium concentration. It appears from the preliminary data shown in Fig. 11 that a variety of erythrocytes show a similar pattern. It would be useful to evaluate whether this is due to the external potassium concentration, although it may be a function of internal potassium content as well. Sheep erythrocytes, for example, can be divided into two distinct categories. Red cells from gentically distinct sheep (LK) contain high concentrations of sodium and low concentrations of potassium as do dog and cat erythrocytes. Erythrocytes of other genetic strains of sheep, however, contain more potassium than sodium (HK cells) as in the case of human and most mammalian red cells (Kerr, 1937). The two sheep cell types are morphologically indistinguishable. The total sodium and potassium content of the two cell types are the same, and the total concentration of alkali metals is also identical (cf. Tosteson and Hoffman, 1960). Differences in cation content appear to be due to differences in flux rates and differences in potassium permeability coefficients of the two cells. If relative K fluxes are independent of external concentration of potassium in the presence of high K and LK sheep cells, it is possible to automatically eliminate the mode of action of *G. breve* toxin as one that would depend upon internal sodium and potassium concentrations. At present, the data do not permit a closer evaluation of the direct effects of prymnesin on ion fluxes. It is clear, however, that at certain concentrations prymnesin is most probably not very specific in enhancing the passage of sodium or potassium through the membrane (Dafni and Giberman, 1972).

D. Antihemolytic Effects of Prymnesin

The technique of hypotonic hemolysis as a measure of the interaction of membrane-modifying compounds was introduced by Seeman several years ago (Seeman, 1966). The practical and theoretical consequences of this technique are considerable, for it permits a rapid and quantitative analysis of the protective action of those chemicals that interact with the hydrophobic elements of the cell membrane. Seeman and co-workers have examined in a recent series of investigations (Seeman and Roth, 1972) the "membrane expanding" properties of volatile anesthetics and solvents in an attempt to correlate an antihemolytic effect (protection from hypotonic hemolysis) with their anesthetic properties. In an earlier study, a wide variety of drugs that intimately interact with the lipid portion of the erythrocyte membrane were also examined (Roth and Seeman, 1971). It was found that the minimal blocking concentrations of lipid-soluble anesthetics are identical with the concentrations required for the reduction of hypotonically induced hemolysis in human erythrocytes (usually expressed as the 50% drop in lysis relative to the controls).

We have examined this effect with prymnesin as well as some of the lipids known to be components of the erythrocyte membrane, and we found that cholesterol and pyrmnesin do not protect the erythrocytes against hypotonic lysis (Rauckman and Padilla, 1970). Figure 12 shows a typical experiment in which human erythrocytes were exposed to varying concentrations of lecithin (phosphatidylcholine), cephalin (phosphatidylethanol amine), prymnesin, cholesterol, and lipids extracted from erythrocyte ghosts. Only lecithin and cephalin are protective at approximately 10^{-5} M concentrations (i.e., the hypotonic lysis of the treated cells as <1 relative to the control exposed for 5 minutes as described in the legend). This is taken to be an indication that prymnesin is a specific hemolysin directly

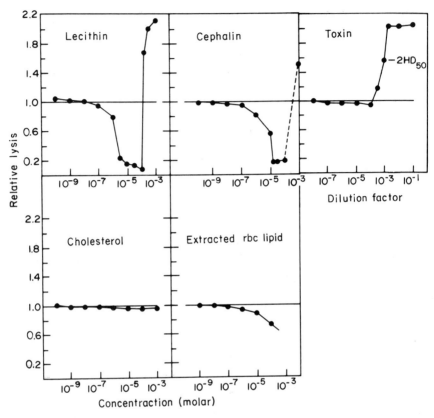

Fig. 12. Hypotonic lysis of human red blood cells (rbc) as a function of lipid and toxin concentration using Seeman's method (Seeman, 1966). Ordinate expresses the relative lysis [Abs (540 nm) experimental/Abs (540 nm) control] where 1.0 = 40–55% hemolysis. Abscissa shows the concentration or dilution factor. (From Rauckman and Padilla, 1970.)

interacting with cholesterol in its initial attack upon the red cell membrane. It thus does not impart a protective or expanding action upon the membrane. Prymnesin is therefore an agent whose ultimate value as a probe of membrane function will be to delineate the interaction and removal of specific membrane components. The results of this analysis also emphasize the need to examine other nonhemolytic bioactive compounds such as *Gymnodinium breve* toxin as potential membrane-expanding agents. In other words, their primary action, as in the case of volatile anesthetics (Seeman and Roth, 1972), may be to expand the membrane and bring about a reduction in the activity of membrane-localized enzymes by inducing a slight but critical volume change or unfolding in their tertiary structure. Prymnesin does not appear to operate in this manner.

IV. Concluding Remarks

In this chapter, we have sought to briefly summarize some of the features of the prymnesin–membrane interaction. Admittedly, we have only begun to bring into focus those parameters that will, in time, allow a quantitative and sequential analysis of the physicochemical events that accompany the destructive action of prymnesin. Because of its potent hemolytic activity, as well as uncertainties regarding its molecular architecture (Paster, 1968; Ulitzur and Shilo, 1970b), it is difficult, if not impossible, to do more than reach a few general conclusions as to how prymnesin brings about cell lysis.

If we may venture a guess, it is through the application of those methods that detect rapid but specific changes in the secondary structure of membrane components under the influence of bioactive compounds that we will make definite progress. These would include measurements of the shift in circular dichroism, electron spin resonance, and x-ray diffraction.

It is in this light that the microcalorimetric measurements assume greater significance. It does not appear accidental that the maximum binding parameter, hemolytic activity, and heat production all occur at the same pH. Considering the magnitude of the heat liberated, the lytic action of prymnesin is considerable in terms of the chemical bonds that are broken. Not only is prymnesin a powerful hemolysin, but it very rapidly disrupts the membrane to such an extent that as shown by Dafni and Giberman (1972) there is rapid loss of not only ions, but amino acids and macromolecules from the cells as hemolysis is initiated. Yet, if prymnesin does react with specific components of the cell membrane, as seems to be the case from the protective influence exerted by cholesterol, cephalin, and *G. breve* toxin, it may be possible to disassemble artificial and natural membranes as we measure, by independent means, the loss of specific biological activities.

ACKNOWLEDGMENTS

This research was supported by Grant SD 00120 from the Food and Drug Administration, Consumer Protection, and Environmental Health Service, United States Public Health Service. One of us (D. F. M.) gratefully acknowledges a Career Development Award (K04-GM 42569-03, National Institute of General Medical Sciences) from the Public Health Service and NIMH Grant MH 20078-01.

REFERENCES

Bergmann, F., and Kidron, M. (1966). Latent effects of haemolytic agents. *J. Gen. Microbiol.* **44**, 233–240.

Beutler, E. (1969). Drug-induced hemolytic anemia. *Pharmacol. Rev.* **21**, 73–103.

Binford, J. S., Jr., Martin, D. F., and Padilla, G. M. (1972). Hemolysis induced by *Prymnesium parvum* toxin. Calorimetric studies. *Biochim. Biophys. Acta* (In press).

Dafni, Z. (1969). The primary effect of *Prymnesium parvum* cytotoxin. *J. Protozool.* **16**, Suppl., 38.

Dafni, Z., and Giberman, E. (1972). Nature of initial damage to Ehrlich ascites cells caused by *Prymnesium parvum* toxin. *Biochim. Biophys. Acta* **255**, 380–385.

Dafni, Z., and Shilo, M. (1966). The cytotoxic principle of the phytoflagellate *Prymnesium parvum*. *J. Cell Biol.* **28**, 461–471.

Danon, D. (1963). A rapid micro method for recording red cell osmotic fragility by continuous decrease of salt concentration. *J. Clin. Pathol.* **16**, 377–382.

Folch, J., Lees, M., and Stanley, G. H. S. (1957). A simple method for the isolation and purification of total lipids from animal tissue. *J. Biol. Chem.* **226**, 497–509.

Ginn, F. L., Hochstein, P., and Trump, B. F. (1969). Membrane alterations in haemolysis: Internalization of plasmalemma induced by primaquine *Science* **164**, 843–845.

Hoffman, P. G., Jr. (1969). "Kinetics of potassium transport in LK and HK sheep red cells." Ph.D. Dissertation, Duke University, Durham, North Carolina.

Kerr, S. E. (1937). Studies on the inorganic composition of blood. VI. The relationship of potassium to the acid-soluble phosphorus fraction. *J. Biol. Chem.* **117**, 227–235.

Kitzinger, C., and Benzinger, T. H. (1960). Principles and methods of heatburst microcalorimetry and the determination of free energy, enthalphy and entropy changes. *Methods Biochem. Anal.* **8**, 309–60.

Loftfield, R. B., and Eigner, E. A. (1969). Molecular order of participation of inhibitors (or activators) in biological systems. *Science* **164**, 305–307.

Marchesi, V. T., and Palade, G. E. (1967). The localization of Mg-Na-K-activated adenosine triphosphatase on red cell ghost membranes. *J. Cell Biol.* **35**, 385–404.

Martin, D. F., and Padilla, G. M. (1971a). Hemolysis induced by *Prymnesium parvum* toxin. Kinetics and binding. *Biochim. Biophys. Acta* **241**, 213–225.

Martin, D. F., and Padilla, G. M. (1971b). Characterization of *Prymnesium parvum* toxin by means of hemolytic kinetics. *Environ. Lett.* **1**, 199–203.

Martin, D. F., Padilla, G. M., and Brown, P. A. (1971). Hemolysis induced by *Prymnesium parvum* toxin. Effect of primaquine treatment. *Biochim. Biophys. Acta* **249**, 69–80.

Martin, D. F., Padilla, G. M., and Dessent, T. A. (1972a). Computer-determined rate constants of hemolysis induced by *Prymnesium parvum* toxin. *Analyt. Biochim.* (In press).

Martin, D. F., Padilla, G. M., Heyl, M. G., and Brown, P. A. (1972b). Effect of *Gymnodinium breve* toxin on hemolysis induced by *Prymnesium parvum*. *Toxicon* **10**, 285–290.

Padilla, G. M. (1970). Growth and toxigenesis of the chrysomonad *Prymnesium parvum* as a function of salinity. *J. Protozool.* **17**, 456–462.

Paster, Z. (1968). Prymnesin: The toxin of *Prymnesium parvum* Carter. *Rev. Int. Oceanogr. Med.* **10**, 249–258.

Ponder, E. (1948). "Hemolysis and Related Phenomena," p. 398. Grune & Stratton, New York.

Rauckman, B., and Padilla, G. M. (1970). The binding and hemolysis of human erythrocytes by prymnesin. *14th Annu. Meet., Biophys. Soc., 1970* Biophys. Soc. Abstracts, p. 73a.

Reed, C. F., Swisher, S. N., Marinetti, G. V., and Eden, E. G. (1960). Studies of the lipids of the erythrocyte. I. Quantitative analysis of the lipids of normal human red blood cells. *J. Lab. Clin. Med.* **56,** 281–289.

Reich, K., Bergmann, F., and Kidron, M. (1965). Studies on the homogeneity of prymnesin, the toxin isolated from *Prymnesium parvum* Carter. *Toxicon* **3,** 33–39.

Repaske, R. (1958). Lysis of gram-negative organisms and the role of versene. *Biochim. Biophys. Acta* **30,** 225–232.

Rose, H. G., and Oklander, M. (1964). Improved procedure for the extraction of lipids from human erythrocytes. *J. Lipid Res.* **6,** 428–431.

Roth, S., and Seeman, P. (1971). All lipid-soluble anaesthetics protect red cells. *Nature (London) New Biol.* **231,** 284–285.

Seeman, P. (1966). A method for distinguishing specific from non-specific hemolysins. *Biochem. Pharmacol.* **15,** 1767–1774.

Seeman, P., and Roth, S. (1972). General anaesthetics expand cell membranes at surgical concentrations. *Biochim. Biophys. Acta* **255,** 171–177.

Shilo, M. (1967). Formation and mode of action of algal toxins. *Bacteriol. Rev.* **31,** 180–193.

Shilo, M. (1971). Toxins of Chrysophyceae. *In* "Microbial Toxins" (S. Kadis, A. Ciegler, and S. J. Ajl, eds.), Vol. VII, pp. 67–103. Academic Press, New York.

Shilo, M., and Rosenberger, R. F. (1960). Studies on the toxic principles formed by the chrysomonad *Prymnesium parvum* Carter. *Ann. N.Y. Acad. Sci.* **90,** 866–876.

Tosteson, D. C., and Hoffman, J. F. (1960). Regulation of cell volume by active cation transport in high and low potassium sheep red cells. *J. Gen. Physiol.* **44,** 169–194.

Ulitzur, S., and Shilo, M. (1964). A sensitive assay system for determination of the ichthyotoxicity of *Prymnesium parvum*. *J. Gen. Microbiol.* **36,** 161–169.

Ulitzur, S., and Shilo, M. (1966). Mode of action of *Prymnesium parvum* ichthyotoxin. *J. Protozool.* **13,** 332–336.

Ulitzur, S., and Shilo, M. (1970a). Effect of *Prymnesium parvum* toxin, cetyltrimethylammonium bromide and sodium dodecyl sulphate on bacteria. *J. Gen. Microbiol.* **62,** 363–370.

Ulitzur, S., and Shilo, M. (1970b). Procedure for purification and separation of *Prymnesium parvum* toxins. *Biochim. Biophys. Acta* **201,** 350–363.

Villamil, M. F., and Kleeman, C. R. (1969). The effect of ouabain and external potassium on the ion transport of rabbit red cells. *J. Gen. Physiol.* **54,** 576–588.

Ways, P., and Hanahan, D. J. (1964). Characterization and quantification of red cell lipids in normal man. *J. Lipid Res.* **5,** 318–328.

Author Index

Numbers in italics refer to the pages on which the complete references are listed.

A

Aaronson, S., 128, 144, *171, 172*
Abbott, B. C., 15, 20, *32, 34*, 49, 51, 52, 54, 74, *83*, 129, 133, 135, 143, 144, 148, 151, 156, 160, 169, *172, 175*, 191, 194, 196, 198, *199, 200, 201*, 242, 254, 255, 256, *262*
Abraham, E., 5, *31*
Ackerman, C. J., 222, 223, 231, *237*
Agin, D., 150, *172*
Aguilar-Santos, G., 12, *31*
Alam, M., 135, 157, 159, 167, 169, *172, 176*, 190, 192, *201*
Albert, A., 110, *124*
Albuquerque, E. X., 10, *31*
Aldrich, D. V., 181, 185, *199, 201*
Alender, C., 3, *31*
Altschule, M. D., 9, *34*
Amakaru, O., 17, *35*
Amatniek, E., 11, *35*, 96, *106*
Andersen, N., 22, *31*
Anderson, N. C., 18, 19, 27, *33*
Arai, H., 75, *84*
Aramaki, Y., 109, 110, 111, *124*
Ariens, E. J., 206, 208, *236*
Armstrong, C. M., 115, *125*
Asano, M., 209, 222, *236*
Aschner, M., 143, *176*, 242, 243, *262, 263*
Augustinsson, K., 214, 216, *236*
Austen, T. S., 129, *173*

B

Bacq, Z. M., 39, 40, 41, 59, 75, *81*
Baddiley, J., 206, 216, *237*
Bailey, R. M., 184, *199*
Baker, H., 128, 144, *171, 172, 174*
Balenovic, K., 220, *236*
Ballantine, D., 129, 133, 135, 144, 148, 156, 160, 169, *172*, 191, 194, 196, *199, 200*
Banister, J., 208, 214, 216, 222, 227, *236*
Bannard, R. A., 235, *237*
Banner, A. H., 134, *172, 174*, 198, *200*
Barnes, W. J., 2, *31*
Bartels, E., 19, 21, *31*
Baslow, M. H., 4, 11, *31*, 128, 129, 131, 134, 135, 161, *172, 175*
Baumann, J. B., 223, *240*
Beadle, G. W., 225, *238*
Beidler, L. M., 79, *81*
Bein, S. J., 131, *175*
Becker, M. C., 150, *173*
Bellenger, N., 205, *236*
Benati, O., 208, 219, 224, *237*
Benson, A. A., 205, 206, 210, *236, 238, 239*
Benzinger, T. H., 282, *294*
Bergmann, F., 242, 243, 245, 248, 253, 254, 258, 259, 261, *261, 262, 263*, 272, 275, *294, 295*
Bergner, A. D., 162, *172*
Bernstein, H. J., 53, *83*

297

Subject Index

A

Acetylcholine, *see also* Choline derivatives, 99–101, 153, 191, 206
  effect on ileum muscle, 254
  iontophoretic application of, 114
  measurement of sensitivity to, 114
  release, 119, 162
Acetylcholinesterase, 191
ACh, *see* Acetylcholine
Action potential, 147–148
  effect of prymnesin on, 256
  of end plate region, 113–114, 117
  monitoring of, 150
  in nerve–muscle preparation, 92–97
  and neuromuscular transmission, 99–102
  and postsynaptic depolarization, 150
  of sciatic nerve, 93–94
Aflatoxin, 234
Algae, *see* Plankton
Algal blooms, 129–130
Alginic acid, 7
  distribution, 27–28
  properties of, 28
Alkaloid derivatives, 199
Amphidinium carteri, 228–233, 235
  active substance from, 165–166
  analysis of extracts, 228–233
  choline content of, 211
  growth curves, 142
Amphiporine, 39–41, 71, 74–75, 79

  discovery of, 54
  induction of repetitive spiking, 40
  nicotinelike contracture, 39
  purification and bioassay of, 41, 49
Amphiporus, 39
  toxic compounds from, 74–75
Amphiporus angulatus, 71, 80
Amphiporus lactifloreus, 71
Amphiporous ochraceus, false anabaseine test in, 73
Anabaena, 130, 138
Anabaseine, 45, 58, 66, 70–74, 80
  biosynthesis, storage, and release, 77–78
  colorimetric determination, 57–59, 80
  compounds related to, 71–73
  distribution of, 70–73
  effect on crustacean axon, 74–75
  identification of, 71
  imine bond in, 74
  induction of contractures, 74
  mass spectra, 53–54
  myosmine analog of, 74
  nicotinelike effects of, 74–75
  proposed structure of, 58, 79
  role in prey paralysis, 76–77
  standard curve for test, 45
  synthesis of, 54–57
Anacystis, 130
Anacystis cyanea, 168
Animal venoms, expression of potency for, 144–145

307

DATE DUE

AP 5'74		
NOV 1 8 1997		
DEC 1 8 2000		

DEMCO 38-297